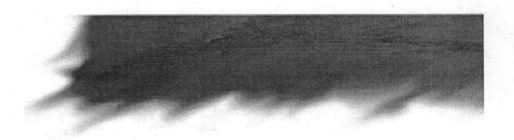

Study Guide for Black, Hawks, Keene

MEDICAL-SURGICAL NURSING

Clinical Management for Positive Outcomes

Sixth Edition

Elizabeth Ann Coleman, PhD, RNP, AOCN
Professor
College of Nursing
University of Arkansas for Medical Sciences
Little Rock, Arkansas

Sue Wyatt Huskey, MSN, RN
Clinical Assistant Professor
College of Nursing
University of Arkansas for Medical Sciences
Little Rock, Arkansas

W.B. Saunders Company
A Harcourt Health Sciences Company
Philadelphia   London   New York   St. Louis   Toronto   Sydney

W.B. SAUNDERS COMPANY
A Harcourt Health Sciences Company
The Curtis Center
Independence Square West
Philadelphia, PA 19106-3399

Nursing is an ever-changing field. Standard safety precautions must be followed, but as new research and clinical experience broaden our knowledge, changes in treatment and drug therapy may become necessary or appropriate. Readers are advised to check the most current product information provided by the manufacturer of each drug to be administered to verify the recommended dose, the method and duration of administration, and contraindications. It is the responsibility of the treating physician, relying on experience and knowledge of the patient, to determine dosages and the best treatment for each individual patient. Neither the Publisher nor the editor assumes any liability for any injury and/or damage to persons or property arising from this publication.

The Publisher

Study Guide for
Medical-Surgical Nursing: Clinical Management for Positive Outcomes (6/e)   ISBN 0-7216-9341-5

Printed in the United States of America.

Last digit is the print number: 9 8 7 6 5 4 3 2 1

Dedications

To my grandchildren: Ella Beatrix Coleman, Taylor Marie Jones, Jessica Nichole LaVergne, Jason Michael Jones, Zachary Christopher LaVergne, and Gary Alan Jones

Ann Coleman

To my husband Harold for 31 years of love and support; to our children Brian and Melissa, they have flown from the nest but land frequently

To my parents Wayne and Olivia Wyatt for their continual encouragement and support

To my sisters: Carol Dean, the other nurse in the family; and Marie Landis and Margaret Capps, the twins, who really are on the same wavelength. We have experienced breast cancer and survived.

To my nursing students—past, present, and future—the real teachers

Sue Huskey

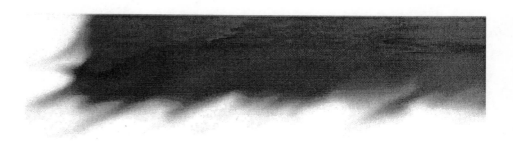

Preface

The purpose of this *Study Guide for Medical-Surgical Nursing* is to help you, the student, focus on important content. Based on research, we know that your learning will be enhanced by reading the textbook before class and by having study questions that will guide your readings. The objectives introduce each chapter and should also help guide you to the important content in the chapter.

The section entitled "Learning the Language," a review of anatomy, physiology, and terminology, will facilitate your understanding of the pathophysiology and the disorders. This understanding will be basic to developing nursing care. Completion of the sections entitled "Thinking Critically" and "Putting It All Together" will enhance learning and test your understanding of the content in an application situation. Some of the chapters have a "Critical Points to Remember" section. You may want to complete a similar section for the other chapters.

Use the *Study Guide* as a review and then concentrate on content areas that are more difficult. If you are certain of the answer to a question or definition, move on to the next one. You may find that what is most efficient for your time and learning is to only write in answers for questions that require you to use the textbook or for which you are not sure of the answer. Answers to all of the questions are included in the back of the *Study Guide* to help you verify your answers.

Case studies are included within some chapters in the *Study Guide*. You can use these to learn care of clients with specific disorders. More complex case studies are presented in the textbook.

The appendixes in the *Study Guide* contain forms or worksheets for organizing information on the classical/textbook picture of any disorder, note-taking outlines/worksheets for arrhythmias, and blank grids for gathering data. These worksheets will help focus your learning in the clinical setting.

We, the authors of the *Study Guide*, enjoy clinical practice and teaching nursing students. We hope that the *Study Guide* will assist you as you learn medical-surgical nursing care and that you too will enjoy your experiences in clinical practice.

Acknowledgments

We offer thanks to the individuals who helped us with this *Study Guide*.

To Norma L. Pinnell, MSN, RN, faculty member with the Colleges of Nursing at Southern Illinois University at Edwardsville and Deaconess Health System in St. Louis, Missouri, who was one of the authors (along with Ann Coleman and Janet Lord) of the third and fourth editions of the *Study Guide for Luckmann and Sorensen's Medical-Surgical Nursing: A Psychophysiologic Approach*. To Janet E. Lord, PhD, RN, faculty member with the College of Nursing at the University of Arkansas for Medical Sciences, who continued as an author (along with Ann Coleman and Sue Huskey) of the 5th edition of the *Study Guide for Black and Matassarin-Jacobs' Medical-Surgical Nursing: Clinical Management for Continuity of Care*. Their valuable contributions are a part of the current work.

To Lisa Hernandez of Editorial & Production Services, who helped design and prepare the final manuscript for production.

To Victoria Legnini, Associate Developmental Editor, W.B. Saunders Nursing Division, who provided support and encouragement and helped keep us on schedule during manuscript preparation and editing.

To Barbara Cullen, Executive Editor, W.B. Saunders Nursing Division, who supervised the acquisition and overall production of the ancillary package.

To Adrienne Simon, Editorial Assistant, W.B. Saunders Nursing Division, who kept the chapters from the textbook coming and supported us during manuscript preparation.

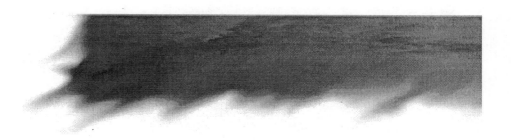

Contents

U N I T

1

Promotion of Self-Care

Theories of Health Promotion and Illness Management

Many theories exist today that attempt to describe the cause of illness. In the late 1800s, scientists relied on the germ theory and the biomedical theory to explain illness and disease. Newer theories use a multicausal approach to illness. These newer theories can be grouped into four major categories: homeostatic theories, psychosocial theories, biobehavioral theories, and mind-body theories.

Regardless of the cause of illness, each client perceives, evaluates, and responds to illness in a different manner. Reactions to illness are influenced by a variety of factors, including culture, knowledge base, and the client's definition of health and illness.

Today, Americans are more aware of health promotion measures and are moving toward greater independence in their self-care role. It is important, therefore, that the nurse address health promotion in every aspect of care and in every care setting.

On the other hand, people with chronic conditions or illnesses are the fastest-growing client population. These clients present a challenge to health care providers and resources. Often, their needs are not well understood in an era of high technology, rapid client discharge, and social attitudes that seem to idealize the healthy, youthful, "perfect" image. It is important for nurses to understand how the needs of these clients may differ from those of clients hospitalized with an acute illness. In order to assist clients with chronic conditions, nurses may need to refocus their assessments and interventions. Evaluation of outcomes may also have to be altered in terms of the long-term nature of the chronic condition.

OBJECTIVES

1.1 Discuss the major theories of disease/illness.

1.2 Describe the concepts of health and illness.

1.3 Define terms associated with health promotion.

1.4 Summarize the evolution of the concept of health promotion.

1.5 Discuss the three levels of prevention and the behaviors associated with each level.

1.6 Identify the six categories of risk factors.

1.7 Describe the impact of environment on health and wellness.

1.8 Discuss the relationship among nutrition, exercise, and health promotion.

1.9 Describe three methods of managing stress.

1.10 Discuss general concepts related to chronic conditions.

1.11 Discuss the processes of adaptation as they relate to chronic conditions.

1.12 Describe various health care facilities that provide care for persons with chronic conditions.

LEARNING THE LANGUAGE: TERMINOLOGY RELATED TO THEORIES OF HEALTH AND ILLNESS

Briefly define the following terms.

1. Signs

2. Symptoms

3. Syndrome

4. Germ theory

5. Multicausal theory

6. Adaptation

7. Psychosocial theory

8. Cognitive appraisal

9. Daily hassles

10. Daily uplifts: breathers, sustainers, restorers

11. Biopsychosociospiritual

■ *Theorist and the Causation of Illness*

Match the theorist in Column A with the appropriate type of theory in Column B.

Column A	Column B
12. _____ Bernard	A. Germ theory
13. _____ Schwartz	B. Homeostatic theory
14. _____ Friedman and Rosenman	C. Psychosocial theory
15. _____ Pasteur	D. Biobehavioral theory
16. _____ Lazarus	E. Mind-body theory
17. _____ Mason	
18. _____ Holmes	
19. _____ Selye	
20. _____ Wolf	
21. _____ Wolff	

Match the terms in Column A with the appropriate theorist in Column B.

Column A

22. _____ Internal milieu
23. _____ Way of life
24. _____ Daily hassles
25. _____ General adaptation syndrome
26. _____ Type A personality
27. _____ Self-regulation
28. _____ Homeostasis
29. _____ Cognitive appraisal
30. _____ Stage of resistance

Column B

A. Selye
B. Wolf
C. Bernard
D. Schwartz
E. Cannon
F. Lazarus
G. Friedman and Rosenman

KNOWLEDGE BUILDING: STUDY QUESTIONS RELATED TO THEORIES OF HEALTH AND ILLNESS

31. Differentiate between general adaptation syndrome (GAS) and local adaptation syndrome (LAS). Describe the three distinct stages associated with these two syndromes.

32. Mr. G. was admitted to the hospital for pneumonia. His serum glucose on admission was 135 mg/dL. He does not have diabetes mellitus. According to Selye's theory, what would be the reason for the above-normal serum glucose?

33. Differentiate between the two basic types of behavior patterns: type A personality and type B personality. Identify diseases that are usually associated with each personality type.

34. Explain what is meant by the term *biocultural factors* in disease.

35. Describe in your own words the definition of *health* and what causes illness.

Briefly define the following terms.

36.   Health

37.   Health promotion

38.   Wellness

39.   Self-responsibility

40.   Primary prevention

41.   Secondary prevention

42.   Tertiary prevention

43.   Risk factors

Match the behavior in Column A with the correct level of prevention in Column B.

Column A	**Column B**
44. _____ Participating in cardiac rehabilitation	A. Primary
45. _____ Maintaining ideal weight	B. Secondary
46. _____ Wearing a seat belt	C. Tertiary
47. _____ Screening for tuberculosis	
48. _____ Getting yearly Papanicolaou (Pap) smears	
49. _____ Participating in speech therapy after a stroke	
50. _____ Maintaining a low-cholesterol, low-fat diet	

Match the descriptive statement in Column A with the correct risk factor category in Column B.

Column A	**Column B**
51. _____ Smoking	A. Genetic
52. _____ Demise of extended family	B. Age
53. _____ At risk for sickle cell anemia	C. Biologic characteristics
54. _____ Excessive noise in work situation	D. Personal health habits
55. _____ Divorce	E. Lifestyle
56. _____ Increased incidence of atherosclerosis	F. Environment
57. _____ Lack of emotional support within family structure	
58. _____ Family history of diabetes	
59. _____ Lack of recreational exercise	
60. _____ Nutritional deficits or excesses	

THINKING CRITICALLY: KNOWING WHAT TO DO AND WHY

■ Study Questions on Health Promotion

61. Describe in your own words what is meant by "To promote health, nurses must understand the complex social, political, and economic forces that shape clients' lives."

63. Discuss the main points of *Healthy People 2000: Health Promotion/Disease Prevention: Objectives for the Nation.*

64. Review the American Nurses Association (ANA) social policy statement and summarize the ANA's definition of nursing as it relates to health promotion.

62. Compare Dunn's concept of wellness and high-level wellness to Travis' wellness model.

■ Creating an Awareness of Health Promotion and the Environment

65. Briefly discuss how individuals can play a role in cleaning, maintaining, and striving to improve conditions of the environment using the chart below.

Recognizing/Believing	Conserving	Water
Consuming	Eating	Moving
Stepping Forward		

THINKING CRITICALLY: CHRONIC CONDITIONS—KNOWING WHAT TO DO AND WHY

66. Describe the stages in which chronic conditions evolve.

67. The major focus of this chapter is on the physical, psychological, and social adaptive changes and challenges that a person with a chronic condition may face. Identify one change and one challenge from each area. Consider what nursing interventions you could implement to assist a client with the changes and the challenges.

You are in a clinical experience with a case manager preceptor. The preceptor receives a consult to assess Mr. J., an 80-year-old widower with a 15-year history of arteriosclerotic health disease and two recent hospitalizations for congestive heart failure. The preceptor assigns you to complete an assessment of Mr. J.

68. Identify specific areas to be included as part of the assessment of the client with a chronic condition.

69. Part of your assessment reveals that Mr. J. is on several medications, including Coumadin, digoxin, Norvasc, nitroglycerin, and Lasix. Based on this data, what further assessments would you make?

70. Data from your assessment leads you to the conclusion that Mr. J. could benefit from an exercise program. What further assessments would you need to make to determine if Mr. J. will be able to carry out an exercise program?

Putting It All Together

■ Case Study #1

Two females of similar backgrounds and academic performance were admitted to a very intense, demanding nursing program. Three weeks into the beginning nursing courses, student A is optimistic and has a positive attitude. She thinks the program is different from regular college courses but she expected it to be hard and demanding. Prior to starting the nursing program she met with her family to develop a plan for managing the changes that would occur because of nursing school. She is always prepared for class and clinical and is very seldom late for class. She has a "B" average in the course.

On the other hand, student B is often late for class and frequently misses class due to illness. Student B very seldom knows the class schedule or what assignments are due and when. She says she sleeps 3 to 4 hours a night and does not do anything but study. She believes the nursing program places impossible demands on her time. She is very negative and says the faculty is trying to flunk her out of the program. She complains about the course being unorganized and the faculty not knowing anything about what they are teaching. She hates any type of active learning and dislikes working in small groups. She complains that the instructor never tells the class what is important or what questions will be on the test. She does not understand why this course is not taught like her anatomy and physiology class. "My anatomy teacher gave us pages of notes and told us what was going to be on the test. I do not understand why nursing does not do the same thing. Why can't the teacher just tell us what is important and what we should study? I spend most of my time trying to figure out what is going to be on the test. It is just not fair." Student B has a "B" average in the course.

71. Use Lazarus' theory of stress response to explain these two nursing students' responses.

72. Which of the two students would be more susceptible to illness?

73. What are some of the daily hassles encountered by beginning nursing students?

74. Discuss some ways to help student B cope with the stressors of nursing school.

■ Creating an Awareness of Personal Health Promotion: Nutrition and Exercise

Nursing programs are demanding and time-consuming. Often, proper nutrition and exercise are given less priority during this time, when they actually should be given higher priority to help nursing students cope with the difficulties of juggling home, school, and work demands.

75. Take a few minutes to evaluate your dietary habits and exercise patterns. Use the food diary on page 649 of the textbook to document three days of your regular food intake. Use the food pyramid in Figure 2-1 in the textbook to analyze your diet. What are your strengths and weaknesses related to food intake? What changes need to be made to improve your health? Will these changes be easy or difficult to introduce into your present lifestyle?

76. Take a few minutes to evaluate your physical exercise habits over the last year. What are your strengths and weaknesses related to exercise? What changes need to be made to improve your health? Will these changes be easy or difficult to introduce into your present lifestyle? Discuss specific strategies to improve your flexibility, muscle strength, and endurance.

■ Case Study #2

Mr. G. is a 78-year-old client with diagnoses of angina, arteriosclerotic heart disease, and cerebrovascular accident. The physician has prescribed diuretic, cardiotonic, and antihypertensive drugs for him. The client is a widower and lives alone on a farm 20 minutes from a small town. His case is being followed by a home health agency.

On this visit, the nurse notes that his house is cluttered. He has difficulty finding his medicines and eventually locates them under some magazines on the floor of the living room. He indicates that he doesn't always remember to take them and sometimes gets the bottles mixed up. When the nurse does a drug count, there are too many diuretics and an insufficient number of cardiotonic drugs. His physical assessment reveals a blood pressure of 150/90, pulse 52, and 2+ pitting edema of the ankles.

77. The facts that Mr. G. is 78 years of age and has arteriosclerotic heart disease fit under which risk factor category?
    A. genetic
    B. lifestyle
    C. biologic characteristics
    D. environment

78. The fact that the client lives alone fits under which risk factor category?
    A. biologic characteristics
    B. lifestyle
    C. personal health habits
    D. age

79. The facts that Mr. G.'s blood pressure is 150/90 and he has 2+ pitting edema fit under which risk factor category?
    A. age
    B. personal health habits
    C. environment
    D. genetic

80. When establishing priorities for Mr. G., which one of the following nursing diagnoses would be ranked first?
    A. High risk for injury related to diminished mental processes
    B. Fluid volume excess related to improper drug therapy
    C. High risk for impaired gas exchange related to excess fluid volume
    D. High risk for impaired skin integrity related to 2+ pitting edema

81. Which one of the following health promotion measures addresses Mr. G.'s priority need?
    A. maintenance of self-responsibility
    B. stress control
    C. maintenance of nutritional intake
    D. identification of support system

■ *Chronic Conditions and Illness*

82. Chronic conditions are increasing in the United States for which of the following reasons?
    A. increased incidence of communicable diseases such as tuberculosis
    B. better survival from acute illnesses that have residual effects
    C. earlier discharge from the hospital
    D. the average age of people in the United States is decreasing

83. Which of the following behaviors would be expected of a client with a chronic illness in the psychological adaptation phase of integration?
    A. preoccupation with self
    B. insistence that nothing is wrong
    C. revising life goals
    D. feelings of guilt

84. Mr. M., age 28, is paralyzed from his waist down due to a car accident six years ago. Which of the following physiologic changes occurring in disuse syndrome would he be most at risk for?
    A. sleep disturbance
    B. pressure sores on his coccyx
    C. decreased lung volume
    D. loss of upper body muscle tone

85. The focus of hospice care for the person with a chronic condition is directed toward care of the client
    A. during the terminal phase of a chronic condition.
    B. during the acute episodes of a chronic condition.
    C. requiring ventilator support in the home.
    D. requiring intravenous therapy in the home.

86. Physiologic adaptive challenges for a person with a chronic condition would include all of the following except
    A. preventing complications of disuse syndrome.
    B. controlling disease manifestations.
    C. learning techniques to substitute for lost function.
    D. dealing with genetic concerns.

CHAPTER 2

Health Promotion in Young and Middle-Aged Adults

It is better to *prevent* diseases and health problems than to *treat* diseases and health problems. If as much money, time, and energy were devoted to health promotion and illness prevention no doubt the health care cost in America would decrease. Health promotion focuses on prevention and self-care. Health promotion activities covered in this chapter are healthy eating, healthy activity, and effective coping. In addition, recommendations for screening for disease are covered. It is important for nurses in all settings to be familiar with current recommendations for disease screening as well as healthy lifestyles. Nurses must "think outside the box," use creative strategies, and take active roles in improving the health of Americans.

OBJECTIVES

1.1   List the leading cause of death for young and middle-aged adults.

1.2   Identify health risks for young and middle-aged adults.

1.3   Discuss health promotion activities for young and middle-aged adults.

KNOWLEDGE BUILDING: STUDY QUESTIONS RELATED TO HEALTH PROMOTION

1.   What is the leading cause of death in young adults?

2.   Discuss two health-related goals of *Healthy People 2000* for young and middle-aged adults.

3.   True or false. The percentage of overweight people is slowly decreasing.

4.   Define obesity.

5.   Obese people have a higher risk to develop serious health problems. List four health risks for obese people.

6.   Your are presenting healthy eating information and the USDAA Food Guide Pyramid to female college students. One student asks you why there are specific guidelines for grains, fruits, and veg-etables; milk products; and protein/meat groups but not for the fats and sweets. How would you respond?

7.   For one day (24 hours) keep a food diary of everything you eat and drink. Read the labels or consult a resource that lists nutritional values. For each food or drink consumed, list the

- number of servings eaten.
- number of calories.
- total fat in grams.
- total carbohydrate count in grams.
- total fiber in grams.
- total protein in grams.

8.   Use the activity pyramid Figure 2-1 to develop an activity plan for a 50-year-old obese female.

9.   What is the purpose of the CAGE and AUDIT Questionnaires?

10.   List three health problems related to smoking.

11.   What would be your response to the following situation? A client tells you, "Every time I come to this clinic the nurse asks me how much I smoke and if I want assistance to stop smoking. Every time I tell them 'no, I don't want to stop smoking.' Can't you people take no for an answer? I am thinking about changing nurse practitioners."

12.   Your client is a 32-year-old female who has come to the clinic on a wellness visit. She tells you her last immunizations were the ones required for college. What immunizations are recommended by the U.S. Preventive Services Task Force (USPSTF)?

Match the barrier to exercise listed in Column A to the suggested nurse's response in Column B.

Column A

13. _____ I am usually too tired to exercise.
14. _____ There is not a convenient place.
15. _____ I am too old.
16. _____ I am too overweight.
17. _____ I do not have time.

Column B

A. I understand, but we are talking about 20 minutes three times a week; you can even break it up into smaller sessions. Let's look at your schedule and see how we can fit this in.

B. I understand, and this is a problem for many people. Let's talk about places and activities that are convenient and try to come up with a plan that will work for you.

C. I understand the feeling. What exercise do you feel you are too overweight to try? Everyone, regardless of size, can benefit from exercise. Walking is the easiest and most convenient to perform. Let's work together to come up with an exercise program that will work for you.

D. It is never too late to start exercising. People of any age can benefit from exercise. Mr. G. (pick someone who is older than the client) would have a good laugh at you saying you are too old to exercise.

E. Exercise actually increases your energy level.

Match the type of stress management in Column A with the description in Column B.

Column A

18. _____ Thought stopping
19. _____ Cognitive reappraisal
20. _____ Effective coping
21. _____ Rational emotive therapy
22. _____ Stress resistance

Column B

A. Decrease the body's response to stress by healthy eating and activities and relaxation techniques

B. Changing the perception of the event or stressor

C. Purposefully interrupting obsessive or negative dialog and replacing it with positive thoughts

D. Based on the premise that much stress is related to common irrational beliefs such as, "I must be perfect at everything I do."

E. Recognizing the problem causing stress and developing ways to cope with or solve the problem

Effective coping involves recognition of the problem causing stress and developing ways to cope with or solve the problem. Give the rationale for each of the following problem-solving skills.

Problem-Solving Skill

23. First, does the problem really exist or is it imagined?

24. Second, is the problem really important or just a nuisance?

25. Third, does the problem have feasible solutions?

Rationale

List the reason for recommended screening for the general population ages 25-64 years.

Screening	Reason	Frequency
Blood pressure	26.	Periodic
Height/weight	27.	Periodic
Total blood cholesterol	28.	Every 5 years
Pap test (Papanicolaou)	29.	At least every 3 years
Fecal occult blood test	30.	Annually
Mammogram and clinical breast exam	31.	Annually
Rubella serologic testing (females)	32.	Once
Assessment for problem drinking	33.	Periodic
Prostate exam Digital exam and PSA	34.	Males over age 50 and African-American males over age 40

3

Health Promotion in Older Adults

Approximately 60% of people entering the hospital are over age 65. Nurses caring for people over 65 need information on the developmental, physical, and psychosocial needs of this population, as well as information about special ethical, legal, and economic issues. Demographics reveal that the elderly population is currently the fastest-growing segment in the nation. This fact, and the special health care needs of this population, have implications for nursing and health care. A plan for these demographic changes is needed to meet the health care requirements of this population.

OBJECTIVES

3.1	Define terminology related to aging.
3.2	Discuss demographics related to persons over 65.
3.3	Discuss health promotion activities for persons over 65.
3.4	Describe physiologic and psychosocial factors influencing functional status of elderly persons.
3.5	Compare and contrast dementia, delirium, and depression.
3.6	Discuss medication use and abuse among persons over 65.
3.7	Describe government support, health care resources, services, and housing options for persons over 65.
3.8	Discuss ethical and legal issues affecting persons over 65.

LEARNING THE LANGUAGE: TERMINOLOGY RELATED TO HEALTH PROMOTION IN OLDER ADULTS

Match the terms in Column A with their descriptions in Column B.

Column A

1. _____ Advance directives
2. _____ Competence
3. _____ Delirium
4. _____ Dementia
5. _____ DETERMINE
6. _____ Gerontic nursing
7. _____ Geriatrics
8. _____ Gerontology
9. _____ Living wills
10. _____ Medicaid
11. _____ Medicare
12. _____ Ombudsman
13. _____ Omnibus Budget Reconciliation Act
14. _____ Patient Self-Determination Act
15. _____ SSI

Column B

A. Ability to adequately fulfill one's role and handle one's affairs

B. Law requiring that long-term care residents be maintained at their highest level of physical, mental, and psychosocial well-being

C. Advocacy organizations for nursing home residents

D. Act designed to protect health care consumers; requires providers to inform patients of right to refuse treatment and provide information about advance directives

E. Legally binding documents that allow competent people to document the medical procedures they want to have done should they be unable to make those decisions in the future

F. Legal documents to allow a person to specify what type of medical treatment is desired if the person becomes incapacitated

G. Government health insurance designed to provide medical care to individuals over 65

H. Government health assistance program to meet the needs of low-income people under 65 and for older people requiring long-term care

I. Clinical syndrome characterized by intellectual deterioration severe enough to interfere with the ability to cope with daily life

J. Syndrome characterized by global cognitive impairment of abrupt onset that is reversible

K. Nutrition assessment acronym

L. Branch of health care concerned with medical problems and care of elderly people

M. Specialized nursing care of elderly people that occurs in any setting

N. Ensures a minimum income to people with limited income who are blind, disabled, or elderly

O. Scientific study of the process and problems of aging

Mark the following statements true or false. Correct the information in the false statements.

16. _____ By the year 2020, people over 65 will make up nearly 22% of the U.S. population.

17. _____ Percentage of older people in minority ethnic groups will decline compared to the total percentage of the elderly population.

18. _____ Life expectancy for men is 78.6 years.

19. _____ Forty percent of women over 65 live with their spouses.

20. _____ Social Security benefits are the main source of income for people over 65.

21. _____ Fifty percent of people over 65 have one or more chronic illnesses.

22. _____ Older people have increased dietary needs for vitamin D, vitamin B$_6$, and calcium.

23. _____ The most common sensory impairments in people over 65 are touch sensations and hearing.

24. _____ Substance abuse in older adults is rare.

25. _____ Over one-half of all people over 65 are living in nursing homes.

26. _____ Ninety percent of people over 65 take an average of five prescriptive and three over-the-counter medications daily.

Briefly answer the following questions.

27. What are the three levels of nursing care provided in nursing homes?

28. What are the physiologic changes that affect the action of medications in people over 65?

29. What are teaching strategies that might have to be considered when teaching people over 65?

30. How do the physiologic changes affecting the action of medications in people over age 65 impact nursing care when giving medications?

31. Your client is a 72-year-old female with newly diagnosed non-insulin–dependent diabetes. You will be teaching your client about diabetes, medication, foot care, hyperglycemia, and hypoglycemia. Before you begin teaching, what assessments would you make of your client that would guide your teaching strategy?

32.   You are assigned a newly admitted client who is 80 years old. Among your assessments you would complete a thorough assessment of your client's sensory abilities. What would you include?

PUTTING IT ALL TOGETHER

33.   Physiologic changes that may affect the nutrition of people over 65 include all of the following except
    A.   loss of taste buds.
    B.   increased hydrochloric acid production.
    C.   decreased colonic peristalsis.
    D.   fat intolerance.

34.   Assisting your older adult client to cope with multiple losses could include which of the following strategies?
    A.   relocation to a new apartment
    B.   getting rid of personal items
    C.   joining groups
    D.   increasing antidepressive medication

35.   Dementia is characterized by which of the following features?
    A.   gradual onset
    B.   reversible state
    C.   fearful or perplexed affect
    D.   poor long-term memory

36.   Congregate housing would be the most appropriate option for a person who needs
    A.   24-hour supervision.
    B.   terminal-care support.
    C.   supervision and assistance with activities of daily living (ADL).
    D.   assistance with meals, transportation, and social and recreational activities.

37.   Approximately half of the physical deterioration in older adults is caused by
    A.   chronic illness.
    B.   normal aging changes.
    C.   osteoporosis.
    D.   disuse.

U N I T

2

Health Care
Delivery Systems

CHAPTER 4

Overview of
Health Care Delivery

The health care system in the United States is large and complex. There are many groups and institutions that affect the structure and function of the system. In addition, these groups and institutions affect the quality and cost of health care.

There are a variety of funding programs that assist with the cost of health care. These programs have changed significantly in the past 75 years in an attempt to meet the needs of society.

Working within the health care system are nurses, the primary care providers. The roles of nurses have also changed. The practice of nursing no longer is limited to the hospital setting. Today, the discipline of nursing offers a variety of career opportunities.

OBJECTIVES

4.1 Discuss the major groups and institutions involved in the United States health care system.

4.2 Describe the various mechanisms available for funding health care.

4.3 Discuss the major focuses of the Period of Expansion, the Period of Regulation and Cost Containment, and the Period of Reform.

4.4 Discuss nursing's role in health care reform.

LEARNING THE LANGUAGE: TERMINOLOGY RELATED TO HEALTH CARE DELIVERY

Match the definitions in Column A with the correct health care funding program in Column B.

Column A

1. _____ A federally funded national health insurance program for citizens over age 65

2. _____ A joint federal and state insurance program for certain low-income citizens

3. _____ The largest private not-for-profit insurance company set up through special legislation in the 1930s

4. _____ The client pays a monthly premium that entitles him or her to health care from a physician within the system

5. _____ For-profit companies that sell insurance to companies or individuals

6. _____ A group of physicians and at least one hospital that link together to form a system of care

7. _____ A federally mandated, state funded and administered insurance program for workers injured on the job

8. _____ A term used to describe clients who have no insurance and are responsible for payment of health care

9. _____ Businesses that develop their own insurance programs for employees

Column B

A. PPO (preferred provider organization)

B. HMO (health maintenance organization)

C. Self-insurance

D. Medicare

E. Medicaid

F. Blue Cross and Blue Shield

G. Commercial insurance companies

H. Workers' compensation

I. Private pay

KNOWLEDGE BUILDING: STUDY QUESTIONS RELATED TO HEALTH CARE DELIVERY

■ Short Answer

10. Explain the major focus of the Period of Expansion, Period of Regulation and Cost Containment, and Period of Reform in health care funding.

Explain the purposes of the following:

11. Social Security Act of 1935

12. Hill-Burton Act

13. National Health Planning Resources Act of 1974

14. Tax Equity and Fiscal Responsibility Act (TEFRA) of 1983

15. Prospective Payment System (PPS) and Diagnostic Related Groups (DRGs)

16. What are the public's health care concerns?

17. What is the largest group of health care providers?

5

Ambulatory Health Care

The period of health care cost containment that began in the mid-1980s has dramatically changed the focus of health care. Mandates from health care payers have caused a shift of health care services from the hospital to community-based settings. Surgeries, treatments, and procedures that once required lengthy hospital stays are now performed in ambulatory care centers. The different types of ambulatory care centers share two common characteristics: they provide care for clients who require less than 24 hours of care and for clients who can manage their self-care after the procedure. The shift in the health care workforce from hospital-based to community-based settings has several implications for nursing. Ambulatory care nurses have many of the same responsibilities for organizing and providing care as hospital-based nurses, but they have less time to provide nursing care. They must be aware of the practice standards and protocols for their setting and be able to quickly assess and prioritize plans of care for clients who remain in their institution for less than 24 hours.

OBJECTIVES

5.1 Define the terms related to ambulatory care.

5.2 Discuss the major changes in health care that have resulted in an increase in ambulatory care services.

5.3 Discuss the general discharge criteria for ambulatory care.

5.4 Discuss the role of the nurse in ambulatory care.

5.5 Discuss the criteria for AAACN (American Academy of Ambulatory Care Nursing) certification.

LEARNING THE LANGUAGE: TERMINOLOGY RELATED TO AMBULATORY HEALTH CARE

Match the definitions in Column A with the appropriate term in Column B.

Column A	Column B
1. _____ Nursing care provided to clients with institutional episodes of less than 24 hours	A. Ambulatory care
2. _____ Includes individualized and standard treatment for a specific client or group	B. Professional nurse
3. _____ Organized services delivered to groups of clients by nursing staff	C. Ambulatory care nursing
4. _____ A registered nurse	D. Family
5. _____ May include individuals related by blood or marriage, or in self-defined relationships	E. Health care team
6. _____ Care delivered to patients who require less than 24 hours of institutional care	F. Patient
7. _____ Includes the patient, family, and other members of the system who are involved in the development and implementation of the care plan	G. Plan of care
8. _____ An individual who requests or receives nursing services	H. Nursing services

Match the descriptions in Column A with the nursing role in Column B.

Column A	Column B
9. _____ Designs and presents in-service education	A. Enabling operation
10. _____ Develops expected client outcomes	B. Technical procedure
11. _____ Assists with procedures	C. Nursing process
12. _____ Promotes positive public relations	D. Telephone communication
13. _____ Calls client with test results	E. Advocacy
14. _____ Instructs client on medical-nursing regimen	F. Teaching
15. _____ Completes client history	G. Care coordination
16. _____ Organizes and maintains work environment	H. Expert practice
17. _____ Finds resources in the community	I. Quality improvement
18. _____ Participates in research of others	J. Research
19. _____ Participates in on- and off-site education	K. Continuing education

THINKING CRITICALLY

Provide short answers to the following questions.

20.   Discuss the main reasons for the shift from hospital settings to ambulatory care settings.

21.   List the two criteria for all ambulatory care settings.

22. List five ambulatory care settings in your area.

24. Discuss the role of the nurse in an ambulatory care setting that uses a medical model versus the nursing model.

23. List the common discharge criteria for ambulatory care.

25. Discuss the criteria for AAACN certification and for maintaining certification.

Acute Health Care

The acute care setting is changing rapidly. Students entering nursing today will be a part of these changes as the role of the professional nurse adapts to the setting changes. Chapter 6 provides an overview of the roles of the nurse in the acute care setting, options for settings for client care, nursing care delivery systems within the acute care setting, and measures to ensure quality delivery of health care.

OBJECTIVES

6.1 Discuss the historical changes that have occurred in relation to hospital nursing.

6.2 Describe hospital facilities available for clients who require acute care and subacute care.

6.3 Describe roles and responsibilities of nurses in hospitals.

6.4 Compare and contrast nursing care delivery systems.

6.5 Discuss the role of the licensed nurse in managing unlicensed assistive personnel.

6.6 Discuss various measures whose purposes are to ensure quality health care delivery.

LEARNING THE LANGUAGE: TERMINOLOGY RELATED TO ACUTE HEALTH CARE

Match the terms in Column A with their description in Column B.

Column A

1. _____ Age Discrimination and Employment Act
2. _____ Case management
3. _____ Clinical pathways
4. _____ Cross-training
5. _____ Diagnosis-related groups
6. _____ Magnet hospital
7. _____ Nursing intensity
8. _____ Occupational Safety and Health Act
9. _____ Primary care
10. _____ Proprietary hospital
11. _____ Rehabilitation Act of 1973
12. _____ Risk management
13. _____ Subacute care
14. _____ Team nursing

Column B

A. For-profit, privately owned hospital

B. Provide medical care for complex problems that require a team of health care providers

C. Designed to fill the gaps between acute and long-term care

D. Length of stay estimates tied to payments

E. System of care in which the RN leads a group of health care personnel in providing care for 10–20 clients

F. Model of care that provides consistent care from an RN when he or she is working

G. Care delivery mode that incorporates continuity and efficiency in addressing long-term needs of clients

H. Guide to direct care and recovery from a predictable problem

I. Combination of the amount of care and skill level at which care is provided

J. Process of preparing nurses to be able to work effectively in more than one unit

K. Law whose purpose was to promote employment of older people based on their ability rather than age

L. Law requiring all employees with government contracts of more than $25,000 to take affirmative action to recruit, hire, and advance disabled people who are qualified

M. Requires a place of employment to be free from recognized hazard

N. Planned program of loss prevention and liability control

■ *Short Answer*

15. What were the major factors in the 1920s, '30s, and '40s that had an impact on hospital nursing?

16. What are the primary reasons that a client requires hospitalization?

17. What are the three types of hospitals?

18. What has been the impetus for the development of subacute care facilities?

19. What are the major roles of nurses within the acute care setting?

20. What are major categories usually included in patient classification systems?

21. What are goals for nurses and other health care workers that will enhance the dimensions of performance and assist with the goal of cost containment?

■ *Multiple Choice*

22. The main disadvantage of team nursing is that it
    A. is expensive because personnel are fragmented.
    B. generates many calls to physicians from one nursing unit.
    C. requires that the nurse be proficient in all nursing tasks.
    D. requires clients to interact with multiple people.

23. You are planning care for your five clients today. You have one unlicensed assistive person working with you. In planning tasks to delegate, which of the following is the most important question?
    A. What is the age of the client?
    B. Is the task one that only an RN can legally perform?
    C. How many clients are you assigned?
    D. Who is the least expensive person who can do the task?

24. Patient classification systems have the purpose of identifying
    A. the acuity level of the clients.
    B. the clients by diagnosis.
    C. clients requiring home health care.
    D. staffing needs for a particular unit.

25. As a beginning professional concerned with risk management, it would be important for you to know that which of the following is in the top five areas of highest risk in the hospital?
    A. medication errors
    B. decubitus ulcers
    C. restraint incidents
    D. sharps injuries

CHAPTER 7

Home Health Care

The term *home health care* is used, along with *community-based nursing*, to describe health care primarily provided to clients outside acute care settings. Rising health care costs and consumer demands for comprehensive and economical services have greatly increased the need for home health care. The shift from acute care to community-based care is expected to increase yearly. Continuity of care is a major theme. In addition to being competent in communication, assessment, and technical skills, home health care nurses must know about reimbursements and the eligibility requirements of Medicare, Medicaid, and third-party providers. The added responsibility of providing care and documenting the care following accreditation and reimbursement guidelines can become overwhelming. The Omaha System, designed by practicing community health nurses, facilitates nursing practice, documentation, and information management. It provides a framework for providing care, documentation of services, and evaluation of outcomes of care. This system is in the public domain; thus, potential users may access it easily.

OBJECTIVES

7.1 Discuss one major trend that affects home healthcare.

7.2 Discuss the eligibility, requirements, and coverage for Medicare and Medicaid.

7.3 Discuss the basic principle of community-based nursing care.

7.4 Discuss the purpose of the Omaha System.

LEARNING THE LANGUAGE: TERMINOLOGY RELATED TO HOME HEALTH CARE

Define the following terms.

1. Acute care/hospital-based nursing

2. Community-based nursing

3. Home health care

4. The Omaha System

5. The Nightingale Tracker

THINKING CRITICALLY

Provide short answers to the following questions.

6. What is the major trend affecting the use of home health care services in the United States?

7. Discuss the basic philosophy of community-focused care.

8. The home health care nurse is scheduled to insert a Foley catheter in a homebound female client. Discuss how planning and implementing this procedure would be different in the home versus the hospital setting.

Use the bridge to home health care on page 109 of the textbook to determine the eligibility for Medicare or Medicaid for the following situations.

9. _____ Mr. J. is a 75-year-old male who suffered a cerebrovascular accident (CVA) two weeks ago. He is paralyzed on his left side and has difficulty with speech and eating.

10. _____ Mr. E. is a 65-year-old male who is recovering from a myocardial infarction he had six weeks ago. He is able to drive himself to the clinic and has resumed moderate activities.

11. _____ Ms. D. is a 55-year-old female with congestive heart failure secondary to cardiomyopathy. She has been disabled for three years and receives Social Security benefits.

12. _____ Mr. K. is a 45-year-old college professor who has recently been diagnosed with insulin-dependent diabetes mellitus.

13. _____ B.L., a 24-month-old male, is ventilator-dependent, secondary to a closed head injury.

CHAPTER 8

Long-Term Care

The nurse's roles and responsibilities in long-term care facilities (LTCFs) are complex, awesome, and rewarding. It is complex and awesome because the residents have multiple physical problems and mental changes. There are no on-site physicians, no diagnostic testing, nor any laboratory. Nurses must recognize subtle signs of change in physical condition or behavior and decide when to contact the physician and family. Caring for residents in LTCFs is often very rewarding because of the long-term relationship with residents and their families.

Residents of LTCFs can be any age; however, the majority are elderly. The risk of being in an LTCFs increases with each decade. The average age of residents is 82 years old. Most residents need assistance with activities of daily living or require interventions that they cannot perform independently. Approximately one-half of the residents of LTCFs have some type of progressive cognitive impairment. This chapter focuses on long-term care facilities; however, the long-term care system also includes subacute or transitional living, assisted living, adult day care, home care and hospice.

OBJECTIVES

8.1 Discuss the historical development of long-term care facilities.

8.2 Discuss the long-term care regulations.

8.3 Discuss the resident's adjustments to long-term care facilities.

8.4 Describe the staffing requirements for long-term care facilities.

THINKING CRITICALLY

1. Discuss the significance of the following on the growth of long-term care facilities.
   - The Social Security act of 1935

   - The 1946 Hill Burton Hospital Survey

   - Counteraction Act, 1965 Medicare and Medicaid

   - The Omnibus Budget Reconciliation Act of 1987

2. What are the staffing requirements for long-term care facilities?

3. Discuss the requirements for the minimum assessment database (MDS).

4. List important resident information that is not assessed on the MDS.

5. Give one example of each regulation included in the Omnibus Budget Reconciliation Act (OBRA). Use Box 8-1 in the textbook.

   A. Residents' rights _____

   B. Admission, transfer, discharge _____

   C. Resident behavior and facility practices _____

   D. Quality of life _____

   E. Resident assessment _____

   F. Quality of care _____

   G. Nursing services _____

   H. Dietary services _____

   I. Physician Services _____

   J. Specialized rehabilitative services _____

   K. Pharmacy services _____

   L. Administration _____

Discuss adjustments of the residents to long-term care facilities related to:

6.   Environment

7.   Routines

8.   People

9.   Independence

10.   Give two examples of how nurses can promote holistic nursing care in long-term care facilities.

Health Assessment

CHAPTER 9

Health History

Health assessment focuses on the individual client. It is divided into two components: the health history and the physical assessment. The health history consists of subjective data while the physical assessment contains objective data. Usually, the health history includes biographic and demographic information, health risk appraisal, psychosocial assessment, and a review of the client's physical health history. In addition, an in-depth nutritional assessment and a spiritual assessment may be included.

OBJECTIVES

9.1   Describe the concept of health assessment.

9.2   Discuss the main components of the health history interview.

9.3   Discuss the importance of psychosocial assessment for clients with medical-surgical problems.

9.4   Discuss the eight psychosocial risk factors.

9.5   Explain the purpose of the review of symptoms and symptoms analysis portion of the physical health interview.

9.6   Record health assessment findings using an organized format.

9.7   Apply the nursing process to health assessment.

LEARNING THE LANGUAGE: TERMINOLOGY RELATED TO HEALTH ASSESSMENT

Match the data in Column A with the correct component of the health history in Column B.

Column A	Column B
1. _____ "I have had a headache for three days."	A. Review of systems
2. _____ White female	B. Family history
3. _____ What makes the headache worse?	C. Symptom analysis
4. _____ Have you experienced any chest pain, shortness of breath, dizziness?	D. Chief complaint
5. _____ Hypertension for two years	E. Past medical history
6. _____ Lives with wife and three children	F. Biographic information
7. _____ Father has diabetes mellitus	G. Psychosocial history

Match the data in Column A with the correct functional health pattern in Column B.

Column A		Column B	
8. _____	Takes a vitamin supplement	A.	Activity and exercise
9. _____	Denies any constipation	B.	Nutrition and metabolic
10. _____	Walks two miles, three days a week	C.	Elimination
11. _____	Yearly Papanicolaou (Pap) smear	D.	Health perception and health management
12. _____	Wears glasses for reading	E.	Cognitive–perceptual

Use textbook Table 9-2, Health Promotion and Risk Management, to complete the following grid.

RISK FACTOR	SCREENING AND PREVENTIVE MEASURES		
Risk Factor	**Potential Health Problem**	**Self-Care Activities**	**Professional Level Activities**
Risk Factor: Race			
13. Black	Hypertension		
	Skin cancer		Monitor lesions
14. Hispanic		Regular exercise Diet with > 30% fat	
15. Native-American	Alcohol abuse		
Risk Factor: Genetic or Family-Related			
16. Heart disease	Cardiovascular disease		
17. Overweight	Obesity-related diseases		
18. Breast cancer in mother or sister		Learn how to perform breast self-examination (BSE)	Mammography as indicated per age
Risk Factor: Age-Related			
19. Falls	Injury or trauma		
20. Self-medication errors		Request or use prepackaged unit dose medications	Careful assessment of medication history
Risk Factor: Biologic			
21. Hyperlipidemia	Cardiovascular disease		
22. Hypersensitivity reactions		Avoid known allergens	

Risk Factor: Personal Habits

23.	Inadequate rest and sleep	Lowered resistance to illness		Complete evaluation of sleep patterns
24.	Inadequate calcium intake		Consume 800 mg of calcium per day; Limit milk sources of calcium	
25.	Tobacco use	Cancer of mouth or lung		Counseling to help stop smoking

Risk Factor: Lifestyle

26.	Stress and coping ability	Many health problems related to high stress levels		
27.	High-risk sexual activity	STDs	Practice safe sex, use condoms; limit sex partners	

Risk Factor: Environment

28.			Limit exposure to loud music and machinery; Wear protective earplugs	Regular, complete audiometric screening
29.	High accident risk activity	Unintentional injury or death		

Risk Factor: Socioeconomic

30.	Recent immigration	Diseases common to locale of origin
31.	Lack of adequate health insurance coverage	Delayed or postponed treatment of health problems

THINKING CRITICALLY: SHORT ANSWER QUESTIONS

32. Differentiate between subjective and objective data.

33. Differentiate between psychological patterns and social experiences.

34. Discuss the nurse's responsibility concerning confidential information.

35. Describe methods the nurse could use to assess the client's health perception.

36. Discuss the purpose of a health risk appraisal.

37. Explain the difference between *affect* and *mood* and how you would assess for each.

38. Give an example of how the nurse would assess recent and remote memory.

PUTTING IT ALL TOGETHER

39. Which of the following is considered biographic information?
    A. 36 years of age
    B. smokes one pack of cigarettes daily
    C. hypertensive
    D. consumes a diet low in fat

40. Which of the following is classified as a biologic risk factor?
    A. sleeps six hours a night
    B. impaired mobility
    C. hyperlipidemia
    D. works in a textile plant

41. Which of the following is classified as a lifestyle risk factor?
    A. consumes six beers a day
    B. consumes 300 milligrams of calcium daily
    C. works in a high-risk environment
    D. participates in high-risk sexual activity

42. Which one of the following is classified as an environmental risk factor?
    A. works in a stress-provoking situation
    B. lacks insurance coverage at work
    C. recently divorced
    D. lacks health-promoting self-care habits

43. A client comes to the clinic complaining of chest pain and shortness of breath. The nurse would prioritize the health history to focus on
    A. activity and exercise patterns.
    B. symptom analysis.
    C. cognitive and perceptual patterns.
    D. health risk appraisal.

44. During a psychosocial assessment, the nurse assesses the client's mental status. Which of the following would give the nurse information regarding a client's mental status? The client
    A. can repeat a series of five to seven numbers.
    B. is highly motivated.
    C. has a strong support system.
    D. is heterosexual.

45. Ms. J., 55, states that she does a monthly BSE. The nurse should recommend a mammogram
    A. every 2-3 years.
    B. every year.
    C. every 3 years.
    D. every 1-2 years.

CHAPTER 10

Physical Examination

The physical examination consists of collecting objective data that is used to validate the client's subjective data. The extent and depth of the physical examination are determined by the client's needs. There are two types of physical examinations: the screening examination and the regional examination. The screening examination is an organized, superficial assessment of all major body systems. The regional examination is an in-depth assessment of a specific body system. The four primary techniques used in a physical examination are inspection, palpation, percussion, and auscultation.

OBJECTIVES

10.1   Discuss the purpose of a physical examination.

10.2   Describe the types of physical examinations.

10.3   Describe the four primary techniques used in a physical examination.

10.4   Define anatomic terms used to describe locations of physical findings.

10.5   Calculate ideal body weight.

10.6   Identify equipment commonly used in a physical examination.

10.7   Discuss the preparation for a physical examination.

10.8   Demonstrate a basic adult screening physical examination.

10.9   Demonstrate ability to process and record data.

LEARNING THE LANGUAGE: TERMINOLOGY RELATED TO PHYSICAL EXAMINATION

Match the definitions in Column A with the correct type of physical assessment in Column B.

Column A

1. _____ A superficial check of the major body systems for detecting possible problems

2. _____ An in-depth assessment of a specific body system

3. _____ An in-depth assessment plus laboratory and diagnostic tests

4. _____ To record baseline data and to assess for changes in the client's health status

Column B

A.   Periodic head-to-toe assessment

B.   Complete physical examination

C.   Screening physical examination

D.   Regional or branching examination

Use textbook Table 10–1 to match the assessment areas in Column A with the client position or activity in Column B. There may be more than one answer.

Column A	**Column B**
5. _____ Prostate	A. Sitting
6. _____ Otoscopic	B. Standing
7. _____ Breast	C. Walking
8. _____ Heart	D. Supine
9. _____ Lungs	E. Left lateral recumbent
10. _____ Peripheral pulses	F. Lithotomy
11. _____ Abdomen	G. Standing and bending over examining table
12. _____ Deep tendon reflexes	H. Sims'
13. _____ Anus and rectum	
14. _____ External eye	

KNOWLEDGE BUILDING: STUDY QUESTIONS RELATED TO PHYSICAL EXAMINATION

Provide short answers to the following questions.

15. List at least four aspects that can be assessed by the inspection technique.

16. Describe when the nurse should use the diaphragm on the stethoscope. When should the bell be used?

Define the following and give one example.

17. Inspection

18. Light palpation

19. Deep palpation

20. Percussion

21. Auscultation

THINKING CRITICALLY: KNOWING WHAT TO DO AND WHY

What would you do if:

22. the client failed the whisper test?

23. bronchial lung sounds were heard in the bases?

24. the client has heard muffled heart sounds?

25. no bowel sounds were auscultated?

26. you were unable to palpate the popliteal pulses?

27. you were unable to elicit deep tendon reflexes?

28. you heard a blowing heart sound?

29. you obtained a sitting BP of 120/80 in the right arm and 140/90 in the left arm?

30. you suspected a yeast infection when examining the oral cavity?

31. you elicited rebound tenderness during the abdomen exam?

32. in the health history, the client reported a productive cough?

33. the client reported difficulty swallowing in the health history?

34.   the client has a strong family history of breast cancer?

39.   Pulses strong in both legs

40.   Bad breath noted

Explain the following:

35.   What is meant by "the client is used as a control or self-standard for comparison during the physical exam"?

41.   Vital signs WNL

42.   Normal bowel sounds

36.   Why does the nurse compare the physical examination to known standards?

43.   Hair color appropriate for age

44.   Can see with both eyes

37.   What is meant by the term *contralateral*?

45.   No problems with hearing

Revise the following physical examination findings.

38.   Lung sounds within normal limits (WNL)

■ *Multiple Choice*

46. Which part of the hand is used to determine skin temperature?
    A.   fingertips
    B.   dorsum
    C.   palmar surface
    D.   ulnar aspect

47. Tympany is the characteristic sound heard with percussion of the
    A.   stomach or bowel.
    B.   chest of a client with emphysema.
    C.   liver.
    D.   lungs of a child.

48. The tubing on a stethoscope should be
    A.   6-8 inches in length.
    B.   less than 6 inches in length.
    C.   no longer than 12-15 inches in length.
    D.   no longer than 20 inches in length.

49. Which anatomic structure or organ is distal to the femur?
    A.   left kidney
    B.   pelvis
    C.   iliac crest
    D.   tibia

50. Which anatomic structure or organ is ipsilateral to the right arm?
    A.   right leg
    B.   nose
    C.   left leg
    D.   mouth

51. The client's pulse is easily palpable, forceful, and not easily obliterated by pressure. The nurse should record the pulse amplitude as
    A.   0
    B.   1+
    C.   2+
    D.   3+

52. The client's respirations are rapid and shallow. Inspirations are prolonged followed by a short, ineffective expiration. The nurse would classify these respiratory patterns as
    A.   Kussmaul's.
    B.   apneustic.
    C.   bradypnea.
    D.   eupnea.

11

Diagnostic Assessment

Diagnostic testing refers to the various methods used to assess body structure and function. Nursing responsibilities include assessing the client's ability to participate in testing, preparing the client for the test, and caring for the client after the test. It also includes interpreting and/or communicating test results and collaborating with other members of the health care team. It is common for the nurse to delegate performing specimen collection, and pre- and postprocedure care to other licensed and unlicensed personnel. Delegation of tasks to other personnel requires clear instructions; therefore, the nurse should be familiar with the various tests and the pre- and postprocedure care.

OBJECTIVES

11.1 Discuss the purpose of diagnostic testing.

11.2 Describe the various types of diagnostic testing.

11.3 Discuss the nursing responsibilities for diagnostic testing.

11.4 Discuss aspects of diagnostic testing that are commonly delegated to other personnel under the supervision of the nurse.

LEARNING THE LANGUAGE: TERMINOLOGY RELATED TO DIAGNOSTIC TESTING

Match the definitions in Column A with the correct diagnostic test in Column B.

Column A	Column B
1. _____ Study of cell function	A. Microbiology studies
2. _____ Diagnostic procedure for study of bones and soft tissue	B. Blood studies
	C. Urine studies
3. _____ Representations produced by all types of x-rays	D. Diagnostic imaging
	E. X-ray studies
4. _____ The use of high-frequency sound waves to visualize soft tissues	F. Contrast x-rays
	G. Computed tomography (CT)
5. _____ Direct visualization of a body system or part by means of a lighted, flexible tube	H. Magnetic resonance imaging (MRI)
	I. Positron emission tomography (PET)
6. _____ Provides information on kidney and lower urinary tract function and systematic disorders that affect urine formation	J. Ultrasonography
	K. Angiography
7. _____ Contrast material is injected into vessels to assess their patency or evaluate blood flow	L. Radionuclide scanning
	M. Endoscopy
8. _____ Used to determine normal, expected abnormal, and unexpected abnormal findings in the blood	N. Cytologic studies
9. _____ Performed to determine whether bacteria are present in a sample of body fluid or tissue	
10. _____ Radiopaque liquid is used to identify defects in the GI system	
11. _____ Scans cross-sectional image differences in bone and soft tissue	
12. _____ Radioisotopes or tracers that are used to visualize organs or body regions that cannot be seen on plain films	
13. _____ Noninvasive test that uses magnetic fields and radiofrequency impulses to produce images	
14. _____ Allows imaging of metabolic and physiologic function	

Match the definitions in Column A with the correct term in Column B.

Column A	Column B
15. _____ A specimen that has been spread across a glass slide	A. International systems of units (SI)
	B. Specificity
16. _____ The use of dyes to help identify microorganisms	C. Noninvasive
	D. Stain
17. _____ Does not require skin to be broken or a cavity or body system to be entered	E. Smear
	F. Sensitivity
18. _____ The ability of a diagnostic test to correctly identify a person who is disease-free	
19. _____ Provides common language for units of measurement	
20. _____ The ability to correctly identify disease	

Give the rationale for the selected nursing intervention.

Diagnostic Procedure	Preprocedure Care	Postprocedure Care
MRI	21. Ask client to remove all metal-containing objects (e.g., brassiere, jewelry, wristwatch).	22. Monitor output if contrast dye was used.
Upper gastrointestinal series	23. Instruct client to abstain from food and drink for 6-8 hours before test.	24. Teach client to drink extra fluids and eat adequate fiber.
Computed tomography (CT)	25. Ask about problems with claustrophobia.	26. Record intake and output.
Positron emission tomography (PET)	27. Sedate agitated clients prior to procedure.	28. Resume normal activities.
Ultrasonography	29. Instruct the client on what to expect during the procedure.	30. Resume normal activities.
Arteriogram	31. Assess for iodine allergies.	32. If femoral approach was used, keep the leg immobile for 12 hours.
Bronchoscopy	33. Assess cranial nerves 9 and 10.	34. Nothing by mouth until gag reflex returns.

Biopsy

35. Allow time for client to express concerns and anxieties.

36. Monitor biopsy site.

Blood cultures

37. Thoroughly clean the puncture site.

38. Administer antibiotics after the specimen is drawn.

24-hour urinalysis

39. Instruct the client on the importance of collecting all of the urine for the specified time.

40. Instruct the client not to place urine in the collection container after the test ends.

UNIT

4

Foundations of Medical-Surgical Nursing

ANATOMY AND PHYSIOLOGY REVIEW: THE CELL

The cell is the basic unit of all living organisms. A basic understanding of cell structure and function enhances understanding of material in later chapters. For example, the effects of a myocardial infarction (heart attack) are directly related to injury at the cellular level and many of the effects and side effects of medications are based on cellular activities, as well as allergic reactions and multiple other pathophysiologic events.

OBJECTIVES

4.1 Compare and contrast the general structure and function of prokaryotic and eukaryotic cells.

4.2 Discuss the structure and function of the major cell components.

4.3 Discuss the process of cell replication.

4.4 Describe alterations in cellular structure and function.

4.5 Discuss various mechanisms of cellular injury.

LEARNING THE LANGUAGE: TERMINOLOGY RELATED TO THE CELL

Match the following descriptors with the correct type of cell.

Column A

1. _____ Cytoplasmic matrix
2. _____ Organelles
3. _____ Minimal infrastructure
4. _____ Produce energy
5. _____ Reproduce themselves

Column B

A. Prokaryotic cells
B. Eukaryotic cells
C. Both

Briefly describe the function of the following.

6. Cell

7. Cell membrane

8. Nucleus

9. Mitochondria

10. Endoplasmic reticulum

11. Golgi complex

12. Lysosomes

13. Microtubules and microfilaments

14. Identify the cell structures:

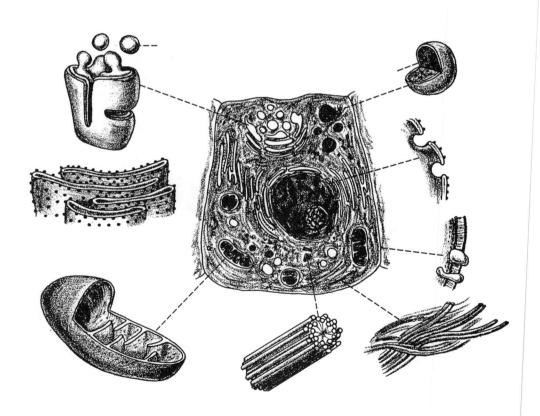

Match the terms in Column A with the definitions in Column B.

Column A

15. _____ Active transport
16. _____ Bulk transport
17. _____ Diffusion
18. _____ Deoxyribonucleic acid (DNA)
19. _____ Facilitated diffusion
20. _____ Osmosis
21. _____ Phagocytosis
22. _____ Pinocytosis
23. _____ Receptor-mediated
24. _____ Ribonucleic acid (RNA)

Column B

A. Movement of water across a cell membrane

B. Mode of entry of gases and smaller, relatively hydrophilic molecules into cells

C. Transport into cells by means of special carrier proteins for small diffusible molecules with electrical charges

D. Expenditure of energy to transport ions or molecules across the membrane against an electrical gradient

E. Method of transport where cells take up substances by trapping the material within the enclosing vesicle

F. Transport that is random, spontaneous, and nonspecific for uptake of small amounts of extracellular fluid

G. A specific receptor on a membrane binds to its ligand and initiates uptake

H. Transmits genetic instructions and determines the structures of cell proteins

I. Contains hereditary transport information

J. Process similar to receptor-mediated transport except material taken up is particulate and the enclosing vesicle much larger

■ *True/False*

Respond to the following true/false questions on cell replication. If a question is false, support your answer with a corrected statement.

25. _____ Skin, mucous membrane, and blood-forming cells are replaced at a rapid rate.

26. _____ Heart and skeletal muscles may reproduce only once or twice in a lifetime.

27. _____ Hepatocytes and differentiated lymphocytes reproduce in response to a stimulus.

28. _____ An injury causing loss of cells in the spinal cord would be permanent.

29. _____ Somatic cells divide exclusively by mitosis.

30. _____ Mitosis and meiosis are both used in the process to produce gametes.

31. _____ Mitosis produces two daughter cells that have gene content identical to the parent cell.

■ *Short Answer*

32. What are the three major causes of cellular alteration?

33. Differentiate among cell changes with atrophy, hypertrophy, precancerous, and neoplastic growth.

■ *Multiple Choice*

34. Your client sustained a gunshot wound to the lumbar spinal cord with loss of sensation below the level of injury. Based on your knowledge of cell replication, you would expect that your client will have
   A. rapid return of function.
   B. no return of function.
   C. slow return of function.
   D. partial return of function.

35. Based on your understanding of cell replication, you would expect recovery of blood-forming cells from chemotherapy (cancer medications) to be
   A. slow.
   B. nonexistent.
   C. fairly rapid.
   D. temporary.

36. Your client is admitted to the hospital with a serious gram-negative infection. The mechanism of cellular damage involves
   A. reduced nutrient absorption.
   B. stasis of blood, clot formation, and ischemia.
   C. mutations, enzyme inactivation, and interruption of cell division.
   D. release of endotoxins that act on macrophages and T lymphocytes.

12

Clients with Fluid Imbalances: Promoting Positive Outcomes

Any client can develop fluid and electrolyte imbalances. It is the nurse's responsibility to assess each client's hydration status, to anticipate potential fluid and electrolyte imbalances, and to prevent associated problems. Fluid and electrolyte balance is essential for life. Therefore, the following principles are important: intake must equal output (the body is mostly water [60%], and most of this water is inside the cells); changes in fluid pressures produce movement of fluid from one fluid compartment to another; and, specifically, hydrostatic pressure – colloid osmotic pressure must equal capillary filtration pressure.

OBJECTIVES

12.1   Define terms related to fluid imbalance.

12.2   Discuss the concepts of fluid pressures resulting in fluid movement and osmolality balance and imbalance.

12.3   Describe the etiologic factors and pathophysiology that underlie fluid volume imbalances, with and without osmolality abnormalities.

12.4   Accurately assess a person's fluid status.

12.5   Identify people who are at risk for developing fluid imbalances and identify the specific imbalances that they are likely to incur.

12.6   Describe the nursing assessment and interventions involved in replacing fluid via the oral route and by parenteral administration.

12.7   Assess for iatrogenic complications arising from intervention in fluid imbalances.

12.8   Prevent fluid imbalance by presenting clear learning/teaching guidelines to the person and significant others.

Learning the Language: Terminology Related to Fluid Disorders

Briefly define the following terms.

Terms Related to Body Water

1.   Intracellular fluid

2.   Extracellular fluid

3.   Interstitial fluid

4.   Plasma

Terms Related to Fluid Movement

5.   Osmolality

6.   Blood hydrostatic pressure

7.   Colloid osmotic pressure (oncotic pressure)

8.   Capillary filtration pressure

Thinking Critically: Knowing What to Do and Why

■ Study Questions Related to Fluid Imbalances

9.   In which of the following compartments is most of the body's water located: intracellular, interstitial, or intravascular? What percentage of water is located in each compartment?

10.   What is the average amount of fluid needed by adults per day? What are the usual sources?

11.   Do cells shrink or swell with a high serum Na^+?

12.   What signs or symptoms are the result of brain cells shrinking or swelling?

13.   Why should normal saline, rather than water, be used to irrigate nasogastric tubes?

14. Why are daily weights a good indicator of fluid balance? How many liters of fluid are represented by a kilogram of body weight?

15. What specific blood pressure changes (in systolic and diastolic readings) indicate that plasma volume is inadequate?

16. What happens to an individual who receives large amounts of IV normal saline (NS), especially over a short period of time?

17. What type of IV fluid is usually given to a person who has an extracellular fluid depletion?

18. Will people with increased antidiuretic hormone (ADH) secretion have low, normal, or high serum Na^+? Why?

Clients with Electrolyte Imbalances: Promoting Positive Outcomes

Four important electrolytes, which are often checked by measuring serum values, are sodium, potassium, chloride, and carbon dioxide. Serum sodium ion (Na^+) usually reflects hydration status because "water goes where salt is." Acute or rapid changes are dangerous, as brain cells cannot adapt to them. The potassium ion (K^+) is known as "king electrolyte," because small changes in the serum level affect muscle functioning, most significantly cardiac functioning. (It is helpful to remember that any lab value that is reported in decimal numbers cannot vary much without accompanying complications.) Chloride ion (Cl^-) and carbon dioxide (CO_2) serum values reflect acid-base balances and will be discussed in the next chapter. Two other important electrolytes are calcium ion (Ca^{++}) and magnesium ion (Mg^{++}). Both affect neuromuscular activity, with electrolyte deficits increasing activity and electrolyte excesses decreasing activity.

OBJECTIVES

13.1 Define terms related to electrolyte imbalances.

13.2 Describe the etiologic factors and pathophysiology that underlie potassium ion imbalances.

13.3 Describe the etiologic factors and pathophysiology that underlie calcium ion imbalances.

13.4 Describe the etiologic factors and pathophysiology that underlie magnesium ion imbalances.

13.5 Accurately assess a person's electrolyte status.

13.6 Identify people who are at risk for developing specific electrolyte imbalances.

13.7 Assess for iatrogenic complications arising from electrolyte imbalances.

13.8 Prevent electrolyte imbalance by presenting clear learning/teaching guidelines to the person and significant others.

LEARNING THE LANGUAGE: TERMINOLOGY RELATED TO ELECTROLYTE IMBALANCES

Briefly define the following terms related to electrolytes.

1. Electrolytes

2. Ions

3. Cation

4. Anion

5. Milliequivalent (mEq)

PUTTING IT ALL TOGETHER

■ *Case Study*

Mr. W., 76, is having surgery for benign prostatic hyperplasia (BPH). The surgeon uses multiple irrigations while performing the transurethral resection of the prostate (TURP) to remove tiny pieces of the resected prostate gland and to control the bleeding. On the afternoon of the first postoperative day, Mr. W. is confused and a check of his serum lab values reveals a serum sodium (Na+) of 124 mEq/L. Because normal serum sodium ranges from 135 to 145 mEq/L, the nurse notifies the physician. The physician orders another check on the serum sodium, and changes the IV from $D_5$1/2 NS to NS. Another specimen is obtained and Mr. W.'s serum sodium is now 116 mEq/L and he is having mild seizures.

6. What is the relationship between Mr. W.'s acute decrease in his serum sodium level and his state of mental confusion?
   A. Water is shifting to the intracellular compartment.
   B. Hyponatremia causes brain cells to shrink causing hypoexcitability.
   C. The decrease in the release of ADH has resulted in dilutional hyponatremia.
   D. Brain cells swell as the serum osmolality increases.

7. Mr. W. needs to be checked for which of the following signs and symptoms because of his hyponatremia?
   A. diminished bowel sounds and abdominal distention
   B. skin dry and flushed
   C. weakness and tremors
   D. peaked narrow T waves on V leads of a 12-lead electrocardiogram (ECG)

8. Normal saline IV fluid has twice the percentage of NaCl as is contained in $D_5$1/2 NS; what percent of $D_5$1/2 NS is NaCl?
   A. 0.33%
   B. 0.45%
   C. 3.0%
   D. 45%

9. Which of the following characteristics accurately describe IV NS?
   A. hypotonic, maintenance fluid
   B. isotonic, maintenance fluid
   C. isotonic, replacement fluid
   D. hypertonic, replacement fluid

10. Because Mr. W.'s condition and latest lab results indicate a severe electrolyte imbalance, the physician orders an IV with more sodium. It is essential that this IV fluid be given very slowly to prevent which of the following most likely complications?
    A. extravasation and tissue necrosis
    B. severe hypernatremia
    C. redistribution of potassium
    D. hypervolemia

Acid-Base Balance

Serum pH must remain within the very narrow range of 7.35-7.45, which is slightly alkaline, for body cells to function normally. The nurse has the responsibility to detect and help correct acid-base imbalances, and when possible, to prevent these disorders. Early recognition of signs and symptoms of acid-base imbalances can prevent complications and the development of severe mixed acid-base imbalances.

OBJECTIVES

14.1   Discuss general concepts of acid-base balance to include regulation and compensation to correct imbalances by the respiratory, urinary, and blood buffer systems.

14.2   Describe the etiologic factors and pathophysiology that underlie respiratory acidosis, respiratory alkalosis, metabolic acidosis, and metabolic alkalosis.

14.3   Describe in detail the nursing assessment, diagnosis, and interventions that relate to each imbalance.

PUTTING IT ALL TOGETHER

■ Etiologies and Manifestations of Acid-Base Imbalances

Match the etiologies of acid-base disturbances in Column A with the resulting specific acid-base disturbance in Column B. Provide a rationale for your answers to 2, 6, 8, and 11.

Column A	Column B
1. _____ Diuretics (loss of K+ and Cl– in urine)	A. Metabolic acidosis
2. _____ Breath-holding	B. Metabolic alkalosis
Rationale:	C. Respiratory acidosis
	D. Respiratory alkalosis

1. _____ Diuretics (loss of K+ and Cl– in urine)
2. _____ Breath-holding
    Rationale:

3. _____ Air hunger (high altitudes)
4. _____ Severe diarrhea (loss of deep GI contents)
5. _____ Renal insufficiency
6. _____ Vomiting or nasogastric suction
    Rationale:

7. _____ Narcotic overdose
8. _____ Early salicylate poisoning
    Rationale:

9. _____ Hysteria/anxiety
10. _____ Hypokalemia
11. _____ Diabetic ketoacidosis
    Rationale:

Column B

A.   Metabolic acidosis
B.   Metabolic alkalosis
C.   Respiratory acidosis
D.   Respiratory alkalosis

Give two clinical manifestations for each of the following acid-base imbalances. Check your answers with those provided in the Critical Monitoring feature in Chapter 14 of the text.

12.   Respiratory acidosis

14.   Respiratory alkalosis

13.   Metabolic alkalosis

15.   Metabolic acidosis

■ *Interpretation of Blood Gases*

Analyze the following blood gas results. Check your interpretation by using the acid-base map in Figure 14-7 in Chapter 14 of the text. The map is an excellent tool to take to clinical as you learn to interpret blood gases.

	pH	pCO_2	HCO_3	pO_2	Analysis
16.	7.40	40	24	95	_____
17.	7.33	33	17	100	_____
18.	7.35	30	16	220	_____
19.	7.48	26	19	105	_____
20.	7.40	60	36	58	_____

CRITICAL POINTS TO REMEMBER

Respiratory Acidosis	Respiratory Alkalosis	Metabolic Acidosis	Metabolic Alkalosis
pH < 7.35, pCO_2 > 45 mm Hg	pH > 7.45, pCO_2 < 35 mm Hg	pH < 7.35, pCO_2 usually < 35 mm Hg, HCO_3 < 22 mEq/L	pH > 7.45, HCO_3 > 26 mEq/L
Due to hyperventilation; e.g., with respiratory infections, chest trauma, depression of medullary respiratory center, neuromuscular diseases affecting the respiratory muscles	Due to hyperventilation; e.g., with anxiety, iatrogenically by ventilator set on high rate or large volume	Due to acid increase or base loss	Due to acid loss (vomiting or gastric suction), or base increase (receiving $NaHCO_3$), or loss of Cl–, which causes a compensatory increase of $NaHCO_3$
Often occurs with chronic obstructive pulmonary disease (COPD)	May occur with hypoxemia	Anion gap is serum Na+ – (Cl– + HCO_3–); normal = 12–14 mEq/L	With hypovolemia or aldosterone excess, alkalosis persists (Na+ retained and H+ excreted)
Carbon dioxide retained	Carbon dioxide exhaled	High anion gap occurs with acid increase; e.g., renal failure, lactic acidosis, ketoacidosis	Volume repletion with normal saline administration often corrects alkalosis, if problem is not aldosterone excess
When compensated, pH normal, pCO_2 > 45 mm Hg, and HCO_3 > 26 mEq/L	When compensated, pH normal, pCO_2 < 35 mm Hg, and HCO_3 < 22 mEq/L	Normal anion gap occurs with loss of base; e.g., diarrhea, enteric drainage	
	Too rapid correction may cause posthypercapnic metabolic acidosis	When compensated pH normal, pCO_2 < 35 mm Hg, HCO_3 < 22 mEq/L	

Clients Having Surgery: Promoting Positive Outcomes

When caring for adult clients, surgery is a frequent treatment the nurse will encounter. While surgery may be a frequent care experience for the nurse, for the client it most likely will be an anxiety-producing situation. In addition to the client's anxiety, the surgery itself carries risks that the nurse must recognize and manage. From the client's perspective there is no minor or routine surgery. From the time the surgery is proposed through discharge, the nurse has an active role requiring sensitive, accurate assessment, analysis, intervention, and evaluation.

OBJECTIVES

15.1 Discuss basic concepts related to perioperative nursing.

15.2 Interview a person who is to undergo surgery, gathering subjective and objective data.

15.3 Discuss the legal aspects of informed consent.

15.4 Discuss the physical, psychosocial, and teaching aspects of preoperative care.

15.5 Describe the roles of health care providers who participate in the intraoperative experience.

15.6 Discuss the implications of the types of anesthesia used in the operating room.

15.7 Discuss the nurse's role in caring for the client in the operating room.

15.8 Describe nursing care of the client in the postanesthesia recovery room.

15.9 Identify elements of client assessment essential upon transfer to the nursing unit after surgery.

15.10 Discuss goals of care during the postoperative phase.

LEARNING THE LANGUAGE: TERMINOLOGY RELATED TO CLIENTS HAVING SURGERY

Column A	Column B

Match the terms in Column A with the definitions in Column B.

1. _____ Anesthesiologist
2. _____ Antiembolism stockings
3. _____ Circulating nurse
4. _____ CRNA
5. _____ General anesthesia
6. _____ Informed consent
7. _____ Incentive spirometry
8. _____ Intraoperative phase
9. _____ Malignant hypertension
10. _____ Patient-controlled analgesia
11. _____ Perioperative nursing
12. _____ Preoperative phase

A. Design, coordinate, and deliver care to clients before, during, and after surgery

B. Time from decision for surgical intervention to transfer of client to the operative suite

C. Time from transfer of client to the OR to transfer of client to the recovery room

D. Legal document for any invasive procedure signifying that the client has received full disclosure about the procedure

E. Device used to promote lung expansion

F. Hose used to prevent thrombophlebitis or thromboembolism

G. Means of delivery of pain medication that the client administers

H. Physician who administers anesthesia

I. A registered nurse with special education who administers anesthesia

J. A registered nurse responsible for safety, sterility, assisting with monitoring the client, documentation, supplies, and client preparation in the OR

K. Drug-induced depression of the central nervous system

L. A genetic disorder characterized by uncontrolled skeletal muscle contraction, leading to potentially fatal elevation of temperature in clients receiving a combination of succinylcholine and inhalation agents

Match the surgical positions in Column A with the descriptions in Column B.

Column A	Column B

13. _____ Dorsal recumbent
14. _____ Laminectomy
15. _____ Lateral
16. _____ Lithotomy
17. _____ Trendelenburg's

A. Side-lying on OR table bent at the waist

B. Legs elevated in stirrups

C. Prone position with OR table at an angle

D. Flat on back (supine)

E. Head is lower than trunk of body

Match the anesthetic agents in Column A with their actions in Column B.

Column A	Column B
18. _____ Cocaine	A. Given IV for short-term general anesthesia
19. _____ Halothane	B. Inhalant with low anesthetic potency
20. _____ Ketamine hydrochloride	C. General anesthesia with mild muscle relaxation
21. _____ Lidocaine	D. Blocks uptake of norepinephrine—topical only
22. _____ Marcaine HCl	E. Blocks nerve impulses—injection
23. _____ Nitrous oxide	F. IV agent with sedative, immobilizing, analgesic, and amnesic effects
24. _____ Pavulon	G. Muscle relaxant
25. _____ Thiopental sodium	H. Local agent, contraindicated in children under 12

■ *Short Answer*

Provide rationales for the following preoperative assessments:

Perioperative Assessment	Rationale
26. Nutrition status	
27. Smoking history	
28. Weight	
29. Age	

■ *Case Study: Postoperative Client*

Ms. W. is a 70-year-old widow who had a cholecystectomy (gallbladder removal) under general anesthesia. She received a combination of Anectine, morphine, and Ethrane for anesthesia. In OR she received 1000 cc D₅LR. The report from the surgery team indicated that the surgery was uncomplicated. She had an estimated blood loss of 500 cc. Ms. W. was extubated in OR; her VS on admission to the recovery room were B/P 130/86, P 88 reg, R 16 reg, moderate in depth, and T 98.4° F. Her color is slightly pale, the IV of D₅LR is infusing at 100 cc/h without difficulty, the abdominal dressing is dry, the Foley is draining clear, light-amber urine and a T-tube line, unclamped, is attached to a drainage bag. Ms. W. responds slightly to her name. She is positioned on her left side. Fifteen minutes later, the VS taken are BP 120/80, P 90 reg, R 12 reg and moderate depth. She does not respond as readily when her name is called and is restless.

The third set of VS are BP 120/78, P 96 reg, R 10 and shallow.

30. What is the nursing action at this point?

Arterial blood gases are ordered STAT. The results are pH 7.32, pCO$_2$ 70, HCO$_3$ 27.

31.   Interpret the ABGs.

32.   What is the most likely reason for these ABGs?

The recovery room nurse notifies the anesthesiologist of the ABG results. The anesthesiologist orders Narcan.

33.   What is the reason for this order?

34.   If Ms. W.'s shallow, slow respirations had not been assessed, analyzed, and reported, what may have occurred?

Ms. W. is eventually transferred back to the surgery unit. A number of nursing actions must take place upon her arrival to the unit.

35.   Number the following elements of the baseline assessment in order of priority:
  _____ Urine output and color
  _____ Bile output from T-tube
  _____ Pulse rate and rhythm, blood pressure, and temperature
  _____ Dressing intactness and drainage
  _____ Level of consciousness
  _____ Respiration rate, depth, and skin color
  _____ Position of person for alignment, safety, and comfort

36.   Justify your selection of number 1 and 2 priority.

Four hours after admission to the surgery unit, the nurse notes that Ms. W.'s total urine output is 100 cc of amber urine.

37.   Check which of the following actions would be most appropriate, then number the actions in order of implementation.
  _____ Check Foley patency.
  _____ Notify the physician.
  _____ Wait 4 hours to see what the urine output is before calling the physician.
  _____ Check mucous membranes and skin turgor.
  _____ Check IV rate, patency, and total intake.
  _____ Give Ms. W. an injection of pain medication.
  _____ Take vital signs.

■ *Multiple Choice*

38.   Which of the following diet selections would be most beneficial for a client preoperatively?
  A.   lean roast beef, orange and spinach salad, and whole-wheat roll
  B.   meatless spaghetti sauce with pasta, green salad, and an apple
  C.   roast chicken, Jell-O and carrot salad, and yogurt
  D.   lean hamburger and bun, lettuce salad, and pear

39.   Preoperative assessment of a client's alcohol habits is important for which of the following reasons?
  A.   assess for possibility of hypercoagulability
  B.   assess for the stability of the blood glucose level
  C.   predict kidney function
  D.   potential for unpredictable reactions to anesthesia

40. When the nurse signs as witness on a surgical permit, he or she is affirming that the
    A. surgeon has given full disclosure about the procedure to the client.
    B. client was mentally able to sign the permit.
    C. signature on the permit is the client's.
    D. client was given alternatives to the surgical procedure.

41. The surgeon orders Demerol 50 mg and Robinul .2 mg IM for preoperative medication. Which of the following effects would the nurse expect to see in the client?
    A. decreased gastric secretion and amnesic effect
    B. sedation and decreased oral-pharyngeal secretions
    C. antiemetic effect and decreased anxiety
    D. pain relief and antiemetic effect

42. Which of the following would be most relevant in assessing the postoperative client for blood loss?
    A. serosanguineous drainage on the dressing
    B. tachycardia, tachypnea, and decreased blood pressure
    C. decreased bowel sounds and vomiting
    D. restlessness and pain

16

Clients with Wounds: Promoting Positive Outcomes

Caring for clients with wounds is a relatively common nursing experience. Wound care requires diverse nursing skills. Assessment skills are needed in the observation of the local wound as well as for signs of systemic involvement. Treatment will encompass a range of skills from selection of appropriate dressings, to wound cleansing and packing, and application of dressings. There will also be preventive aspects built into the nursing care including the prevention of complications of wound healing. With clients being discharged from the hospital with increasingly complex wounds to care for, nurses also need to be able to adapt wound care to the client's home environment and self-care abilities. Terminology and content of this chapter is the foundation of many aspects of nursing and will be used by many nurses on a daily basis.

OBJECTIVES

16.1 Describe the processes involved in the phases of normal wound healing.

16.2 Describe the types of wound healing intention.

16.3 Discuss the functions of various nutrients needed in wound healing.

16.4 Describe management of the client with an inflammation, incision, chronic inflammation, and open wound.

LEARNING THE LANGUAGE: TERMINOLOGY RELATED TO CLIENTS WITH WOUNDS

Match the terms in Column A with the correct definition in Column B.

Column A

1. _____ Adenosine diphosphate (ADP)
2. _____ Angiogenesis
3. _____ Bands
4. _____ Basophils
5. _____ Chemotaxis
6. _____ Complement system
7. _____ Cytokines
8. _____ Collagen
9. _____ Epithelialization
10. _____ Free radicals
11. _____ Granulation tissue
12. _____ Growth factors
13. _____ Histamine
14. _____ Inflammation
15. _____ Keloids
16. _____ Kinins
17. _____ Leukotrienes
18. _____ Macrophages
19. _____ Mast cells
20. _____ Monocytes
21. _____ Neutrophils
22. _____ Prostaglandins
23. _____ Wound contraction

Column B

A. WBC which arrives at site of injury following the neutrophils and phagocytose bacteria

B. Monocytes that enter tissues and phagocytose bacteria

C. Cells filled with histamine and neutrophil chemotactic factors

D. A matrix of collagen, capillaries, and cells that fill the wound with new connective tissue

E. Formation of new blood vessels

F. Migration of epithelial cells

G. A type of scar tissue that extends well over the suture line

H. An unstable form of oxygen having an unpaired electron

I. Promotion of movement of leukocytes into the area of injury

J. Mediators of wound healing that regulate the mobility, differentiation, and growth of leukocytes

K. Catalysts for wound healing released by platelets and macrophages that prime other cells to enter the growth phase

L. Reconstructs connective tissues and adds strength to the wound

M. WBCs that arrive first at the injury site and phagocytose foreign agents

N. A series of physiologic responses to injury that is nonspecific and occurs in the same way regardless of the type of injury

O. Drawing in of the edges of the wound

P. Chemical causing the same reaction as histamine, but the response lasts longer

Q. Plasma protein that increases vascular permeability and allows leukocytes to enter the tissue

R. Stimulates cells lining the capillaries to constrict

S. Immature neutrophils

T. WBCs that secrete histamine

U. Chemical released by platelets to promote clotting

V. Group of plasma proteins activated by microorganisms that promotes inflammation

W. Chemicals released by mast cells that act the same as histamine and cause pain

KNOWLEDGE BUILDING: STUDY QUESTIONS RELATED TO CLIENTS WITH WOUNDS

Determine whether each of the following statements is true or false. Correct any false statements.

24. _____ Neutrophils are also called "polys" and "segs."

25. _____ Eosinophils help control the inflammatory response by secreting antihistamine.

26. _____ Basophils increase during the healing phase of inflammation.

27. _____ Lymphocytes increase during chronic inflammation.

28. _____ Neutrophils increase during chronic inflammation.

29. _____ Lymphocytes are formed in lymphoid tissue.

30. _____ Monocytes act as scavengers at the inflammatory site.

31. _____ Neutrophils normally comprise the largest percent of defensive cells.

32. _____ Epithelialization can be hastened if a wound is kept moist.

Match the descriptions of exudate in Column A with the correct type of inflammatory exudate in Column B.

Column A	**Column B**
33. _____ Bright or dark red	A. Serous
34. _____ Thin, clear, yellow	B. Hemorrhagic
35. _____ Thick, partly liquefied necrotic tissue	C. Serosanguineous
36. _____ Blood-tinged yellow or pink, usually thin	D. Purulent

■ Components of Wound Healing

37. List factors that are likely to have an adverse effect on wound healing.

38. The important concepts in Chapter 16 on wound healing involve the process of normal wound healing. To be sure you understand this process, outline the key components of each phase of wound healing.

I.   Vascular Response Phase

III.   Proliferative (or Resolution) Phase

IV.   Maturation Phase

II.   Inflammation Phase

THINKING CRITICALLY

■ Understanding Rationales

Provide the rationales for using the following wound dressings.

Dressing and Use	Rationale
39. Wet-to-dry debridement with gauze	
40. Transparent film over an abrasion	
41. Hydrocolloid for shallow ulcer	
42. Hydrogel for pressure ulcer	
43. Exudate absorber for deep wound with eschar	
44. Calcium alginate for wound with profuse drainage	

■ *Knowing What to Do and Why*

45. You are completing discharge planning for your client who is postop an open cholecystectomy. In providing information to your client about wound care and when to return for wound suture removal, what teaching needs to be included?

46. Your client has a moist-to-dry dressing for a 3-cm-wide by 10-cm-long open abdominal wound. What is the most commonly used and least detrimental topical agent to use to moisturize the dressing? Why?

47. What type of dressing would you use to pack the wound described in Question 46?

48. What is the purpose of wet-to-dry dressing?

49. What aspects of the wound will you assess and document?

50. Identify nutrients that would be included in interventions for a nursing diagnosis of At risk for impaired wound healing related to poor nutritional intake.

PUTTING IT ALL TOGETHER

■ *Case Study*

Mr. E. is a 79-year-old client admitted to the hospital for a colon resection for cancer. Mr. E. is a widower who lives alone. His activity is limited to walking very short distances because of an arthritic hip. He states that his appetite is poor. He is 5'10" tall and weighs 135 pounds. Mr. E. takes an antihypertensive medication—clonidine hydrochloride (Catapres)—0.1 mg, twice daily. Three weeks ago he completed a course of a steroid (Decadron) for an acute episode of his arthritis.

51. Factors in Mr. E.'s history that place him at risk for delayed wound healing include which of the following?
    A. nutritional status and antihypertensive medication
    B. Decadron and arthritis
    C. nutritional status and Decadron
    D. age and antihypertensive medication

Mr. E. has a partial colectomy and an end-to-end anastomosis. The surgery and recovery room periods are uneventful. Mr. E.'s postoperative orders include nothing by mouth (NPO), IV $D_5$1/4 NS at 100 cc/hour, sit up in chair 3x/day on postop day one; ambulate with assistance 3x/day on postop day two; turn, cough, and deep-breathe q2 hours, and nasogastric to low suction. Mr. E. is alert, but only moves when the nurse assists him. On the second postop day he develops a temperature of 101.1° F. The physician orders aspirin gr. 10 per rectal suppository, which lowers his temperature to 99.0° F. Mr. E. becomes quite diaphoretic as his temperature decreases.

52. Mr. E. develops a wound infection. Which of the following findings would be expected in his WBCs and differential?
    A. WBC—8000
    B. monocytes—15%
    C. eosinophils—10%
    D. neutrophils—80%

53. The physician orders a normal saline wet-to-dry dressing change every shift for Mr. E. The purpose of this type of dressing is that the wound requires
    A. cleaning.
    B. topical antibiotics.
    C. protection.
    D. application of cold.

54. Which of the following would indicate a wound infection as opposed to normal inflammation?
    A. erythema around the entire wound
    B. serosanguineous drainage
    C. pain at the site
    D. swelling of wound edges

55. Which of the following items would be highest priority for assessment of a client who had an open reduction of a fractured tibia and is at risk for compartmental syndrome?
    A. pulses distal to the fracture
    B. circumference of the extremity
    C. capillary refill
    D. movement of proximal joints

17

Perspectives on Infectious Disorders

When possible, we need to prevent infection rather than rely on treating it. Prevention requires an understanding of the infection process, the transmission chain, and the control measures that break the chain. Nurses have an obligation to remain current on research regarding infectious diseases and are responsible for taking appropriate precautions in caring for all clients. Preventing cross-contamination by assigning a nursing team to a group of clients for the necessary period of care and appropriate hand-washing prevents infections, decreases mortality, and saves health care dollars.

OBJECTIVES

17.1 Discuss factors involved in the transmission and development of infectious disease.

17.2 Obtain a nursing history that will help to identify the person at risk for developing an infectious disease.

17.3 Perform specific preventive nursing measures in the health care setting to decrease the incidence of nosocomial infections.

17.4 Discuss universal precautions and the two tiers of isolation strategies: standard precautions and transmission-based precautions.

17.5 Discuss Occupational Safety and Health Administration (OSHA) guidelines for protecting health care workers exposed to blood and other potentially infectious materials.

17.6 Discuss OSHA guidelines for preventing the spread of tuberculosis in hospitals.

17.7 List recommendations for adult immunizations.

PUTTING IT ALL TOGETHER

Provide short answers to the following questions.

1. What are the five components in the chain of infection and what role does each play in infectious disease?

6. What is the established protocol for management of needlestick injuries at your clinical site?

7. What does being "colonized with methicillin-resistant *Staphylococcus aureus*" mean?

2. One of the most common sites of nosocomial infections (infections acquired in health care agencies) is the urinary tract. What specific nursing interventions will decrease this risk?

8. What is the Center for Disease Control's (CDC) recommendation for hepatitis immunization for health care workers?

3. Results of studies have shown a relationship between invasive devices and an increased risk of infection. What are some nursing interventions that can decrease this risk for clients who must have invasive devices?

9. What is the CDC's recommendation for measles immunization for health care workers?

4. *Escherichia coli* is the organism often responsible for nosocomial infections. What implications does this have for teaching females good hygiene practices?

10. How often should people age 65 and older receive an influenza vaccine?

5. What is the correct technique for implementing the single most important procedure for limiting the spread of microorganisms and nosocomial infections?

THINKING CRITICALLY: BRIDGE TO HOME HEALTH CARE: INFECTION CONTROL

Give the rationales for the following home health care nursing interventions.

Intervention	Rationale

11. Store hand-washing supplies in an outside pocket of the nursing bag.

12. Use a waterproof nursing bag or one that has a plastic liner.

13. For clients with MRSA or VRE, take into the home only the supplies needed for the visit.

14. Teach clients and family to add one cup of full-strength bleach to laundry of soiled linens and clothing.

15. Place old dressings/wound-care supplies in a plastic bag, tie the bag closed, and dispose of it in the family garbage. Double-bag if there is a danger of the bag ripping or tearing.

CHAPTER 18

Perspectives in Oncology

Cancer is the second leading cause of death in the United States. This fact alone emphasizes the importance of nurses learning about these complex disorders. There are many issues surrounding cancer that concern nurses.

OBJECTIVES

18.1 Discuss basic concepts related to cancer.

18.2 Discuss factors predisposing a person to cancer and the impact of cancer.

18.3 Compare and contrast characteristics of normal cells and cancer cells.

LEARNING THE LANGUAGE: TERMINOLOGY RELATED TO NEOPLASTIC DISORDERS

Define the following terms.

1. Cancer

2. Malignant

3. Neoplasm

4. Benign

5. Incidence rate

6. Differentiation

7. Contact inhibition

8. Metastasis

9.   Carcinogens

10.   Papanicolaou (Pap) test

11.   Tumor staging

12.   Tumor grading

13.   Oncogene

14.   Label the following neoplasms as **B** for benign or **M** for malignant.
   A. _____ Meningioma
   B. _____ Fibrosarcoma
   C. _____ Leiomyoma
   D. _____ Melanoma
   E. _____ Osteoma
   F. _____ Adenoma
   G. _____ Multiple myeloma
   H. _____ Glioblastoma
   I. _____ Papilloma
   J. _____ Glioma
   K. _____ Adenocarcinoma
   L. _____ Fibroma
   M. _____ Dermoid cyst
   N. _____ Teratocarcinoma
   O. _____ Nevus
   P. _____ Lymphosarcoma
   Q. _____ Lymphangioma
   R. _____ Lipoma
   S. _____ Leukemia
   T. _____ Basal cell
   u. _____ Liposarcoma

Match the neoplasms in Column A with their tissue of origin in Column B.

Column A	**Column B**
15. _____ Leiomyosarcoma	A. Connective tissue
16. _____ Carcinoma	B. Endothelium
17. _____ Papilloma	C. Epithelium
18. _____ Glioma	D. Gonads
19. _____ Adenocarcinoma	E. Muscle tissue
20. _____ Meningioma	F. Nerve tissue
21. _____ Nevus	
22. _____ Leukemia	
23. _____ Melanoma	
24. _____ Basal cell carcinoma	
25. _____ Squamous cell carcinoma	
26. _____ Fibroma	

Compare the following characteristics of malignant cells with normal cells; list a similar characteristic for a normal cell.

27. Cancer cells are anaplastic.

28. Cancer cells lose contact inhibition.

29. Cancer cells grow in presence of necrosis.

30. Cancer cells invade adjacent tissue.

31. Cancer cells serve no useful purpose.

32. Cancer cells proliferate in response to abnormal stimuli.

33. Cancer cells have an erratic growth rate.

34. Cancer cells' birthrate exceeds the cells' death rate.

Clients with Cancer: Promoting Positive Outcomes

While survival statistics for people diagnosed with cancer are improving, cancer remains the second leading cause of death in the United States. For primary prevention, nurses can have an active role in teaching people about lifestyle changes that will decrease their chances of developing certain cancers. For secondary prevention, nurses can teach them about the warning signs of cancer and encourage people to have checkups and to follow the American Cancer Society's recommendations for early detection measures. Once clients are in the health care system, for instance in the diagnostic phase, the nurse will be assessing them and preparing them for tests. The nurse will also be supporting clients and their families throughout this stressful period.

OBJECTIVES

19.1 Discuss the nurse's role in cancer prevention and screening.

19.2 Discuss general and specific techniques involved in cancer diagnosis and the nurse's role.

19.3 Discuss the role of surgery in cancer treatment and diagnosis.

19.4 Discuss radiation therapy as a treatment modality for neoplastic disorders, its potential side effects, and nursing care.

19.5 Discuss chemotherapy as a treatment modality for neoplastic disorders, its side effects, and nursing care.

19.6 Discuss bone marrow transplantation and biologic response modifiers used as cancer treatment modalities.

LEARNING THE LANGUAGE: TERMINOLOGY RELATED TO TREATMENT MODALITIES FOR NEOPLASTIC DISORDERS

Match the terms in Column A with the correct definition in Column B.

Column A	Column B
1. _____ Advance directive	A. Radiation delivered from a source placed some distance from the target site
2. _____ Alopecia	
3. _____ COBRA	B. An indeterminate period after curative treatment has been completed
4. _____ External radiation therapy	
5. _____ Extravasation	C. A philosophy of care that emphasizes symptom control, pain management, and providing comfort and dignity for the client during the dying process
6. _____ Hospice	
7. _____ Internal radiation	D. Legislation that protects insurance coverage for 18 months following employment termination
8. _____ Myelosuppression	
9. _____ Nadir	E. Care aimed at improving the quality of the client's life for as long as possible
10. _____ Palliative care	
11. _____ Survivorship	F. A statement made by a competent individual directing his or her medical care in the event he or she is unable to make health care decisions
12. _____ Vascular access devices	
	G. Infusions of chemotherapy that become exuded (dislodged) and cause tissue damage
	H. Catheters placed into one of the major veins of the upper chest
	I. Placement of specially prepared isotopes directly into or near the tumor itself or into the systemic circulation
	J. Loss of hair
	K. The time after chemotherapy administration when the white blood cell or platelet count is at the lowest point
	L. Depression of white blood cell, platelet, and red blood cell production

Match the types of bone marrow transplants in Column A with the correct description in Column B.

Column A	Column B
13. _____ Allogeneic	A. The marrow donor is an identical twin.
14. _____ Autologous	B. The marrow donor is usually a sibling or parent.
15. _____ Syngeneic	C. The recipient is also the donor.

Match the following biologic response modifiers (BRMs) in Column A with the correct description in Column B.

Column A		**Column B**

16. _____ Interferon (IFNa)

17. _____ Colony-stimulating factors (CSFs)

18. _____ Erythropoietin (EPO)

19. _____ Granulocyte CSF (G-CSF)

20. _____ Granulocyte-macrophage CSF (GM-CSF)

21. _____ Interleukins

22. _____ Monoclonal antibodies (MoAbs)

A. Substances produced by mononuclear phagocytes whose function is to promote normal hematopoiesis

B. Specific antibodies directed against a single antigenic determinant on the cell surface; may be used to deliver immunotoxins to the tumor site

C. Naturally occurring factors that stimulate hematopoiesis

D. BRM used to treat anemia

E. Small proteins with antiviral, immunomodulatory, and antiproliferative cellular activity

F. CSFs that stimulate granulocytes

G. CSFs that stimulate macrophages and granulocytes

THINKING CRITICALLY: KNOWING WHAT TO DO AND WHY

For each of the following situations, give the nursing intervention and its rationale.

23. Ms. J. is receiving Adriamycin, which will likely cause alopecia. What are appropriate nursing interventions in relation to the client's impending hair loss?

24. Mr. C., who has Hodgkin's disease, has severe pruritus all over his body. What can be done to minimize the sensation of pruritus?

25. Mr. B. is taking prednisone as a part of his chemotherapy protocol and has developed neutropenia. What nursing interventions are necessary?

26. Ms. S. is receiving chemotherapy that is known to cause stomatitis. What are appropriate nursing interventions?

27. Mr. C. is receiving a course of radiation therapy and has erythema and some dry desquamation over his chest. He asks the nurse what kind of lotion he can use. What is the nurse's best intervention? Why?

28. How should the nurse respond to Mr. J.'s comment that he is feeling very tired since he has been receiving radiation therapy?

29. How can the side effects of nausea and vomiting be minimized for a client receiving a chemotherapy drug that is highly emetic?

30. Ms. D. is undergoing diagnostic tests for suspected cancer of the colon. What are the supportive nursing interventions for a client during the diagnostic phase of the cancer continuum?

31. Ms. J. is on chemotherapy and her platelet count is 20,000/mm³. What are the appropriate nursing assessments?

■ *Case Study*

Ms. R. is 33 years old and comes to the gynecology clinic for a check-up. Her examination will include a pelvic with a Pap smear. Ms. R. reports that she has not had a Pap smear before. The nurse explains the pelvic examination to her and then includes some client teaching. The nurse shares with Ms. R. the American Cancer Society's guidelines for early detection of cervical cancer.

32. Which of the following would be the correct guideline to share with Ms. R.? A Pap test should be performed
    A. every three years for sexually active women.
    B. annually for three years and, with negative results, performed as the physician advises.
    C. annually for sexually active women over age 40.
    D. every two years regardless of sexual activity.

Ms. R. received a notice from the clinic that her Pap smear was suspicious and that she needed to return to the clinic. The physician explained to Ms. R. that the examination of the cells from her cervix showed Class IV cells.

33. The nurse would understand this to mean that Ms. R.
    A. has cervical cancer.
    B. possibly has cervical cancer.
    C. has mild to moderate dysplasia.
    D. has a severe inflammatory process.

34. Ms. R. is scheduled for a biopsy. The nurse explains to her that this procedure will likely involve
    A. removal of her cervix for microscopic examination.
    B. a needle aspiration of some tissue for microscopic examination.
    C. removal of a piece of tissue for microscopic examination.
    D. removal of the tumor for microscopic examination.

Ms. R.'s biopsy turns out to be negative; however, after this scare she is very interested in cervical cancer and cancer risks in general.

35. The nurse discusses risk factors for cervical cancer with Ms. R. Which of the following contains the most complete and accurate information about risk factors?
    A. over 30, sexually active
    B. multiple sex partners, chronic cervicitis, history of Human papilloma virus (HPV)
    C. nonparous, overweight, and sexually active
    D. sexually active at early age, intercourse with a circumcised male

CLIENT EDUCATION: KNOWING WHAT TO TEACH AND WHY

■ Guidelines for Early Detection of Cancer

Indicate whether each of the following statements is True (T) or False (F). If the statement is False, provide the correct answer.

36. _____ An annual chest x-ray is recommended for heavy smokers.

37. _____ Mammography is recommended every other year for women over 50 years of age.

38. _____ A complete physical exam is recommended every year for people over age 40.

39. _____ The Pap test should be performed on women every year for two years and, if normal, then every three years.

40. _____ A stool guaiac is recommended yearly for everyone over age 35.

41. _____ A sigmoidoscopy is recommended at age 50 and then every 3-5 years.

42. _____ Breast self-exam (BSE) should be practiced routinely every two weeks in high-risk groups.

43. _____ An annual oral exam is recommended.

PUTTING IT ALL TOGETHER

■ Case Study

Mr. A., 70, is admitted to the urology unit with suspected cancer of the prostate. The diagnosis is confirmed after a biopsy and Mr. A. is started on treatment.

44. During the diagnostic phase of the cancer continuum, which of the following nursing actions would be most appropriate?
    A. giving the client and his family simple explanations about the tests and treatments
    B. helping the client return to his previous level of functioning
    C. providing options for the client and family to deal with the terminal phase of the disease
    D. helping the family to contact a hospice

45. Mr. A. will be treated with a combination of external beam radiation therapy and chemotherapy. While teaching the client and family about the effects of external beam radiation, the nurse would know that more teaching is necessary if a family member stated:
    A. "The radiation rays will help to destroy the cancer cells."
    B. "We will have to be careful to limit the time we spend close to him."
    C. "The line marks on his body should not be washed off."
    D. "He may lose his hair only in the genital area."

46. Mr. A. will also be treated with intravenous (IV) and oral chemotherapy. When preparing the IV chemotherapy, safety precautions recommend that the nurse
    A. stay in the client's room for less than 30 minutes per shift.
    B. wear gloves and a gown when entering the client's room.
    C. request that the family handle all bedpans and urinals.
    D. empty bedpans and urinals wearing gloves and gown for 48 hours after chemotherapy administration.

47. Mr. A. is receiving chemotherapy drugs that potentially cause myelosuppression. The nursing implications of this toxic effect are to
    A. place the client on neutropenic precautions.
    B. assess the client's temperature, throat, gums, and stools.
    C. pad the patient's side rails.
    D. begin the client on mouth rinses every 4 hours.

48. Mr. A. is started on G-CSF. Nursing implications for this medication include which of the following?
    A. teaching the client about the potential severe side effects
    B. starting the medication IV with saline
    C. following the client's red blood cell count
    D. assessing the client for bone pain

20

Clients with Psychosocial and Mental Health Concerns: Promoting Positive Outcomes

Some clients with medical-surgical problems have pre-existing serious mental disorders. Effective communication is an essential skill in providing care for these clients. Family, culture, spirituality, and sexuality are psychosocial concepts that affect clients and therefore impact nursing care. Universal psychosocial concepts include anxiety, stress, coping mechanisms, and self-esteem. Examination of these concepts is necessary to providing holistic nursing care.

OBJECTIVES

20.1   Identify the basic principles of communication pertinent to addressing the psychosocial and mental health concerns of clients.

20.2   Review the concepts of anxiety, stress, coping mechanisms, and self-esteem.

20.3   Discuss culture, spirituality, and sexuality as important considerations for providing holistic nursing care.

20.4   Describe how nursing care plans must be altered to meet the needs of clients with medical disorders and serious mental illnesses.

THINKING CRITICALLY: KNOWING WHAT TO DO AND WHY

■ Short Answer

1.   What four psychosocial concepts are considered to be universal?

2.   How long does an acute mild stress response usually last?

3.   What physiologic response usually ends an acute mild stress response?

4.   List two nursing interventions to decrease a client's anxiety.

5. What is the difference between a flat affect and an inappropriate affect?

7. If verbal and nonverbal behavior do not agree, which is more likely to reflect the client's true feelings?

6. How can communication serve as the first clue that a client has a psychiatric illness?

8. What are three components of basic teaching for every client?

■ Matching

Match the following psychiatric manifestation in Column A with the causative medications in Column B. The types of medications in Column B may be used more than once as they may cause more than one type of psychiatric manifestation.

Column A	Column B
9. _____ Depression	A. Beta-adrenergic blocker
10. _____ Anxiety	B. Narcotics
11. _____ Paranoia	C. Anticholinergics
12. _____ Agitation	D. Digitalis glycosides
13. _____ Mania	E. Corticosteroids
14. _____ Delusions	F. Cephalosporins
15. _____ Hallucinations	G. Salicylates

■ Short Answer

16. Why do extrapyramidal symptoms such as stiffness or tremor in arms and legs occur with antipsychotic medications?

18. What is neuroleptic malignant syndrome?

19. List five risk factors for suicide.

17. What is the usual treatment for these extrapyramidal symptoms?

Your client is hospitalized for a relapse of lymphoma. You know that the client and family live 200-plus miles from the hospital and that your client's wife has been sleeping in the client's room. One afternoon you find the client's wife in the dayroom crying.

20.   Describe your initial steps in this situation.

While talking with her, your client's wife tells you that her husband gets angry with her when she does anything, that he won't talk with her, and that she is worried about a 3- and 5-year-old back home staying with her mother. She would like to go home to see the children, but she is afraid to leave her husband.

21.   You are considering a nursing diagnosis of Altered family processes. What additional data would you need to confirm this diagnosis?

22.   You confirm the diagnosis of Altered family processes. One intervention you include in your plan of care is improving communication between the patient and his wife. How would you proceed?

23.   Explain how you would apply the nursing process to a client who does not speak or understand English.

24.   Describe nursing interventions that would promote sexual health.

Putting It All Together

25.   A client who is hospitalized for a myocardial infarction (heart attack) asks the nurse, "Do you think my heart attack is a punishment from God for my sins?" The nurse's best response would be which of the following?
   A.   "No, my belief is that God loves us and forgives us."
   B.   "You're just worried because of your heart attack; you'll feel better tomorrow."
   C.   "Would you like to talk to someone from the chaplain's office?"
   D.   "You're concerned that God may be punishing you for something you've done in the past?"

26.   In assessing a client with Spiritual distress, which of the following questions would provide the most information?
   A.   "What is your religion?"
   B.   "What helps you the most when you have special needs?"
   C.   "Would you like to see a chaplain?"
   D.   "Do you attend church regularly?"

27.   Spirituality can best be defined as
   A.   an organized set of beliefs.
   B.   encompassing values, meaning, and purpose.
   C.   regular church attendance.
   D.   belief in a specific religion.

28. The nursing diagnosis Altered family processes is used when
    A. family behavior is considered destructive.
    B. a healthy family is challenged by the stress of a chronic illness.
    C. family behavior is interfering with treatment.
    D. family behavior suggests that there is abuse.

29. A cultural assessment would include all of the following except
    A. preferred foods.
    B. body space/comfort zone.
    C. religious practices.
    D. a genogram.

30. The most important first step for the nurse to take in working with sexuality and sexual issues is to
    A. clarify personal values in relation to sexual health.
    B. identify and understand sexual problems.
    C. assist clients in dealing with sexual problems.
    D. know the subject matter related to sexuality.

21

Clients with Sleep and Rest Disorders and Fatigue: Promoting Positive Outcomes

Sleep is defined as a state of unconsciousness during which time the cerebrum rests. During this state of unconsciousness, the individual can be aroused by external stimuli. Sleep is characterized by a sleep-wake cycle. The sleep-wake cycle is one of the circadian rhythms of the body. It is divided into four stages; each stage is characterized by specific physiologic changes.

There are a variety of sleep disorders. In some sleep disorders, the client has difficulty initiating or maintaining sleep (dyssomnias). Other disorders occur during sleep but usually do not produce insomnia or excessive sleepiness (parasomnias). There are also sleep disorders associated with medical and psychiatric diseases. In addition, many drugs influence the sleep-wake cycle.

Clients also can have sensory/perceptual disorders. These disorders are produced by excessive and/or inadequate environmental or internal stimuli. Each individual has an optimal level of sensory input that facilitates his/her sense of well-being. When this optimal level is not maintained, the individual demonstrates physiologic and psychological changes.

OBJECTIVES

21.1 Define terms associated with sleep and sensory disorders.

21.2 Discuss the physiology of sleep and arousal.

21.3 Discuss the clinical manifestations and medical management of dyssomnias.

21.4 Discuss the clinical manifestations and medical management of parasomnias.

21.5 Discuss sleep disorders associated with medical and psychiatric diseases.

21.6 Describe the impact of drugs on the sleep-wake cycle.

21.7 Discuss hospital-acquired sleep disturbances.

21.8 Describe hospital-acquired sensory disturbances.

21.9 Demonstrate appropriate nursing management of the client with a sleep disorder.

LEARNING THE LANGUAGE: TERMINOLOGY RELATED TO SLEEP AND SENSORY DISORDERS

Match the descriptive statements in Column A with the appropriate sleep disorder in Column B.

Column A   **Column B**

1. _____ Repeated episodes of drowsiness followed by   A.   Insomnia
brief naps   B.   Sleep apnea

2. _____ Semi-purposeful behavior during sleep, such   C.   Narcolepsy
as sleepwalking   D.   Sleep starts

3. _____ Persistent difficulty initiating or maintaining E.   Central sleep apnea
sleep
                                                        F.   Nightmares
4. _____ Recurrent periods of cessation of breathing   G.   Somnambulism
for 10 seconds; occurs at least five times per
hour

5. _____ Sudden jerking movement of the legs as a
person is falling asleep

6. _____ Apneic periods; no apparent respiratory
effort

7. _____ Frightening dreams arising in rapid eye
movement (REM) sleep

THINKING CRITICALLY

8. List at least six aspects that should be included in a   11. Describe the four stages of sleep.
sleep history.

12. Differentiate between dyssomnias and
parasomnias.

9. What type of objective data would you expect a
client with a sleep disorder to be experiencing?

13. Describe changes in the sleep cycle that are the
result of aging.

10. During the transition from the awake state to non-
REM (NREM) sleep, concentration levels of three
neurotransmitters decrease. Identify these three
neurotransmitters.

14. List factors that predispose a hospitalized client to sensory overload.

16. A client is taking furosemide (Lasix) 40 mg p.o., b.i.d., for treatment of congestive heart failure (CHF). How could this drug cause a sleep pattern disturbance?

15. List factors that predispose a hospitalized client to sensory deprivation.

PUTTING IT ALL TOGETHER

17. Develop a care plan for a client with Sleep pattern disturbance related to change in sleep environment secondary to hospitalization.

Goals and Outcome Criteria	Nursing Interventions

Perspectives on End-of-Life Care

Hospice care and *palliative care* are terms used for end-of-life care. Hospice began in the United Kingdom in the 1960s and has been slow to move to the United States. Almost 60% of the Americans who die each year spend their final days in a hospital and less than 15% of those receive hospice care. Someone who is dying requires a lot of individualized care. Nursing care includes psychosocial support, teaching the client and family, and managing symptoms. Pain, dyspnea, delirium, depression, fatigue, and sleep disturbances are some of the symptoms requiring management. Care and support for the caregivers and the grieving family are also very important components of end-of-life care.

OBJECTIVES

22.1   Discuss the hospice movement.

22.2   Discuss the differences between palliative care and hospice.

22.3   Describe symptoms often experienced at the end of life.

22.4   Discuss nursing interventions for each of these symptoms at the end of life.

22.5   Describe possible interventions to help the caregivers.

22.6   Discuss the phases of grief.

22.7   Discuss support for the grieving family.

THINKING CRITICALLY

Provide short answers to the following questions.

1.   When is hospice care appropriate for a client?

2.   What is the drug of choice for control of severe pain?

3.   Which classifications of adjuvant medications enhance pain control?

4.   Give an example of a physical and a behavioral intervention that may be used in addition to pharmacologic therapy to control pain.

5.   What are some barriers to adequate pain control?

6.   What is meant by "round-the-clock" dosing for pain control?

7.   How does morphine help relieve dyspnea?

8.   When should oxygen be used to relieve dyspnea?

9.   What are some of the signs of imminent death?

10.   How can the nurse help the family and the dying person with the death event?

11.   What are the normal phases of grief?

12.   How can the nurse assist the family to cope with their grief?

23

Clients with Pain: Promoting Positive Outcomes

Pain is a frequent symptom for which nurses assess and intervene. The subjective, personal nature of the pain experience has been strongly emphasized in the textbook. The nurse's skilled assessment and understanding of pain will assist the nurse in making appropriate clinical judgments in the treatment of clients with pain.

OBJECTIVES

23.1   Discuss the multidimensional phenomenon of pain.

23.2   Discuss physiologic, psychosocial, and theoretical aspects related to the process of pain.

23.3   Discuss the types of pain and pain syndromes.

23.4   Describe the process of pain assessment.

23.5   Discuss nursing interventions for the person with pain.

23.6   Compare and contrast analgesics and various methods of analgesic administration.

23.7   Describe surgical procedures directed at relieving pain.

23.8   Describe stimulation therapies used in pain control.

LEARNING THE LANGUAGE: TERMINOLOGY RELATED TO PAIN

Match the terms in Column A with the definitions in Column B.

Column A

1. _____ Acute pain
2. _____ Chronic pain
3. _____ Neuropathic pain
4. _____ Nociceptors
5. _____ Pain threshold
6. _____ Phantom pain
7. _____ Referred pain
8. _____ Somatic pain
9. _____ Tolerance for pain
10. _____ Visceral pain

Column B

A. Free nerve endings
B. Pain in one area of the body; for example, in the viscera or a deep somatic structure, that is perceived in another area of the body
C. Usually of short duration (less than 6 months), has an identifiable cause, and immediate onset
D. Lowest intensity of a painful stimulus that can be perceived as pain
E. Amount of pain a person is willing to endure
F. Pain that lasts more than 6 months and has no foreseeable end
G. Pain of body wall (muscles and bone) that is poorly localized, may produce nausea, and is frequently associated with blood pressure changes
H. Pain in large interior organs which tends to be diffuse, poorly localized, vague, and dull
I. Severe pain caused by nervous system damage when the flow of afferent nerve impulses has been partially or completely interrupted
J. Pain following amputation that is felt in the body part that was removed

Match the noninvasive therapies in Column A with the descriptions in Column B.

Column A

11. _____ Acupressure
12. _____ Biofeedback
13. _____ Cutaneous stimulation
14. _____ Guided imagery
15. _____ Hypnosis
16. _____ Meditation
17. _____ Progressive relaxation therapy
18. _____ Rhythmic breathing
19. _____ Therapeutic touch

Column B

A. A group of techniques taught to clients with pain in order to gain control over physiologic variables that relate to pain
B. Used by clients as a pain treatment to decrease anxiety, muscle contraction, and induce sleep by learning to tighten and relax muscle groups
C. Focuses attention away from pain. The technique involves sitting comfortably and quietly and focusing attention to flow of breath, a mantra, and a picture or mental image of a peaceful place.
D. Focuses attention away from pain and onto breathing and its rhythm; combines relaxation and distraction
E. Combines relaxation, distraction, and diminishing the source of pain; requires the person to focus on a complex scene
F. Way of realigning energy fields to relieve pain. The technique involves the nurse focusing in a meditative state; assessing the client's energy fields; and rearranging the energy fields by passing hands over the client's body.
G. Stimulation of skin to relieve pain
H. Based on suggestion and the process of focusing attention
I. Pressure applied over acupuncture points

■ *Short Answer*

Provide rationales for the therapeutic nursing interventions listed below.

20. You write in your nurse's notes "client complains of pain." The nurse working with you requests that you cross out "complains," note error with your initials, and write in the word "reports." Why?

21. Your client is 76 years old, is exhibiting some signs of confusion, and requests pain medication. You ask the nurse working with you whether to administer the pain medication. The nurse responds that you need to give the pain medication and then carefully observe your client. Why?

22. Your client is two days postoperative from a colon resection. In preparing him for sleep, you assess his pain level. He rates his pain as a 4 on a scale of 10 but does not wish any pain medication. After discussing this with your instructor, you decide to offer him a back rub. Why?

23. Your client is postoperative for a hysterectomy. You are assessing her pain medication requirements. She rates her pain as a 7 on a scale of 10. She is smiling at you as she relates this information and is visiting with her husband. What is your assessment of her pain on a scale of 1 to 10? Why?

Ms. A. is admitted to the hospital unit with the chief complaint of severe abdominal pain. You have been assigned to complete her admission assessment.

24. What history questions would you ask Ms. A. specifically directed toward the location of her pain?

25. How would you determine the intensity of her pain?

The physician orders meperidine hydrochloride (Demerol) 75 mg IM q3–4h for Ms. A.

26. What preadministration factors would you assess before administering this medication?

27. For which effects would you assess Ms. A. postadministration of the meperidine?

28. Meperidine 75 mg is equivalent to what other medications and doses?

29. What additional nonpharmacologic interventions would you include in your plan of care for Ms. A.?

■ *Multiple Choice*

30.   *Pain threshold* can best be defined as
   A.   the amount of pain a person is willing to endure.
   B.   a person's experience with pain in the past.
   C.   an interpretation of the pain experience.
   D.   the lowest perceivable intensity of stimuli transmitted as pain.

31.   The gate-control theory of pain posits that
   A.   transmission cells (T cells) in the SG may open the gate (transmit pain) or close the gate (inhibit pain).
   B.   factors such as attention memory, thinking, and emotion do not influence the gate mechanism.
   C.   the transmission cells (T cells) are primarily located in the midbrain.
   D.   brain fibers in the medulla, cerebrum, and hypothalamus have little influence on the gate mechanism.

32.   Chronic pain differs from acute pain in that chronic pain
   A.   usually has a sympathetic nervous system response.
   B.   is useful in locating the injury.
   C.   may be associated with withdrawal and depression.
   D.   has the characteristics of fast pain.

33.   A thorough pain assessment will be enhanced by which of the following facts?
   A.   Pain that is real may not have an observable cause.
   B.   The person with real pain will have an elevated BP and pulse.
   C.   Postoperative pain is gone by the third day after surgery.
   D.   If people can sleep they are not in pain.

34.   Teaching guided imagery will help to relieve pain by which of the following mechanisms?
   A.   teaching self-control over physiologic measures that relate to pain
   B.   producing a response that relaxes muscles
   C.   withdrawing positive reinforcement for behaviors related to pain
   D.   focusing attention away from the pain and onto breathing and rhythm

Clients with Substance Abuse Disorders: Promoting Positive Outcomes

Substance use/abuse is a problem in our society today. Clients with substance use/abuse problems enter the acute care setting as a direct result of the substance. That is, for complications, overdose, or emergencies such as auto accidents or they may be in the acute care setting for other medical/ surgical problems that may be complicated by the effects of the substance use/abuse. Careful social history-taking may be the first clue of a potential problem. Care of clients undergoing withdrawal from or treatment for complications of substance abuse can be complex for both physiologic and psychological interventions; it also requires that the nurse be alert while assessing for complications. It is another situation that requires a nonjudgmental caring approach.

OBJECTIVES

24.1   Discuss the heath problem of substance abuse.

24.2   Define terms related to substance abuse.

24.3   Discuss theories about the causes of substance abuse.

24.4   Describe assessment for and the effects of psychoactive substances.

24.5   Discuss the nursing care of clients with substance abuse.

24.6   Discuss the effects of use and abuse of alcohol.

24.7   Discuss the effects of use and abuse of stimulants.

24.8   Discuss the effects of use and abuse of cannabis.

24.9   Discuss the ethical issues of the chemically impaired coworker.

LEARNING THE LANGUAGE: TERMINOLOGY RELATED TO SUBSTANCE ABUSE

Match the descriptions in Column A with the framework for explaining addictive behavior in Column B.

Column A   **Column B**

1. _____ Attempts to explain the variables that may predispose an individual to substance abuse

2. _____ Substance abuse is determined by factors in a person's background.

3. _____ A physiologic condition that can be diagnosed and treated

4. _____ Genetic predisposition

5. _____ Defects in metabolism

6. _____ Neurobiologic abnormalities

7. _____ Abnormal levels of chemicals in the body

8. _____ Fixated in the oral stage of development

9. _____ Intrapersonal and interpersonal difficulties

10. _____ Addiction is a learned behavior that can be unlearned

11. _____ Views substance abuse from cultural and social norms within various groups

A.   Biologic
B.   Psychological
C.   Sociocultural

Match the descriptions in Column A with the correct term in Column B.

Column A   **Column B**

12. _____ Concurrent use of multiple drugs

13. _____ A compulsion, loss of control, and progressive pattern of drug use

14. _____ Affects a person's mood or behavior

15. _____ Continued use of a psychoactive substance despite occurrence of physical, psychological, social, or occupational problems

16. _____ A range of symptoms indicating that a person persists in using a substance, ignoring serious substance abuse-related problems

17. _____ The body's physical adaptation to a drug, whereby withdrawal symptoms will occur if the drug is not used

18. _____ The emotional need or craving for a drug

19. _____ Any use of a drug that deviates from medical or socially acceptable use

A.   Psychoactive substance
B.   Substance abuse
C.   Physiologic dependence
D.   Psychological dependence
E.   Addiction
F.   Polysubstance abuse
G.   Drug misuse
H.   Substance dependence

Match the definitions in Column A with the correct term in Column B.

Column A

20. _____ The ability of one drug to increase the activity of another drug

21. _____ The body's reaction to a drug declines and a larger dose is needed to achieve the same effect

22. _____ Greater amounts of a drug are needed because of tolerance to a similar drug

23. _____ An altered physiologic state

24. _____ The amount of a drug that produces a poisonous effect

25. _____ Accidental or deliberate consumption of a drug in a larger than normal dose

Column B

A. Intoxication

B. Overdose

C. Tolerance

D. Cross-tolerance

E. Potentiation

F. Toxic dose

Match the descriptions in Column A with the correct term in Column B.

Column A

26. _____ The tendency to relapse

27. _____ Return to a normal state of health and behaviors

28. _____ Complete abstinence from drugs while developing a satisfactory lifestyle

29. _____ Voluntarily refraining from activities or use of substances

30. _____ The process of withdrawing a person from an addictive substance in a safe manner

31. _____ Discontinuation of a substance by a person who is dependent on it

32. _____ A period of memory loss for activities as a direct result of using drugs or alcohol

Column B

A. Blackout

B. Withdrawal

C. Detoxification

D. Recidivism

E. Recovery

F. Sobriety

G. Abstinence

Match the descriptions in Column A with the type of substance in Column B (DSM IV's 11 most commonly abused).

Column A

33. _____ Chemical that gives off fumes or vapors that produce an alteration in consciousness

34. _____ A CNS stimulant and the leading cause of preventable death in the United States

35. _____ Interferes with the natural opioid system, which causes a disruption of the neurotransmitters in the brain

36. _____ A drug that has stimulant, depressant, and hallucinogenic properties

37. _____ CNS depressant absorbed directly into the bloodstream from the gastrointestinal system

38. _____ CNS depressant absorbed from the stomach and small intestines

39. _____ Stimulates the CNS and accelerates the activity of the heart and brain

40. _____ The most commonly used CNS stimulant

41. _____ The most widely used illegal drug in the United States

42. _____ Stimulates the CNS and cardiovascular system and blocks peripheral nerve impulses

43. _____ Produces illusions, delusions, and hallucinations and alterations in thought, perceptions, and feelings

Column B

A. Alcohol
B. Amphetamine
C. Caffeine
D. Cannabis
E. Cocaine
F. Hallucinogen
G. Inhalant
H. Nicotine
I. Opioid
J. Phencyclidine (PCP)
K. Sedative, hypnotic, or anxiolytic

THINKING CRITICALLY: UNDERSTANDING RATIONALES

Listed below are components of a client and family education plan. Provide the rationale for each component.

Component	Rationale
44. Concept of addiction	
45. Physical health problems associated with addiction	
46. Nutritional status	
47. Feelings and behaviors of all family members associated with addiction	
48. Areas of life affected by substance abuse: family, social, spiritual, sexual, occupational, financial, legal, and leisure	
49. Roles family members play in addiction	
50. Treatment options and treatment process	
51. Aftercare, self-help groups, and community resources	
52. Skill building in the areas of communication, expression of feelings, socialization, and coping strategies	
53. Impact of both addiction and the recovery process on the roles and responsibilities of all family members	
54. Client confidentiality and right to privacy protected under the 1975 Federal Drug and Alcohol Abuse Act	

THINKING CRITICALLY: KNOWING WHAT TO DO AND WHY

55. What blood level of alcohol is the legal definition for intoxication in most states?

56. What is the effect of tolerance on the relationship of blood alcohol level and behavior?

57. What are the personality characteristics that seem to be common for persons with substance abuse problems?

58. What are delirium tremens (DTs)? When are they most likely to occur?

59. Describe the behavior of stimulant abusers.

60. What are some of the long-term health effects of the use of marijuana?

61. What are the direct and indirect effects of alcohol on the heart?

62. Why is the inhibition of folate metabolism by alcohol a critical problem?

63. How does disulfiram (Antabuse) discourage drinking?

64. What are some of the implications of flunitrazepam (Rohypnol) use in young adults?

65. What are some of the ethical issues of chemically impaired coworkers?

PUTTING IT ALL TOGETHER

■ Case Study: Alcohol Abuse

Mr. H. is a 45-year-old businessman admitted to the hospital for a cholecystectomy. His vital signs are within normal limits, his height is 5'10" and he weighs 145 lbs. In the social history Mr. H. reports smoking up to 40 cigarettes per day and drinking a 6-pack of beer and a "couple of high balls" per day for "many" years. He also notes that he eats two light meals a day. Mr. H.'s chief complaint is severe right, upper-quadrant pain. Presence of gallstones was confirmed with x-ray prior to admission.

66. It would be most important for the nurse to obtain which of the following additional pieces of information?
    A. what kind of "hard" liquor he drinks
    B. when he had his last drink
    C. what brand of cigarettes he smokes
    D. what type of foods he eats

67. The physician orders chlordiazepoxide (Librium). The rationale for administering this drug during Mr. H.'s hospitalization is to
    A. facilitate the withdrawal process.
    B. prevent delirium tremens (DTs).
    C. decrease anxiety prior to surgery.
    D. enhance wound healing.

68. Mr. H.'s history leads the nurse to the conclusion that his surgical risk is increased because of his alcohol use. General factors associated with long-term excessive alcohol use/abuse that place a surgical client at increased risk include which of the following?
    A. impaired liver metabolism
    B. hypervitaminosis
    C. central nervous system stimulation
    D. hypermagnesemia

69. Neurologic deficiencies associated with long-term alcohol abuse are typically caused by
    A. nervous system damage by the alcohol.
    B. alcohol's interference with folate delivery.
    C. impaired metabolism.
    D. poor general nutrition.

70. Postoperatively, the nursing approach to Mr. H.'s alcohol use should be to
    A. not bring it up unless he does.
    B. not bring it up because he did not have delirium tremens.
    C. encourage him to consider referral to a community agency for follow-up.
    D. explain to him that he is an alcoholic and needs treatment.

U N I T 5

Mobility Disorders

ANATOMY AND PHYSIOLOGY REVIEW: THE MUSCULOSKELETAL SYSTEM

The musculoskeletal system enables movement of body parts, with the skeletal system providing support and the musculature facilitating movement. The functional unit of the system is the joint. This chapter provides an overview of the anatomy and physiology of the musculoskeletal system, which is pertinent to understanding assessment of clients with musculoskeletal disorders. Of particular importance are the types of joint movements.

OBJECTIVES

5.1 Identify parts of the axial and appendicular skeleton.

5.2 Describe the general structure of bone.

5.3 Describe bone classification according to shape.

5.4 Identify five major functions of the skeletal system.

5.5 Describe joint categorization according to the degree of movement.

5.6 Identify movements possible for synovial joints.

5.7 Describe three types of muscles.

5.8 Discuss briefly the physiology of the muscular system to include muscle tone and oxygenation.

5.9 Discuss briefly bone remodeling and bone repair.

THINKING CRITICALLY: KNOWING WHAT TO DO AND WHY

■ *Movements Possible by Synovial Joints*

Label the following diagram with the correct names of the movements illustrated.

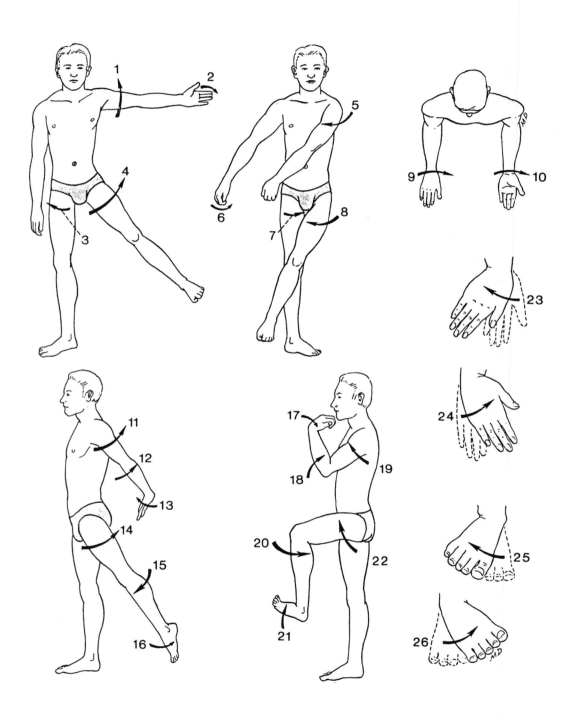

25

Assessment of the Musculoskeletal System

Assessment of the musculoskeletal system may be general or specific depending on whether the assessment is done for screening purposes or for a specific problem or injury. A health history is always included but may be brief or deferred as circumstances dictate, for example, if the injury is extensive or associated with multiple trauma. Biographic and lifestyle data give many leads, for example, persons who work with computer keyboards are more likely to have carpal tunnel syndrome, long-distance truck drivers are prone to lower back pain, the elderly to osteoarthritis. The physical examination needs to include assessment of structure and function.

OBJECTIVES

25.1   Collect pertinent health history and subjective data regarding symptoms related to musculoskeletal problems.

25.2   Obtain objective data in a systematic manner for a general and focal musculoskeletal assessment.

25.3   Describe neurologic assessment of the peroneal, tibial, radial, ulnar, and median nerves.

25.4   Describe the types and degrees of range of motion possible with each joint.

25.5   Provide information about the following diagnostic procedures to the clients having the procedures: x-rays, tomography, dural-energy x-ray absorptiometry, arthrogram, bone scans, indium imaging, biopsy, arthroscopy, and electromyography.

25.6   Describe nursing interventions specific to pre- and postprocedure care for the following diagnostic procedures: bone or muscle biopsy, arthroscopy, arthrocentesis, and electromyography.

THINKING CRITICALLY: KNOWING WHAT TO DO AND WHY

■ Study Questions Related to Musculoskeletal Assessment

1. Is bone pain more likely to be described as throbbing or aching?

2. Is joint pain more likely to be poorly localized or pinpoint in nature?

3. Does the pain associated with osteoarthritis often increase in cold, damp weather?

4. Does pain from bursitis typically increase or decrease at night?

5. What effect does excessive weight gain have on the musculoskeletal system?

6. Name and describe three spinal deformities.

7. Should muscle strength be tested during active or passive range of motion (ROM) or both?

8. How should muscle strength be graded?

9. What is "crepitus"?

■ Diagnostic Tests

10. What are tomograms?

11. How long does it take to have a bone scan?

12. How long will the client need to be inside the cylinder for a magnetic resonance imaging (MRI) test?

16. How can osteoporosis be detected early?

17. What injury is indicated if the client has pain over his lateral epicondyle of his humerus when you pronate his forearm, flex his wrist fully, and extend his elbow with your thumb on his lateral epicondyle?

13. What is an arthroscopy?

14. When is arthroscopy contraindicated?

18. Is serum calcium usually normal, elevated, or decreased with osteoporosis?

15. List client instructions regarding exercise for signs and symptoms of infection, which are usually appropriate following an arthroscopy.

■ *Neurovascular Assessment*

Match the assessments of sensory and motor function in Column A with the nerve tested in Column B. (See Figure 25-6 in Chapter 25 of the textbook.)

Column A	Column B
19. _____ Check web space between thumb and index finger	A. Median
20. _____ Check sole of foot	B. Peroneal
21. _____ Check web space between great and second toe	C. Radial
22. _____ Check pulp of small finger	D. Tibial
23. _____ Check pulp of index finger	E. Ulnar
24. _____ Flex toes	
25. _____ Extend toes	
26. _____ Hyperextend wrist or thumb	
27. _____ Oppose thumb and little finger	
28. _____ Abduct all fingers	

29. Use the Neurovascular Check Sheet below to practice recording assessments in laboratory practice and in the clinical setting with your client who requires neurovascular assessment. Check for pain on passive stretch in the client's lower extremity by dorsiflexing the client's foot, or in the client's upper extremity by flexing the client's wrist. It is important to check for pain on passive stretch because this can be one of the earliest indicators of compartment syndrome. Compartment syndrome is a serious complication and could result in the loss of a limb; therefore early signs of compartment syndrome must be reported to the physician.

EXTREMITY TO BE ASSESSED:					FREQUENCY OF ASSESSMENT:		
DATE & TIME	COLOR	CAPILLARY FILLING	MOTION	SENSATION	PAIN ON PASSIVE STRETCH	IS EXTREMITY ELEVATED?	INITIAL
REPORT ANY SIGNIFICANT CHANGE TO PHYSICIAN							

Color: Pink, Pale, Cyanotic, Black
Capillary Filling: Rapid, Sluggish
Motion: Present, Decreased, Absent

Sensation: Present (with or without stimuli—specify) Decreased, Absent
Pain on Passive Stretch: Present, Absent
Extremity Elevated?: Yes, unless ordered otherwise

26

Management of Clients with Musculoskeletal Disorders

Metabolic bone disease, bone tumors, and musculoskeletal deformities cause discomfort, pain, and disability; affect body image; and may result in fractures and death. The incidence of bone cancer is increasing in the elderly. Osteoporosis among the elderly results in conditions such as hip fractures, which cost more than $10 billion each year. Nurses can help prevent some of these conditions, detect some disorders early for optimal outcome, and minimize the untoward effects of other disorders through support and health teaching.

OBJECTIVES

26.1 Compare and contrast the pathophysiology of osteoporosis, Paget's disease, and osteomalacia.

26.2 Discuss risk factors for osteoporosis and preventive measures.

26.3 Describe diagnostic assessment and treatment including discharge teaching for osteoporosis.

26.4 Identify drug therapy for Paget's disease.

26.5 Describe pain and orthopedic complications that may occur with Paget's disease.

26.6 Describe dietary supplements as an intervention for osteomalacia.

26.7 Compare and contrast the etiology and pathophysiology of osteoarthritis and gouty arthritis.

26.8 Describe the main clinical manifestations and diagnostic findings for osteoarthritis and gouty arthritis.

26.9 Identify medical treatment for osteoarthritis and gouty arthritis.

26.10 Discuss surgical management of the client with arthritis to include indications, techniques, and complications.

26.11 Describe nursing management for the client having a total knee replacement.

26.12 Describe nursing management for the client having a total hip replacement.

26.13 Describe adult scoliosis and surgical management.

26.14 Describe the etiology, diagnosis, and management of osteomyelitis.

OBJECTIVES (*CONTINUED*)

26.15 Differentiate between the terms for benign and malignant bone tumors.

26.16 Describe in general terms the diagnosis and treatment of bone tumors.

26.17 Describe the following common hand and foot disorders as to definition, assessment findings, and treatment: carpal tunnel syndrome, Dupuytren's contracture, ganglion, hallux valgus, hammer toe, and Morton's neuroma.

THINKING CRITICALLY: KNOWING WHAT TO DO AND WHY

■ *Study Questions Related to the Nursing Care of Clients with Musculoskeletal Disorders*

1. What is the difference between primary and secondary osteoporosis?

2. Identify three alterations that usually are needed in the home of a client with severe osteoporosis.

3. Which type of exercises are most effective in preventing bone loss?

4. How should you describe a dual-energy x-ray absorptiometry test to a client?

5. Identify four specific foods high in calcium.

6. What is the recommended daily calcium intake?

7. What is a major complication of untreated scoliosis in an adult?

8. What is the difference between acute and chronic osteomyelitis?

9.   Give four assessment findings associated with osteomyelitis.

10.   Define sequestrectomy and saucerization.

11.   Name five primary malignancies that commonly metastasize to the bone.

12.   Give three characteristics of benign bone tumors.

13.   What is the most common type of primary malignant bone tumor?

14.   List three other types of primary malignant bone tumors.

15.   Why is chemotherapy given preoperatively (neoadjuvant therapy) to treat primary malignant bone tumors?

16.   What is Tinel's sign?

17.   What is the most common benign soft tissue mass in the hand?

18.   Briefly describe a simple bunionectomy.

19.   Describe nonsurgical treatment for hammer toe.

20.   Describe the pain associated with Morton's neuroma.

27

Management of Clients with Musculoskeletal Trauma or Overuse

Musculoskeletal injuries are common and range in severity from relatively minor soft tissue injuries to severe fractures that could result in hemorrhagic shock or chronic infection. Most injuries occur as a result of accidents. The elderly are especially prone to fractures because of osteoporosis and diminished sensory and motor functioning. Sports medicine has emerged as a new specialty because many musculoskeletal injuries occur during sport and recreational activities. The nurse's responsibilities in orthopedic nursing include client education to prevent injuries and accidents, as well as providing care to promote healing, prevent complications, and facilitate rehabilitation to the greatest extent possible. Providing common musculoskeletal interventions, such as rest, physical therapy, assistive devices, casts, traction, and surgery, requires a team approach to identify and meet the client's needs, prevent complications, and minimize disabling effects. Complications could occur with any of these interventions. For example, loss of movement is difficult to cope with and while therapeutic rest promotes healing, it can also produce muscle weakness and joint stiffness. Therefore, the physician applies the cast in such a way that only those joints that must be immobilized to stabilize the fracture are inside the cast. The nurse provides range of motion exercises, which help reduce complications. Physical therapy is often necessary to avoid the problems associated with deconditioning (bone demineralization, decreased range of motion, and decreased muscle mass).

OBJECTIVES

27.1 Identify common types of fractures from a diagram or descriptions.

27.2 Identify signs and symptoms indicative of a fracture.

27.3 Describe the stages of fracture healing.

27.4 Discuss first aid for clients with fractures.

27.5 List the primary goals of treatment for a client with a fracture.

27.6 Describe three basic methods of reducing a fracture.

27.7 Describe the purposes of various types of traction.

27.8 Discuss nursing interventions for clients in traction.

27.9 Discuss potential complications of fractures and give the interventions useful in preventing each complication.

27.10 Describe the purposes of various types of casts.

27.11 Assist with the application and removal of a cast.

27.12 Discuss nursing interventions for clients with casts.

27.13 Discuss nursing care for the client with a fracture treated with external fixation.

27.14 Describe the types of "hip fractures" (fractures of the proximal end of the femur).

27.15 Identify usual signs and symptoms of a fractured hip.

OBJECTIVES (*CONTINUED*)

27.16 Describe potential complications of proximal femur fractures.

27.17 Plan nursing interventions for the client who has undergone surgery to repair a hip fracture.

27.18 Discuss the incidence and type of injuries resulting from sport injuries.

27.19 Describe specific ways to minimize the risk for overuse injuries.

27.20 Discuss common overuse sport injuries as to cause, assessment, and intervention.

27.21 Discuss the goals of physical therapy for clients with musculoskeletal impairment.

27.22 Discuss the application of heat and cold, and the use of massage and exercise.

27.23 Discuss the use of the following assistive devices: crutches, canes, walkers, and supports.

LEARNING THE LANGUAGE: TERMINOLOGY RELATED TO MUSCULOSKELETAL INJURIES

Match the definitions in Column A with the correct term in Column B.

Column A

1. _____ Grating sensation when moving fractured extremity

2. _____ Failure of fracture site to heal after 4-6 months

3. _____ Crippled hand or forearm resulting from compartmental syndrome

4. _____ Muscle injury

5. _____ Partial loss of contact between articulating surfaces of joint

6. _____ Ligament injury

7. _____ Used with pelvic traction

8. _____ "Tennis elbow"

9. _____ Manipulating fractured bones to restore alignment without surgery

10. _____ Knee ligament most frequently injured

11. _____ Potentially life-threatening complication of long-bone and pelvic fractures occurring 24-48 hours after injury, like adult respiratory distress syndrome (ARDS)

12. _____ Realignment of bones during surgery requiring incision

13. _____ Serious complication resulting from compression of the duodenum

14. _____ Fourth stage of bone healing, resulting in new bone

15. _____ Third stage of bone healing, serving as a temporary splint

Column B

A. Anterior cruciate

B. Bivalve

C. Buck's traction

D. Callus formation

E. Callus ossification

F. "Cast syndrome"

G. Closed reduction

H. Compartment syndrome

I. Compound fracture

J. Crepitus

K. Fat embolism

L. Internal fixation

M. Lateral epicondylitis

N. Nonunion

O. Open reduction

P. Osteomyelitis

Q. Rotator cuff tear

R. Sprain

S. Strain

T. Subluxation

U. Volkmann's (ischemic) contracture

V. Williams' position

16. _____ Skin traction used to immobilize a lower
    extremity
17. _____ Splitting cast along both sides to relieve
    excessive pressure
18. _____ Serious complication of fractures resulting
    from compression of nerves and blood
    vessels
19. _____ Injury to shoulder muscles
20. _____ Severe bone infection
21. _____ Realignment of bone ends with hardware
    during surgery
22. _____ A break in the skin or wound over fracture
    site, same as open fracture

THINKING CRITICALLY: UNDERSTANDING RATIONALES

Give the rationale for each of the following nursing interventions for clients with musculoskeletal injuries.

Intervention	Rationale

23. Elevate the client's injured extremity.

24. Use the term "closed" rather than "simple" or
    "uncomplicated" when talking with the injured
    client with a fracture of this type.

25. Tell the client after hip surgery to sit with both feet
    on the floor.

26. Teach the client after hip surgery quadriceps and
    gluteal setting exercises.

27. Check for temperature elevation daily in the
    injured client.

28. Provide and encourage a diet high in vitamins,
    protein, iron, and calcium.

29. Check peripheral neurovascular status bilaterally
    even though only one extremity is in a cast or
    traction.

Nutritional Disorders

ANATOMY AND PHYSIOLOGY REVIEW: THE NUTRITIONAL (GASTROINTESTINAL) SYSTEM

Understanding the pathophysiology of the disorders of the gastrointestinal (GI) tract will be greatly enhanced if you have a basic understanding of its structure and function. Read the following objectives. If you can respond to these correctly, you are ready to progress to the rest of the GI unit. If you cannot respond correctly to the objectives, you would benefit from spending some time reviewing the structure and function of the GI tract and then answering the Study Guide questions.

OBJECTIVES

6.1   Describe the structure and function of the digestive system.

6.2   Describe the normal structure and function of the mouth, esophagus, stomach, and small and large intestines.

6.3   Discuss the effects of aging on the gastrointestinal tract.

6.4   Describe the vomiting reflex.

LEARNING THE LANGUAGE: TERMINOLOGY RELATED TO STRUCTURE AND FUNCTION OF THE GASTROINTESTINAL SYSTEM

Briefly describe or define the following terms.

1.   Lower esophageal sphincter (LES)

2.   Achalasia

3.   Fundus of the stomach

4.   Pyloric sphincter

5.   Chyme

6.   Intrinsic factor

7.   Ileocecal valve

8.   Gut-associated lymphoid tissue

Match the stomach glands in Column A with the product they secrete in Column B. (Answers may be used more than once.)

Column A	**Column B**
9. _____ Cardiac glands	A. Mucus
10. _____ Peptic (chief) cells	B. Gastrin
11. _____ Parietal (oxyntic) cells	C. Pepsinogen
12. _____ Neck cells	D. Hydrochloric acid
13. _____ Pyloric glands	E. Intrinsic factor

Match the segments of the GI tract in Column A with the digestive action that occurs in that segment in Column B.

Column A	**Column B**
14. _____ Colon	A. Beginning starch breakdown
15. _____ Jejunum	B. Final absorption of water, chloride, and sodium
16. _____ Stomach	C. Vitamin B_{12} absorption
17. _____ Mouth	D. Glucose, water-soluble vitamins, protein, and fat are absorbed
18. _____ Ileum	E. Secretes intrinsic factor

THINKING CRITICALLY: UNDERSTANDING RATIONALES

Indicate whether each of the following statements is True (T) or False (F). Provide correct answers for the False statements.

19. _____ Dysphagia means indigestion.

20. _____ Saliva contains the enzyme gastrin.

21. _____ The pH of the gastric contents can reach 1.5.

22. _____ The sympathetic nerves promote gastric secretion and motility.

23. _____ The small intestine is approximately 12 feet in length.

24. _____ The absorbed products of digestion from the small intestine leave via the superior mesenteric vein, which unites with the inferior mesenteric, splenic, and the gastric veins, which leads into the portal systems and to the liver.

25. _____ The primary function of the large intestine is absorption of fats.

26. _____ One effect of aging on digestion is decreased absorption of fat-soluble vitamins.

■ *Understanding the Vomiting Reflex*

Number the sequence for the vomiting reflex.

27. _____ Forced inspiration against a closed glottis decreases intrathoracic pressure.

28. _____ Forceful contraction of abdominal muscles increases intra-abdominal pressure.

29. _____ Gastric contents enter the esophagus.

30. _____ Retching occurs when upper esophageal sphincter remains closed.

31. _____ Reverse peristalsis is initiated in the middle of the small intestine.

32. _____ The lower esophageal sphincter relaxes, and the pylorus and antrum contract.

33. _____ The pyloric sphincter and stomach relax to receive duodenal contents.

34. _____ The trachea closes, as in normal swallowing to prevent aspiration.

35. _____ Vomiting occurs when the upper esophageal sphincter opens.

36. How do emetics work?

CHAPTER 28

Assessment of Nutrition and the Digestive System

A thorough understanding of skills needed for assessment of nutrition and the gastrointestinal (GI) tract facilitates nursing assessments and forms a basis for making nursing judgments—from the initial admitting health assessment to the many daily client assessments. In addition, the nurse caring for adults are frequently involved in preparing them for diagnostic examinations of the GI tract. This requires understanding the tests in order to prepare the client for the pretest and post-test interventions.

OBJECTIVES

28.1 Discuss the importance of a nutritional history.

28.2 Discuss the indications for a nutritional screening and a nutritional assessment.

28.3 Identify elements of a complete history and physical examination for the upper GI system.

28.4 Describe common diagnostic tests used for clients with disorders of the upper GI system.

LEARNING THE LANGUAGE: TERMINOLOGY RELATED TO ASSESSMENT OF CLIENTS WITH GASTROINTESTINAL DISORDERS

Match the types of malnutrition in Column A with the correct definition or description in Column B.

Column A	Column B
1. _____ Kwashiorkor	A. Inadequate calorie and protein intake with increased nutritional requirements
2. _____ Mixed	B. Inadequate protein intake with adequate calorie intake
3. _____ Marasmus	C. Inadequate calorie and protein intake

Match the terms in Column A with the correct definition or description in Column B.

Column A	Column B
4. _____ Anorexia	A. Present in smoked and preserved meats
5. _____ Borborygmi	B. Loss of appetite
6. _____ Dyspepsia	C. Difficulty swallowing
7. _____ Dysphagia	D. Bloody stools
8. _____ Hematemesis	E. Grayish or white spot or patch found on the oral
9. _____ Leukoplakia	mucosa
10. _____ Melena	F. Indigestion
11. _____ Nitrosamines	G. Rapid, high-pitched, loud bowel sounds
	H. Vomiting of blood

THINKING CRITICALLY: KNOWING WHAT TO DO AND WHY

Briefly describe the process or technique used for assessing the following.

12. Chief complaint

13. Abdomen (physical examination)

14. Bowel sounds

Give the rationale for the following.

15. Completing a nutritional screening.

16. Examining the abdomen using the following sequence: inspection, auscultation, percussion, and palpation.

17. Asking the client about family history related to GI disorders.

18. Asking the client about frequency and dose of aspirin or nonsteroidal anti-inflammatory drugs.

19. Asking the client about taking iron supplements.

20. Assessing the client's use of caffeine, alcohol, and cigarettes.

21. Assessing the client for a change in bowel habits.

22.   Assessing the total lymphocyte count (TLC).

24.   Your client tells you he has been taking 3 mg of Coumadin every day for 5 years.

23.   During the health history your client tells you, "I take a multivitamin plus other nutritional supplements."

25.   Your client tells you, "I take meal supplements every day—either a protein shake or protein bars."

List the possible drug-nutrient interaction.

Drug	**Possible Nutrient Interaction**
26. Antacids	
27. Diuretics	
28. Cholesterol-reducing drugs	

UNDERSTANDING CULTURAL FOOD PRACTICES AND RELIGION

For each religion's food restriction list one nursing implication.

Religion	Restriction	Implication
29. Church of Jesus Christ of Latter-Day Saints (Mormon)	No stimulants	
30. Judaism	Kashrut (dietary laws) Meat and diary products cannot be served at the same meal.	
31. Islam	Alcohol strictly forbidden.	
32. Roman Catholics	Abstinence from meat products during Lent.	
33. Seventh Day Adventists	Snacking between meals is discouraged.	

THINKING CRITICALLY: KNOWING WHAT TO DO AND WHY

Use Chapter 28 Boxes 28-2 and 28-3 and Table 28-7 to calculate the ideal body weight (IBW) for the following:

34. Adult female, 5' 5" tall with a 7" wrist circumference, and an R value of 10

35. Adult male, 5' 8" tall, and has a large frame.

Calculate the BMI (body mass index) using one the following formulas:

Body Mass Index (BMI)

$$BMI = \frac{Weight\ (kg)}{height\ (M^2)}$$

$$BMI = \frac{Weight\ (lb)}{height\ (inches)^2 \times 705}$$

A BMI > 27 indicates obesity

36. Female: 5' 4"; 185 pounds

37. Male: 6'; 192 pounds

*Calculate the normal daily protein requirements using the following formula: **0.5 g/kg/day**.*

38. Female: 5' 4"; 185 pounds

39. Male: 6'; 192 pounds

■ *Diagnostic Tests*

	Test	Informed Consent	Pretest Nursing Care	Post-Test Nursing Care
40.	Upper GI series			
41.	Flat plate of the abdomen			
42.	Endoscopy EGD (Esophagogastro-duodenoscopy)			

Management of Clients with MalnutrItion

The concept of malnutrition broadly describes undernutrition or overnutrition related to dietary intake. Protein-energy malnutrition (PEM) results when the body's need for protein and/or energy (glucose and fat) is not supplied by dietary intake. In acute care settings over 40% of hospitalized clients admitted with medical-surgical problems develop PEM during their hospitalization. Compounding the problem is the fact that more clients are being admitted with malnutrition. Thus, nurses deal with the effects of PEM everyday. In addition, many acute and chronic diseases and treatments can affect the ability to ingest or digest foods. Nutritional demands increase in response to critical, chronic, infectious disease. Problems with nutrition can affect wound healing, immune function, medication metabolism and excretion, and overall functional status. Management of clients with malnutrition is truly a multidisciplinary approach between the client and his/her family, nurse, dietitian, physician, occupational therapist, speech therapist, and other members of the health care team. Nurses must have a broad understanding of the concepts of nutrition and malnutrition to identify clients at nutritional risk and to manage clients with malnutrition.

OBJECTIVES

29.1 Identify clients who are at risk for malnutrition and protein-energy malnutrition (PEM).

29.2 Plan and implement nursing care for clients with nutritional problems.

29.3 Discuss nutritional support for clients with malnutrition.

THINKING CRITICALLY: UNDERSTANDING RATIONALES

Provide the rationales for the therapeutic nursing interventions listed below.

Intervention   **Rationale**

Client with Decreased Appetite

1.   Create a pleasant environment during mealtime.

2.   Ensure adequate pain relief before meals.

3.   Provide good oral hygiene.

4.   Increase social interaction at mealtime.

Client with Impaired Swallowing

5.   Place food on the unaffected side.

6.   Once food is at the pharynx, ask the client to tilt his/her chin down.

7.   Have suction equipment available.

8.   Check the client's mouth for lingering food pockets.

9.   Teach family members the Heimlich maneuver.

10.   Maintain high Flower's position for 30 minutes after the meal.

Client Receiving Enteral Feedings

11.   Elevate head of bed (HOB) 30 degrees.

12.   Assess residual volume.

13.   Assess for dehydration.

14.   Flush the tube with water.

Intervention	**Rationale**

Client with Nasogastric Tube

15. Irrigate with normal saline (NS).

16. Measure pH of the aspirant.

17. Administer frequent oral hygiene.

Client Receiving Total Parenteral Nutrition (TPN)

18. Use meticulous aseptic technique.

19. Use an IV pump to administer.

20. Assess for hyperglycemia.

21. Taper TPN when discontinuing.

Client with Eating Disorders

22. Remain with the client for one hour after eating.

23. Assess for dysrhythmias.

Differentiate between Anorexia Nervosa (A) and Bulimia Nervosa (B) by placing the appropriate letter beside each of the following physical manifestations. (Use C to indicate if the characteristic applies to both.)

24. _____ Salivary gland enlargement
25. _____ Poor dental status
26. _____ Low blood pressure and pulse
27. _____ Esophagitis
28. _____ Normal or underweight
29. _____ Cachexia
30. _____ Calluses on fingertips
31. _____ Edema
32. _____ Diarrhea
33. _____ Dysrhythmias
34. _____ Dry, brittle hair
35. _____ Lanugo-type hair
36. _____ Decreased WBC and glucose
37. _____ Osteoporosis
38. _____ Growth retardation
39. _____ Increased potassium and amylase

A   Anorexia Nervosa
B.   Bulimia Nervosa
C.   Both

THINKING CRITICALLY

Use the Admission Nutrition Screening tool on page 666 (Box 29-1) to determine the nutritional risk for the following

patients.

40.   48-year-old white male with history of end-stage liver disease

41.   42-year-old female admitted to the hospital with hypotension following a laparoscopic gall bladder removal; 5' 6" and 150 pounds

42.   62-year-old male with NIDDM who had coronary artery bypass grafting 3 months ago

43.   49-year-old female, 5' 6", 165 pounds, who has lost 25 pounds in the last 2 months on a low carbohydrate diet

44.   34-year-old male, 6', 254 pounds, admitted for evaluation of GERD-like symptoms

CHAPTER 30

Management of Clients with Ingestive Disorders

A healthy oral cavity is the basis of sound nutrition that in turn impacts the total health of the individual. Therefore, teaching primary prevention of disorders of the mouth is a concern for nurses. The secondary prevention focus for nurses involves a thorough assessment of the oral cavity to identify problems early. The tertiary care focus is on nursing care of clients with disorders of the oral cavity.

Disorders of the esophagus are not as clear-cut in terms of known risk factors that primary prevention could affect; therefore, most nursing care will focus on secondary and tertiary care.

OBJECTIVES

30.1 Discuss disorders associated with the mouth, and medical treatment, associated nursing care, and appropriate primary prevention of these disorders.

30.2 Describe disorders associated with the esophagus, and medical treatment, associated nursing care, and appropriate primary prevention of these disorders.

LEARNING THE LANGUAGE: TERMINOLOGY RELATED TO INGESTIVE DISORDERS

Match the terms in Column A with the correct definition in Column B.

Column A

1. _____ Aphthous
2. _____ Avulsed tooth
3. _____ Calculus
4. _____ Candidiasis
5. _____ Dental caries
6. _____ Dental plaques
7. _____ Erythroplakia
8. _____ Gingivitis
9. _____ Herpes labialis
10. _____ Leukoplakia
11. _____ Parotitis
12. _____ Periodontitis
13. _____ Root canal
14. _____ Vincent's angina
15. _____ Xerostomia

Column B

A. Soft mass of proliferating bacteria with other cells in a sticky polysaccharide matrix that adheres to the teeth

B. Tooth decay

C. Removal of the pulp portion of the tooth

D. Hardened plaque

E. Inflammation of the gingiva

F. The most serious form of gum disorder; also called pyorrhea

G. Tooth loss due to trauma

H. Small recurrent ulcerated lesions on the soft tissue of the mouth; canker sore

I. Fever blister or cold sore caused by herpes simplex virus

J. Acute bacterial infection of the gingiva

K. Fungal infection of mouth caused by *Candida albicans*; thrush

L. Precancerous, yellow-white or gray lesion of the oral mucous membranes

M. Red, velvety-appearing patch indicating early squamous cell cancer

N. Dryness of the mouth

O. Inflammation of the parotid glands; surgical mumps

Match the terms in Column A with the correct definition in Column B.

Column A

16. _____ Achalasia
17. _____ Bougienage
18. _____ Cachexia
19. _____ Dysphagia
20. _____ Esophageal reflux
21. _____ Heartburn
22. _____ Odynophagia

Column B

A. Pain on swallowing that affects the mucosa

B. Severe malnutrition

C. Forceful dilation of the lower esophagus and sphincter

D. Gastric contents returning to the esophagus

E. Difficulty in swallowing

F. Progressively increasing dysphagia; "feels like something is stuck in the throat"

G. Sensation of warmth and burning in the lower retrosternal midline; pyrosis, indigestion, or dyspepsia

THINKING CRITICALLY: UNDERSTANDING RATIONALES

Provide the rationales for the therapeutic nursing interventions listed below.

Intervention	Rationale
23. Encouraging brushing teeth after ingestion of caramels or other sticky substances.	
24. Encouraging daily flossing.	
25. Discouraging use of commercial mouthwashes for the client with painful oral lesions.	
26. Discouraging the use of chewing tobacco.	
27. Positioning the client with a tracheostomy in a semi- to high-Fowler's position.	
28. Check pH of stomach contents before PEG feeding.	
29. Teach clients with gastroesophageal reflux disease (GERD) to drink adequate fluids with meals.	
30. Careful assessment of the oral cavity of immuno-suppressed clients.	

■ Medications

Listed below are specific medications used to treat GERD (gastroesophageal reflux disease). Provide the rationale for each medication.

Medication	Rationale
31. Bethanechol (Urecholine)	
32. Metoclopramide (Reglan)	
33. Cisapride (Propulsid)	
34. Omeprazole (Prilosec)	
35. Misoprostol (Cytotec)	

PUTTING IT ALL TOGETHER

■ *Case Study*

Ms. L., 69, presents at the clinic with signs and symptoms of severe heartburn after eating, mild substernal chest pain that is worse when she lies down, and a feeling of fullness. After completing an analysis of the client's symptoms, the nurse finds that Ms. L. takes antacids to help relieve the pain, that sitting up helps relieve the pain, and that the symptoms are much worse after a large meal. The physician orders a barium swallow and other diagnostic tests that result in a diagnosis of hiatal hernia.

36. In teaching Ms. L. about hiatal hernias, the nurse could include which of the following facts?
    A. Hiatal hernias are very rare in women over 65 years of age.
    B. Hiatal hernias are caused by part of the stomach entering the chest cavity due to a muscle weakness.
    C. Hiatal hernias are caused by an inappropriate relaxation at the end of the esophagus.
    D. Hiatal hernias are most common in men in their late forties and early fifties.

37. Ms. L. will be treated medically for the hiatal hernia. Teaching for Ms. L. would most likely include which of the following?
    A. Decrease liquid intake with meals.
    B. Lie flat for 30 minutes after meals.
    C. Take prescribed Reglan 30 minutes after meals.
    D. Eat small, frequent meals (4–6per day).

Ms. L. does not respond to medical therapy and is scheduled for surgery using a thoracic approach.

38. The postoperative nursing care plan will include which of the following in relation to the nursing diagnosis High risk for injury related to surgical procedure and presence of chest tubes?
    A. Clamp chest tubes when ambulating client.
    B. Milk the chest tubes every two hours.
    C. Avoid coughing and deep breathing.
    D. Keep drainage system below the level of the client's chest.

Management of Clients with Digestive Disorders

Gastric disorders include those with a mixed psychological and physiologic basis to those with a purely physiologic basis. Treatments for gastric disorders, therefore, cover a broad range that includes psychiatric, medical, and/or surgical interventions. This broad range of disorders and therapies naturally results in a range of client responses that will challenge the nursing student from assessment through evaluation.

OBJECTIVES

31.1 Identify general clinical manifestations of gastric disorders.

31.2 Discuss types of gastric tubes and care of clients with these tubes.

31.3 Discuss nutritional support for clients with gastric disorders.

31.4 Describe the clinical problems most frequently associated with the stomach and their medical, surgical, and nursing management.

LEARNING THE LANGUAGE: TERMINOLOGY RELATED TO NURSING CARE OF CLIENTS WITH GASTRIC DISORDERS

Match the tubes in Column A with their length in Column B and purpose in Column C.

Column A	Column B	Column C
1. _____ Cantor	A. 125 cm (50 in)	a. Remove gas or fluid from the stomach; obtain specimen of gastric contents
2. _____ Dobbhoff	B. 300 cm (10 ft)	
3. _____ Harris	C. 180 cm (6 in)	
4. _____ Levin Type	D. 120 cm (48 in)	b. Double-lumen tube for emptying or decompressing the stomach
5. _____ Miller-Abbott	E. 160–175 cm (60–66in)	
6. _____ Salem		c. Short-term enteral feeding
		d. Suction and irrigation of intestines
		e. Aspiration of intestinal contents

Match the following gastric surgical procedures in Column A with the descriptions in Column B.

Column A	Column B
7. _____ Antrectomy	A. Removal of distal portion of stomach and anastomosis to the duodenum
8. _____ Billroth I	B. Removal of antrum of stomach and anastomosis with the duodenum
9. _____ Billroth II	C. Removal of stomach with anastomosis of esophagus to the jejunum
10. _____ Gastroenterostomy	D. Surgery creates a passage between the bottom of the stomach and the duodenum
11. _____ Proximal vagotomy	E. Nerve fibers to parietal cells are severed
12. _____ Pyloroplasty	F. Removal of distal segment of stomach and anastomosis to the jejunum
13. _____ Total gastrectomy	G. Provides larger opening from the stomach to the duodenum
14. _____ Truncal vagotomy	H. Vagal nerve fibers to stomach, as well as hepatic and celiac branches, are severed

Match the data in Column A with the correct type of ulcer in Column B.

Column A	Column B
15. _____ Increased acid secretion	A. Gastric
16. _____ 4 to 1; more common in men	B. Duodenal
17. _____ 10% malignancy	C. Stress
18. _____ Pain at night	
19. _____ Associated with severe burns	
20. _____ Vomiting may relieve the pain	
21. _____ Melena more common	
22. _____ Pain may lessen with eating	
23. _____ Normal to decreased acid secretion	
24. _____ Also called stress-erosive ulcers	
25. _____ Large percentage caused by *Helicobacter pylori*	

THINKING CRITICALLY: UNDERSTANDING RATIONALES

Listed below are nursing interventions for clients with ulcers. Provide the rationales for the nursing interventions.

Intervention	**Rationale**
26. Assist the client to rest.	
27. Avoid medications containing aspirin, nonsteroidal anti-inflammatory drugs (NSAIDs), adrenocorticosteroids, and adrenocorticotropic hormone (ACTH).	
28. Assess the abdomen for rigidity.	
29. Assess for B_{12} deficiency after total gastrectomy.	

■ Medications

Listed below are specific medications and their nursing implications. Provide the rationales for the nursing implications.

Implication	Rationale

Clarithromycin (Biaxin), metronidazole (Flagyl), and Omeprazole (Prilosec)

30.   Use in treatment of peptic and duodenal ulcers.

Ranitidine hydrochloride (Zantac)

31.   Give antacids at least one hour before or two hours after administration.

Cimetidine (Tagamet)

32.   Assess mental status of older clients.

Misoprostol (Cytotec)

33.   Give to clients taking long-term aspirin and NSAIDs.

Dicyclomine hydrochloride (Bentyl)

34.   Do not give to clients with BPH, GI obstruction, ulcerative colitis, unstable cardiovascular status; use carefully in clients with narrow-angle glaucoma.

Magnesium oxide, aluminum-mg combinations, calcium carbonate

35.   Do not use in clients with renal disease.

Sucralfate (Carafate)

36.   Give one hour before meals.

CLIENT EDUCATION : KNOWING WHAT TO TEACH AND WHY

List rationales for the following teaching points for clients with dumping syndrome.

Teaching Point	Rationale

37. Eat in a recumbent or semi-recumbent position.

38. Lie down after meals.

39. Increase fat content in meals.

40. Avoid liquids one hour before, during, and after meals.

PUTTING IT ALL TOGETHER

■ *Case Study*

Mr. C. is a 49-year-old salesman who presents at the emergency room with complaints of acute abdominal pain. He gives a 5- to 6-year history of being treated for gastric ulcers with cimetidine (Tagamet), which he takes episodically depending on his pain. His vital signs are B/P 130/70, P 120, R 22, and T 98.4° F. Before any diagnostic tests can be completed, Mr. C. has an emesis of 300 cc of bright red blood. An IV of 1000 cc of lactated Ringer's solution is started, a nasogastric tube is put in place, and saline lavage is ordered.

41. Saline lavage procedure involves which of the following?
    A. instilling and withdrawing iced saline through a nasogastric tube
    B. instilling and withdrawing cooled saline through a nasogastric tube
    C. instilling and withdrawing warmed saline through a nasogastric tube
    D. instilling cooled saline through a nasogastric tube and clamping the tube

Mr. C. is stabilized and admitted to the surgical unit. The nurse on the unit identifies a collaborative diagnosis of High risk for injury R/T complications of perforation.

42. In order to assess for perforation which of the following observations would the nurse need to make?
    A. Assess for soft, tender abdomen.
    B. Assess for hyperactive bowel sounds.
    C. Assess for sudden, sharp, severe pain.
    D. Assess for elevated blood pressure and decreased pulse.

Mr. C. recovers from the acute episode of gastric bleeding and is discharged from the hospital on medical therapy. Six months later he is readmitted with another acute hemorrhage and the decision is made for surgical intervention. Mr. C. is scheduled for a subtotal gastrectomy (Billroth I procedure).

43.   With a Billroth I procedure, which of the following procedures is performed?
   A.   The vagus nerves are surgically severed.
   B.   The pyloric valve is widened.
   C.   The proximal remnant of the stomach is anastomosed to the jejunum.
   D.   The duodenum is anastomosed to the proximal remnant of the stomach.

44.   Nutritional problems that Mr. C. might face after the Billroth I surgery include which of the following?
   A. B_{12} and folic acid deficiency
   B.   iron and vitamin C deficiency
   C.   protein and fat deficiency
   D.   protein and carbohydrate deficiency

45.   Should Mr. C. develop dumping syndrome, which of the following recommendations would the nurse make?
   A.   Take 300 cc of fluids with each meal.
   B.   Sit up for one hour after each meal.
   C.   Eat three regular meals a day.
   D.   Increase the fat content in the diet.

Elimination Disorders

ANATOMY AND PHYSIOLOGY REVIEW: THE ELIMINATION SYSTEMS

The urinary system is composed of the kidneys, ureters, bladder, and urethra. The functioning unit of the kidney is the nephron. Each kidney contains more than one million nephron units. Urine formation occurs in the nephrons through the processes of filtration, reabsorption, and secretion. Once urine formation has occurred, it is excreted from the body; the ureters, bladder, and urethra play a role in this process. In addition to urine formation, the urinary system assists in the regulation of fluids and electrolytes, hydrogen ion balance, and blood pressure. Knowledge of this information is essential for nursing care of clients with disorders of the urinary system.

OBJECTIVES

7.1 Describe the structure and function of the normal urinary tract.

7.2 Identify the two main functions of the urinary system.

7.3 Describe the process of urine formation.

7.4 Describe the regulation of fluids and electrolytes by the kidneys.

7.5 Describe the regulation of hydrogen ion balance by the kidneys.

7.6 Describe the regulation of blood pressure by the kidneys.

7.7 Identify other metabolic and endocrine functions of the kidneys.

7.8 Describe the process of micturition.

7.9 Discuss how aging affects urinary function.

Label the missing parts of the kidney in the diagram below.

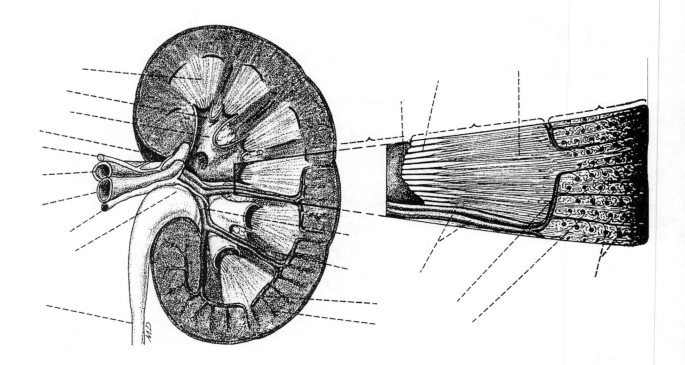

Label the missing parts of the nephron in the diagram below.

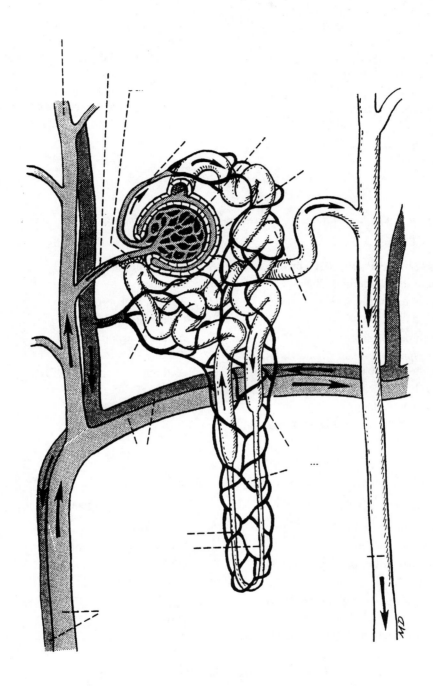

LEARNING THE LANGUAGE: TERMINOLOGY RELATED TO URINARY STRUCTURE AND FUNCTION

Fill in the blanks.

1. The urinary system is composed of _____, _____, _____, and _____.
2. The functioning unit of the kidney is the _____. Each kidney contains more than _____ million nephrons.
3. Urine formation occurs through the process of _____, _____, and _____.
4. Ureters connect the _____ and _____.

5. The bladder holds approximately _____ mL of urine. The _____ extend from the bladder to the external opening. The external opening is called the _____.
6. The main functions of the kidneys are to remove _____ and to regulate fluid and _____, _____, _____, and _____ _____.

Match the descriptions in Column A with the correct kidney function in Column B.

Column A		Column B	
7.	_____ Stimulates red blood cell (RBC) production	A.	Reabsorption
8.	_____ The amount the glomerulus filters	B.	Filtration
9.	_____ 99% of glomerular filtrate is reabsorbed	C.	Tubular reabsorption
10.	_____ Taking back of fluids	D.	Glomerular filtration rate
11.	_____ Regulates blood pressure	E.	Active transport
12.	_____ Active transport of certain chemicals from bloodstream into the tubules	F.	Tubular secretion
		G.	Antidiuretic hormone (ADH)
13.	_____ Passage of liquid through a membrane	H.	Renin
14.	_____ Regulates water balance	I.	Erythropoietin
15.	_____ Requires energy to move solutes across a membrane		

Match the descriptions in Column A with the correct term in Column B.

Column A		Column B	
16.	_____ Adult glomerular filtration rate	A.	Micturition
17.	_____ Normal bladder capacity	B.	Countercurrent mechanism
18.	_____ Amount kidneys filter per day	C.	Ultrafiltration
19.	_____ Urination, voiding	D.	125 mL/minute
20.	_____ High hydrostatic pressure in kidneys causes filtration	E.	80 L/day
		F.	400–500 mL
21.	_____ Allows for production of hyperosmolar urine		

Match the descriptions in Column A with the correct urinary structure in Column B.

Column A		Column B	
22.	_____ Urine excretion pathway	A.	Ureter
23.	_____ Transports urine to bladder	B.	Bladder
24.	_____ External opening	C.	Urethra
25.	_____ Stores urine until it is excreted	D.	Meatus

THINKING CRITICALLY: NORMAL URINARY FUNCTION

Provide short answers to the following questions.

26. Describe the most important factor influencing glomerular filtration rate.

27. Explain how medications can alter the normal glomerular filtration rate.

28. Approximately how much of the glomerular filtrate becomes urine?

29. How much urine can the adult renal pelvis hold? The adult bladder?

30. Explain how the aging process affects urinary function.

CHAPTER

32

Assessment of Elimination

Managing the care of a client with an elimination disorder requires accurate assessment data. Assessment of the upper gastrointestinal and urinary tract may produce embarrassment for some clients, making them hesitant to give information. Use of proper communication techniques is important. The nurse must also be supportive of the client. In addition, the nurse caring for clients with elimination disorders is frequently involved in preparing them for diagnostic examinations of the GI and urinary system. This requires the understanding of the tests in order to prepare the client for the pretest and post-test interventions.

OBJECTIVES

32.1   Identify elements of a complete history and physical examination of the upper gastrointestinal (GI) tract.

32.2   Describe common diagnostic tests and nursing responsibilities for clients with disorders of the upper GI system.

32.3   Identify elements of a complete history and physical examination of clients with urinary disorders.

32.4   Discuss the invasive and noninvasive diagnostic studies used to evaluate urinary function.

32.5   Discuss nursing responsibilities related to selected diagnostic procedures used to evaluate elimination disorders.

32.6   Recognize abnormal findings in a routine urinalysis.

THINKING CRITICALLY: KNOWING WHAT TO DO AND WHY

Give the rationale for gathering data on the following during the health history.

Data	Rationale
1. Biographical and demographic data	
2. Chief complaint	
3. Childhood and infectious diseases	
4. Immunizations	
5. Geographic location/travel history	
6. Nutrition	
7. Habits	
8. Family history related to GI disorders	
9. Bowel elimination pattern	
10. Medications both prescribed and over the counter	

Briefly describe the process or technique used for assessing the following.

11. Abdomen (physical examination)   12. Bowel sounds

13. List four nursing interventions that incorporate the assessment of the anus and rectum.

   Most nurses perform only the inspection of the anus and rectum and do not perform a complete digital exam. However, there are nursing actions and situations where nurses can incorporate some of the exam with other nursing interventions.

THINKING CRITICALLY: KNOWING WHAT TO DO AND WHY

■ *Diagnostic Tests*

	Test Purpose	Informed Consent	Pretest Nursing Care	Post-Test Nursing Care
14.	Carcinoembryonic antigen			
15.	Guaiac			
16.	Stool for ova and parasites			
17.	Flat plate of the abdomen			
18.	Lower gastrointestinal series			
19.	Colonoscopy			

LEARNING THE LANGUAGE: TERMINOLOGY RELATED TO ASSESSMENT OF THE URINARY SYSTEM

Match the descriptions in Column A with the sign or symptom in Column B.

Column A		**Column B**
20. _____ Indicates kidney pain	A.	Casts in urine
21. _____ Ineffectual attempts to void with painful straining	B.	Costovertebral angle pain
	C.	Hesitancy
22. _____ Frequent, painful voiding, small amounts, with bladder spasm	D.	Urgency
	E.	Water diuresis
23. _____ Indicate tubular or glomerular disease	F.	Incontinence
24. _____ Impaired urinal absorption of a solute	G.	Solute diuresis
25. _____ Low specific gravity, low osmolarity, normal serum sodium	H.	Dysuria
	I.	Strangury
26. _____ Painful urination	J.	Tenesmus
27. _____ Difficulty controlling voiding		
28. _____ Trouble starting or maintaining stream		
29. _____ Loss of control over the release of urine from bladder		

Match the descriptions in Column A with the urine abnormality in Column B.

Column A		**Column B**
30. _____ Blood in the urine	A.	Anuria
31. _____ Painful voiding	B.	Benign proteinuria
32. _____ Voiding more than twice a night	C.	Crystalluria
33. _____ Urine output less than 100 mL per day	D.	Dysuria
34. _____ Significant increase in urine output	E.	Hematuria
35. _____ Total urine output less than 400 mL per day	F.	Oliguria
36. _____ Glucose in the urine	G.	Polyuria
37. _____ Protein in urine caused by stress, exercise, fever	H.	Nocturia
	I.	Glycosuria
38. _____ Usually indicates extrahepatic biliary tract obstruction	J.	Bilirubinuria
39. _____ Predisposing factor for kidney stones		

THINKING CRITICALLY

Match the possible etiologies in Column A with the urine color in Column B.

Column A		**Column B**
40. _____ Bleeding from the upper tract	A.	Blue-green
41. _____ Bleeding from the lower tract	B.	Smoky gray
42. _____ Urobilinogen or bilirubin	C.	Red-brown, tea colored
43. _____ *Pseudomonas*	D.	Dark yellow-green
44. _____ Myoglobin/muscle damage	E.	Red

Match the medications in Column A with the urine color change in Column B.

Column A	Column B
45. _____ Amitriptyline (Elavil)	A. Bright orange-red
46. _____ Rifampin	B. Red, red-brown, pink
47. _____ Phenothiazines (Thorazine)	C. Blue or green
48. _____ Multivitamins with riboflavin	D. Colorless or pale yellow
49. _____ Nitrofurantoin (Macrodantin)	E. Bright yellow
50. _____ Diuretics (Lasix)	F. Dark brown-black

Give the rationale for selected components of a focused urological health history.

■ *Functional Health Pattern-Focused Health History*

Health Perception– Health Management

51. Family history

52. Past history

53. Current medications

Nutrition–Metabolic

55. High calcium, high purine

Elimination

57. Urine elimination history

Activity–Exercise

Sleep–Rest

54. Interrupted sleep because of nocturia

Cognitive–Perceptual

56. Pain analysis

Self-Perception–Self Concept

58. Changes in body image

Role–Relationship

59. Occupation

Sexuality– Reproductive

Coping–Stress Tolerance

Values–Beliefs

KNOWLEDGE BUILDING: STUDY QUESTIONS RELATED TO ASSESSMENT OF THE URINARY SYSTEM

60. Explain why the specific gravity of a client's urine might be tested before surgery.

61. Differentiate between urine osmolality and urine specific gravity.

62. Explain the significance of protein in the urine.

63. Explain the significance of an elevation of the blood urea nitrogen (BUN) level.

Indicate whether the following findings are normal (N) or abnormal (A). Provide the correct findings for those that are abnormal.

64. _____ Specific gravity: 1.002–1.035

65. _____ pH: 3.5–7.7

66. _____ Osmolality: 150–250 mOsm/L

67. _____ Color: Amber

68. _____ WBCs: TNTC (Too numerous to count)

69. _____ RBCs: Present

THINKING CRITICALLY: KNOWING WHAT TO DO AND WHY

Test	Informed Consent	Pretest Nursing Care	Post-Test Nursing Care
Clean catch urine	70.	71. Instruct females and uncircumcised males to cleanse meatus. 72. Instruct client to catch about 50 mL of urine after they have started the stream.	
Renogram	73.	74. Explain the purpose of the test.	75. Resume normal activities.
Intravenous pyelography (IVP)	76.	77. Assess for allergies to shellfish. 79. Assess serum creatinine levels.	78. Force fluids. 80. Monitor intake and output.
Uroflowmetry	81.	82. Instruct the client of the purpose of the test.	
Cystoscopy	83.	84. Instruct the client that he/she must remain still during the test.	85. Instruct the client that pink-tinged urine is common.

Management of Clients with Intestinal Disorders

Disorders of the intestinal tract are relatively common. Colon cancer, when both sexes are considered together, is the second most common cancer in terms of morbidity and mortality. Gastroenteritis is an intestinal disorder that most people will experience at some time. Appendicitis is another common disorder. The implication for nurses who care for adults is that they will likely care for clients with some of these disorders. The nurse caring for clients with intestinal disorders will need to develop a variety of assessment, psychomotor, and analytical skills.

OBJECTIVES

33.1 Identify common assessment data for various disorders of the intestinal tract.

33.2 Describe inflammatory disorders of the small and large intestines, medical and surgical management, and nursing care.

33.3 Discuss neoplasms of the intestines, medical and surgical management, and nursing care.

33.4 Describe various ostomy procedures and their nursing management.

33.5 Discuss other disorders of the small and large intestines.

33.6 Describe the effects of blunt or penetrating trauma on the intestines, and medical and nursing management.

33.7 Describe the effects of intestinal obstruction, medical and surgical management, and nursing care.

LEARNING THE LANGUAGE: TERMINOLOGY RELATED TO INTESTINAL DISORDERS

Match the gastrointestinal disorders in Column A with the correct description in Column B.

Column A

1. _____ Amebiasis
2. _____ *Clostridium difficile*
3. _____ Dysentery
4. _____ Gastroenteritis
5. _____ Schistosomiasis
6. _____ Staphylococcus

Column B

A. A blood fluke that eventually settles in the veins of the large bowel or bladder

B. Inflammation of stomach and intestinal tract that primarily affects the small bowel

C. Gastrointestinal infection which develops in 2–4 hours

D. Bacterial dysentery seen in persons receiving large doses of antibiotics

E. Inflammatory condition affecting the colon characterized by severe bloody diarrhea and abdominal cramping

F. Diarrhea results when a protozoan invades the lining of the colon

Match the surgeries in Column A with the correct description in Column B.

Column A

7. _____ Colostomy
8. _____ Ileorectal anastomosis
9. _____ Ileo pouch–anal anastomosis
10. _____ Kock pouch
11. _____ Total proctocolectomy

Column B

A. The colon and rectum are removed, the anus is closed, and a permanent ileostomy is formed

B. A reservoir or pouch is constructed from a loop of ileum; also called continent ileostomy

C. Colon is resected leaving an anal stump and the terminal ileum is anastomosed to this stump

D. Colon is removed and an ileoanal reservoir is created in the anal canal; an ostomy is not needed

E. Colon is resected and an opening between the colon and abdominal wall is created; may be temporary or permanent

Match the diagnoses in Column A with the correct definition in Column B.

Column A	**Column B**
12. _____ Abdominal angina	A. Occurs at the base of the sacrum, usually contains hair, can become infected forming an abscess and then a sinus tract
13. _____ Anal fissure	
14. _____ Anal fistula	
15. _____ Anorectal abscess	B. Abscess that begins as cryptitis with the formation of cysts that extend through the tubular ducts into the submucosal spaces
16. _____ Hirschsprung's disease	
17. _____ Intussusception	
18. _____ Meckel's diverticulum	C. Hypertrophy of the colon due to absence of ganglion nerves in the distal large intestine; congenital megacolon
19. _____ Mesenteric infarction	
20. _____ Pilonidal cyst	
21. _____ Volvulus	D. Ulceration or tear in the lining of the anal canal
	E. Any occlusion in the arterial blood supply to the bowel
	F. Sinus tract that develops from the anal canal to the skin outside the anus or from an abscess to either the anal canal or the perianal area
	G. Partial occlusion of the mesenteric arteries, usually from atherosclerosis
	H. Twisting of the bowel that can cause infarction or obstruction
	I. Telescoping of the bowel into the adjacent bowel
	J. A vestige of embryonic development that results in an outpouching of the bowel

Differentiate between regional enteritis (Crohn's disease) (A) and ulcerative colitis (B) by placing the appropriate letter beside each of the following characteristics. (Use C to indicate if the characteristic applies to both.)

22. _____ Malignancy may result	A, Crohn's disease
23. _____ Remissions and exacerbations	B. Ulcerative colitis
24. _____ Involves all layers of the submucosa	C. Both
25. _____ Segmental lesions	
26. _____ Slowly progressive	
27. _____ Rectal bleeding common	
28. _____ Nutritional deficits	
29. _____ Arthritis can accompany	
30. _____ "Colicky" abdominal pain	
31. _____ Anal abscess common	

THINKING CRITICALLY: UNDERSTANDING RATIONALES

Provide the rationales for the therapeutic nursing interventions listed below.

Intervention	Rationale

Client with Clostridium difficile

32.   Do not give antidiarrheal medications.

Client with Appendicitis

33.   Do not give enema or laxatives.

34.   Report increase in temperature, and change in
       pulse or blood pressure.

Client with Crohn's Disease or Ulcerative Colitis

35.   Assess the stoma's color postproctocolectomy.

36.   Use meticulous skin care after ileostomy.

37.   Cut pouch 1/16" larger than stoma.

Client with Colon Cancer

38.   Teach clients about early detection guidelines for
       colon cancer.

39.   Assess client after abdomino-perineal resection for
       phlebitis.

Client with Obstruction

40.   Assess client for hypotension, hypovolemia, and
       shock.

41.   Assess for increased or absent bowel sounds.

42.   Assess for hypoxia.

■ *Medications*

Listed below are specific medications used with certain disorders. Provide rationales for their use.

Implication for Use	Rationale

Loperamide (Imodium)

43.　With Crohn's disease

Adrenal Steroids

44.　With inflammatory bowel syndrome

Mercaptopurine (6-MP)

45.　Use with Crohn's disease

Sulfasalazine (Azulfidine)

46.　Use with inflammatory bowel syndrome

Neomycin

47.　Use preop with colon surgery

CLIENT EDUCATION: KNOWING WHAT TO TEACH AND WHY

List rationales for the following teaching points.

48.　Ileostomy care
　　Teaching: Change pouch when bowel is least
　　active.
　　Rationale:

49.　Diet with an ileostomy
　　Teaching: Avoid or limit, at least initially, popcorn,
　　peanuts, tough fibrous meats, vegetables with skin,
　　rice, bran, and coconuts.
　　Rationale:

50.　Nutrition with an ileostomy
　　Teaching: Chew food well.
　　Rationale:

51.　Ileorectal anastomosis
　　Teaching: Defecate 4–5 times a day.
　　Rationale:

52.　Colostomy management
　　Teaching: Empty pouch when half full.
　　Rationale:

53.　Colostomy management
　　Teaching: Use karaya gum or powder on skin.
　　Rationale:

54.　Colostomy management
　　Teaching: Report diarrhea to physician.
　　Rationale:

55. Diet education with colostomy
     Teaching: Avoid gas-producing foods.
     Rationale:

56. Diet education with diverticulosis
     Teaching: Follow a high-fiber diet.
     Rationale:

57. Hemorrhoids
     Teaching: Follow a high-fiber diet.
     Rationale:

58. Hemorrhoids
     Teaching: Do not sit on the toilet any longer than
     necessary.
     Rationale:

PUTTING IT ALL TOGETHER

■ Case Study

Ms. C., 55, presents at the clinic with symptoms of intermittent rectal bleeding and constipation. She is unclear
about how long she has had rectal bleeding. Her hemoglobin is 6.5 g/dl and hematocrit is 26%. Ms. C. is admitted to
the hospital for a diagnostic work-up.

59. Known risk factors for colon cancer include which
     of the following?
     A.   Crohn's disease, high-fat, low-residue diet
     B.   adenomatous polyps, living in rural areas
     C.   familial polyposis, high-fat, low-residue diet
     D.   under age 40, ulcerative colitis, high-fat diet

60. Ms. C. is diagnosed as having colon cancer. In
     terms of frequency, the most common site of colon
     cancer is in which of the following?
     A.   rectal area
     B.   sigmoid area
     C.   ascending colon
     D.   descending colon

61. The American Cancer Society's guidelines for
     early detection of colon cancer include which of
     the following?
     A.   annual digital rectal examinations beginning
          at age 50
     B.   annual sigmoidoscopy examinations begin-
          ning at age 50
     C.   annual stool guaiac tests beginning at age 40
     D.   sigmoidoscopy beginning at age 50, then
          after two negative tests, every 3 to 5 years

62. A colostomy has to be performed on Ms. C.
     because of the location of the tumor. In the
     postoperative period, the nurse assesses Ms. C.'s
     stoma. Which of the following would the nurse
     report to the physician?
     A.   stoma red and moist
     B.   stoma dusky or bluish
     C.   stoma swollen and red
     D.   stoma slightly bloody

63. In teaching Ms. C. how to care for her colostomy,
     which of the following statements by Ms. C. would
     indicate the need for more teaching?
     A.   Clean the skin around the stoma with mild
          soap.
     B.   Irrigate the colostomy with 500 cc warm
          water.
     C.   Change the pouch every 4–5 days as needed.
     D.   Empty the pouch when full.

Management of Clients with Urinary Disorders

The principal function of the ureters, bladder, and urethra is to transport urine from the kidneys. Anything that obstructs the flow or interferes with the neuromuscular ability to move and expel urine reduces the ability of these organs to fulfill their role. Urinary system disorders can be extremely problematic for clients, and the nurse can play a major role in the prevention and treatment of these disorders.

OBJECTIVES

34.1   Describe the etiology and pathophysiology of selected disorders of the ureters, bladder, and urethra, including infections, bladder cancer, urinary tract stones, urinary incontinence, and trauma.

34.2   Summarize the clinical manifestations and medical-surgical management of selected disorders of the ureters, bladder, and urethra.

34.3   Assess clients for clinical manifestations of selected disorders of the ureters, bladder, and urethra.

34.4   Plan individualized nursing interventions for clients with both acute and chronic disorders of the ureters, bladder, and urethra.

34.5   Perform nursing interventions appropriate for clients with urinary tract disorders.

34.6   Evaluate effectiveness of nursing care of clients with urinary tract disorders.

LEARNING THE LANGUAGE: TERMINOLOGY RELATED TO URINARY DISORDERS

Match the terms related to infectious processes in Column A with the correct definition in Column B.

Column A	Column B
1. _____ Urosepsis	A. Inflammation of the bladder wall
2. _____ Urinary tract infections (UTIs)	B. An infection within the urinary tract
3. _____ Pyuria	C. Pus in the urine
4. _____ Urethritis	D. Inflammation of the urethra
5. _____ Dysuria	E. Pain upon voiding
6. _____ Cystitis	F. A gram-negative bacteremia originating in the genitourinary tract

Match the terms related to bladder cancer in Column A with the correct description in Column B.

Column A	Column B
7. _____ Hemorrhagic cystitis	A. Blood in urine
8. _____ Intravesical instillation	B. Topical chemotherapy
9. _____ Hematuria	C. Major side effect of chemotherapy
10. _____ Ileal conduit	D. Urinary diversion using a segment of the ileum to attach the ureters and create a stoma
11. _____ Vesicovaginal fistula/colovesical fistula	E. Common complication of radiation
12. _____ Continent ileal reservoir	F. Removal of bladder
13. _____ Cystectomy	G. A pouch created from distal ileum or ascending colon to collect urine
14. _____ Ureterostomy	H. Insertion of a catheter into the renal pelvis
15. _____ Percutaneous nephrostomy	I. Ureters are attached to the surface of the abdomen

Match the terms related to urinary stones in Column A with the correct description in Column B.

Column A	Column B
16. _____ Urolithiasis	A. Calcification or stone
17. _____ Calculi	B. Stones within the urinary system
18. _____ Uric acid stones	C. Cannot be seen on x-ray
19. _____ KUB	D. X-ray of kidney, ureter, and bladder
20. _____ Intravenous pyelography (IVP)	E. Injection of contrast medium to locate stones
21. _____ Cystoscopy	F. Direct visualization of the urinary tract
22. _____ Lithotripsy	G. A procedure in which sound waves are applied externally to break up stones
23. _____ Ureterolithotomy	H. Surgical removal of stones in the ureters

Match the terms related to urinary retention in Column A with the correct definition in Column B.

Column A	Column B
24. _____ Suprapubic	A. Benign prostatic hypertrophy
25. _____ Urethroplasty	B. Urination or voiding
26. _____ Micturition	C. Dilation of urethra either by inserting progressively larger indwelling catheters or a dilating instrument
27. _____ Urinary tract dilation	D. Repair of the urethra
28. _____ BPH	E. Above the symphysis pubis

Match the terms related to urinary incontinence in Column A with the correct definition in Column B.

Column A	Column B
29. _____ Enuresis	A. Dysfunction of the muscle that moves urine from the bladder
30. _____ Paradoxical or overflow incontinence	B. Bed-wetting
31. _____ Detrusor instability	C. Retention with overflow of small amounts of urine
32. _____ Urge incontinence	D. Dysfunction of the bladder caused by a lesion of the central or peripheral nervous system
33. _____ Stress incontinence	E. Inability to hold back the flow of urine when feeling the need to void
34. _____ Reflex incontinence	F. Increased intra-abdominal pressure caused by activities such as coughing and sneezing
35. _____ Urodynamic evaluation	G. Loss of voluntary control of bladder
36. _____ Kegel exercises	H. A series of procedures to evaluate the motor and sensory functions of the bladder and efficiency of micturition
37. _____ Neurogenic bladder	I. Strengthens pelvic muscles to improve retention of urine

THINKING CRITICALLY: UNDERSTANDING RATIONALES

Provide the rationales for the therapeutic nursing interventions listed below.

Intervention	Rationale

Client with Cystitis
38. Teach female client to void immediately after intercourse.

39. Teach female client to cleanse genital area from front to back.

40. Drink at least 3000 mL of fluids per day.

Client with a Urinary Diversion
41. Measure urine every hour for the first 24 hours after surgery.

42. Note the stoma's size and color.

Intervention	**Rationale**
43. Teach client to maintain daily fluid intake of 3000 mL.	
44. Use nonkaraya barrier.	

Client with Urinary Bladder Calculi

45. Encourage fluids up to 4000 mL per day.	
46. Strain all urine.	
47. Teach dietary modifications: calcium and uric acid stones.	
48. Encourage ambulation.	
49. Teach the postcystolithotomy client the care of a suprapubic catheter.	

THINKING CRITICALLY: KNOWING WHAT TO DO AND WHY

Listed below are specific medications and nursing implications associated with the medications. Provide the rationales for the nursing implications. Use a drug handbook as a reference.

Implication	**Rationale**
Anti-infective: trimethoprim, sulfamethoxazole (Bactrim, Septra)	
50. Assess for rash.	
51. Stop prophylactic urine acidification.	
Antispasmodic: oxybutynin chloride (Di-tropan)	
52. Do not administer to client with narrow-angle glaucoma.	
53. Do not administer to client with myasthenia gravis.	
Analgesic/anti-infective: phenazopyridine hydrochloride; sulfisoxazole (Azo-Gantrisin)	
54. Teach client that urine may be dark-brown to red.	
55. Give with full glass of water.	
Sulfonamides: Co-trimoxazole, sulfamethoxazole; trimethoprim (Bactrim, Septra)	
56. Administer with large amount of fluids.	
57. Teach ways to maintain alkaline urine.	

THINKING CRITICALLY

Your client is 12 hours post-op from a total cystectomy with an ileal conduit. On your initial assessment you find that the client's temperature is 100.8° F, pulse 110, and B/P 140/80. The client complains of increasing abdominal pain not relieved by analgesics. Using this information, provide short answers to the following questions.

58.   What additional assessments would you make?

60.   If the stoma was dark and dusky versus red and moist, what would you do?

59.   If your assessment includes absent bowel sounds in all four quadrants of the abdomen with a rigid abdomen, what nursing action would you take?

■ Caring for Clients with Urinary Retention or Incontinence

61.   Which drug classifications contribute to urinary retention?

63.   Discuss how the nurse could distinguish among urinary retention, oliguria, and anuria.

62.   Summarize the potential effects of urinary tract obstruction.

PUTTING IT ALL TOGETHER

■ Case Study

Ms. F., a 24-year-old newly married white female, comes to the clinic with complaints of burning on urination, frequency, urgency, inability to void, and incomplete emptying of the bladder. An assessment reveals cloudy urine, abdominal and flank pain, malaise, and nausea. Ms. F. indicates that she drinks at least 24 ounces of soda per day and approximately four cups of coffee. A urine culture determines that the client has *Escherichia coli* in the urine. Based on her clinical manifestations and urine culture findings, a diagnosis of cystitis is made. The physician prescribes

cinoxacin (Cinobac), 1 gram daily for 14 days and starts the client on an acid-ash diet.

64.   The probable cause for Ms. F.'s cystitis is

A.   use of perfumed toilet paper.

B.   frequent tub baths.

C.   excessive coffee intake.

D.   sexual intercourse.

65. The nurse instructs Ms. F. to
    A. void immediately after intercourse.
    B. use a spermicide to decrease the risk of infection.
    C. increase her coffee intake.
    D. clean her perineal area from back to front.

66. The client is instructed that her medication
    A. may cause hypotension.
    B. should be taken with meals.
    C. should be taken one hour before meals.
    D. may cause peripheral neuropathies.

67. Which of the following food combinations are allowed on an acid-ash diet?
    A. milk, hard cheese, potatoes
    B. cabbage, spinach, bananas
    C. fish, cereals, plums
    D. cottage cheese, cauliflower, apricots

CHAPTER 35

Management of Clients with Renal Disorders

By producing urine, the kidneys regulate the body's fluid, electrolyte, and acid-base balance. The kidneys also play an important role in erythropoietin and prostaglandin synthesis. Therefore, any renal disorder can be potentially dangerous and cause systemic effects. To assess the client accurately, the nurse must know the usual clinical manifestations of renal disorders. Nursing care will be directed by the findings during the assessment.

OBJECTIVES

35.1 Describe the etiology, risk factors, and pathophysiology of selected renal disorders.

35.2 Summarize the clinical manifestations, complications, and medical-surgical management of renal disorders.

35.3 Plan individualized nursing interventions for clients with renal disorders.

35.4 Evaluate the effectiveness of nursing care of clients with renal disorders.

LEARNING THE LANGUAGE: TERMINOLOGY RELATED TO RENAL DISORDERS

Match the descriptions in Column A with the correct renal disorder in Column B.

Column A

1. _____ Immunologic, inflammatory, and proliferative glomerular changes
2. _____ Serous-, blood-, or urine-filled grapelike cysts replace kidney tissue
3. _____ Inflammation of the kidney caused by bacteria
4. _____ Stones formed in the kidneys
5. _____ Progressive reduction of kidney function
6. _____ Abrupt loss of kidney function
7. _____ Protein wasting secondary to diffuse glomerular damage caused by numerous etiologies

Column B

A. Nephrotic syndrome
B. Acute renal failure
C. Chronic renal failure
D. Pyelonephritis
E. Glomerulonephritis
F. Renal calculi
G. Polycystic kidney

THINKING CRITICALLY: KNOWING WHAT TO DO AND WHY

Provide the rationales for the following nursing interventions.

Intervention	**Rationale**

Client with Acute Glomerulonephritis

8.   Instruct client on low-protein, high-calorie diet.

9.   Monitor daily weights.

10.   Provide client with hard candy or lemon slices.

Client with Nephrotic Syndrome

11.   Provide meticulous skin care.

12.   Measure girth daily.

13.   Instruct client on high-protein diet

Client After a Nephrolithotomy

14.   Use sterile technique for dressing changes.

15.   Instruct client to increase fluid intake to 3000–4000 mL daily.

16.   Instruct client to maintain fluid intake throughout the 24-hour period.

17.   Using the illustration below, explain the staging system for renal carcinoma.

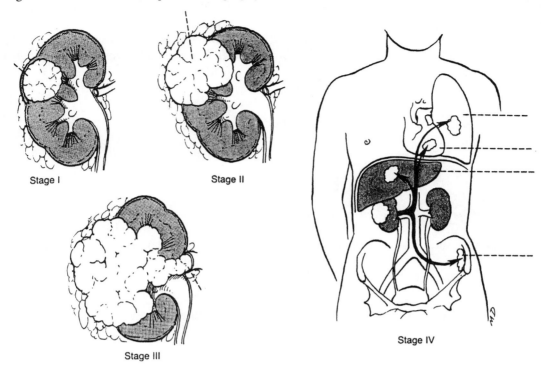

Stage I

Stage II

Stage III

Stage IV

Putting It All Together

■ Clients with Renal Disorders

Provide short answers to each of the following questions related to situations involving clients with various renal disorders.

18.   Ms. J. is receiving intravenous gentamycin and a cephalosporin. Her renal function tests are within normal limits. What nursing interventions will decrease the risk of nephrotoxicity?

20.   Mr. C.'s intravenous pyelogram confirms the suspected diagnosis of renal calculi with renal colic. He is told to drink a lot of liquids. How much fluid should he drink?

19.   After two episodes of acute pyelonephritis within a year, Ms. S. is in the health care facility with signs and symptoms of another infection. She says she doesn't understand why she can't stay well since she took all her medicines. What questions would be important to include when taking her history?

21.   When Mr. C. is instructed to strain his urine, he says he doesn't "understand why I need to go to all that trouble to save a stone I don't want." What response from the nurse would be most helpful to Mr. C.?

22. Ms. S. has a nephrostomy tube. What should the nurse do when the tube quits draining the second postoperative day?

23. Mr. D. has been managing his ileal conduit without difficulty. During this hospitalization for a work-up to rule out a recurrence of cancer, he doesn't want to care for his conduit and has developed a skin irritation around the stoma. What nursing interventions would be appropriate?

Select the best answer for the following questions.

24. Which organism usually causes acute glomerulonephritis?
  A. gram-positive bacilli
  B. beta-hemolytic streptococci
  C. alpha-hemolytic streptococci
  D. gram-negative diplococci

25 Which of the following diets is ordered for the client with acute glomerulonephritis?
  A. high sodium
  B. low calorie, high protein
  C. high calorie, low protein
  D. high fat

26. If a client has an oxalate renal stone, which of the following should be avoided?
  A. water
  B. cola drinks
  C. cheese
  D. milk

36

Management of Clients with Renal Failure

By producing urine, the kidneys regulate the body's fluid, electrolyte, and acid-base balance. The kidneys also play an important role in erythropoietin and prostaglandin synthesis. Therefore, any renal disorder can be potentially dangerous and cause systemic effects. The management of clients with renal failure requires nurses to have a solid understanding of renal function. There are two types of renal failure: acute renal failure (ARF) and chronic renal failure (CRF). Nurses are an important part of the multidisciplinary team caring for clients with renal failure.

OBJECTIVES

36.1   Compare and contrast acute and chronic renal failure.

36. 2   Discuss the outcomes management of renal failure

36.3   Plan individualized nursing interventions for clients with acute and chronic renal failure.

36.4   Compare and contrast peritoneal dialysis and hemodialysis.

36.5   Evaluate the effectiveness of nursing care of clients with renal failure.

LEARNING THE LANGUAGE: TERMINOLOGY RELATED TO CLIENTS WITH RENAL FAILURE

Match the pathophysiologies in Column A with the clinical manifestation of chronic renal failure (CRF) in Column B.

Column A	Column B
1. _____ Impaired insulin production and metabolism	A. Hypernatremia
2. _____ Kidney's inability to excrete hydrogen ions	B. Hyponatremia
3. _____ Rises inversely with calcium	C. Hypocalcemia
4. _____ Kidneys unable to excrete protein waste products	D. Hyperphosphatemia
5. _____ Salt and water retention	E. Carbohydrate intolerance
6. _____ Decreased conversion of 25-hydroxycholecalciferol	F. Elevated serum creatinine
7. _____ Response to high glucose and insulin levels	G. Hyperlipidemia
8. _____ Salt-wasting effect, vomiting, and diarrhea	H. Hypercalcemia
9. _____ Occurs late in the disease from a variety of sources: catabolism, medications, blood transfusion	I. Metabolic acidosis

Match the pathophysiologies in Column A with the clinical manifestation of chronic renal failure (CRF) in Column B.

Column A	Column B
10. _____ Uremic toxins excreted via the skin	A. Pericarditis
11. _____ Phosphate-binding agents and reduced fluid intake	B. Anemia
	C. Constipation
12. _____ Increased secretion of gastric acid	D. Peptic ulcer disease
13. _____ Accumulation of uremic toxins	E. Immunosuppression
14. _____ Reduced erythropoiesis	F. Medication toxicity
15. _____ Physiologic and psychological factors	G. Hypertension
16. _____ Decreased absorption, distribution, metabolism, and excretion of medications	H. Bone demineralization
	I. Decreased libido
17. _____ Fluid and sodium retention, atherosclerosis	J. Neurologic changes
18. _____ Delayed antibody formation, decreased function of leukocytes	K. Severe, intractable pruritus
19. _____ Accumulation of toxins in the body	
20. _____ Kidney–bone–parathyroid and calcium/phosphate/vitamin D interactions	

THINKING CRITICALLY: KNOWING WHAT TO DO AND WHY

Provide the rationales for the following nursing interventions.

Intervention	Rationale

Client with Acute Renal Failure

21. Maintain strict intake and output measurements.

22. Provide range of motion exercises.

23. Use proper medical asepsis.

24. Monitor heart and lung sounds and mental status.

THINKING CRITICALLY

25. What are the goals of dialysis therapy?

26. Identify two complications associated with peritoneal dialysis.

27. Compare the external arteriovenous shunt and the internal arteriovenous fistula used in hemodialysis.

28. Explain why the client on hemodialysis may require water-soluble vitamins.

29. Explain why polystyrene sulfonate (Kayexalate) may be administered to the client with chronic renal failure.

30. Ms. S. asks why her daughter is so anemic. The daughter is in chronic renal failure and is managed on hemodialysis. What would be an appropriate response?

31. Ms. S. also wants to know how to help her daughter with the "itching and rash." What should Ms. S. be told?

32. Describe the symptoms of graft rejection experienced by clients with kidney transplants.

33. Using the illustration below, explain the prerenal, renal, and postrenal causes of acute renal failure.

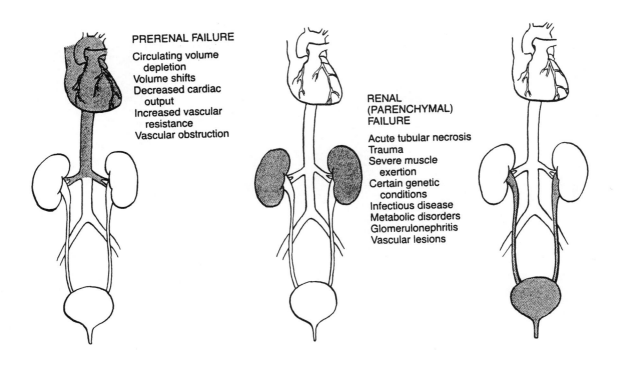

PRERENAL FAILURE
Circulating volume depletion
Volume shifts
Decreased cardiac output
Increased vascular resistance
Vascular obstruction

RENAL (PARENCHYMAL) FAILURE
Acute tubular necrosis
Trauma
Severe muscle exertion
Certain genetic conditions
Infectious disease
Metabolic disorders
Glomerulonephritis
Vascular lesions

Putting It All Together

34. Which of the following is the primary cause of end stage renal disease?
    A. chronic glomerulonephritis
    B. congestive heart failure
    C. diabetes mellitus
    D. acute pyelonephritis

35. Which of the following is considered a prerenal cause of acute renal failure?
    A. obstruction of the urinary tract
    B. increased vascular resistance
    C. trauma to the kidneys
    D. glomerulonephritis

36. Which of the following is a common cause of chronic renal failure?
    A. diabetes
    B. congestive heart failure
    C. hypotension
    D. repeated bouts of cystitis

37. Which of the following drugs is administered to reduce the client's phosphorus level?
    A. calcium gluconate
    B. sorbitol
    C. calcium lactate
    D. aluminum hydroxide

Sexuality and Reproductive Disorders

ANATOMY AND PHYSIOLOGY REVIEW: THE REPRODUCTIVE SYSTEMS

A basic understanding of the structure and function of the male and female reproductive systems will facilitate your learning of the content in Chapters 37 through 41. Defining the following terms and answering the questions should serve as a guide as to how much time you need to spend reviewing these systems before proceeding to the next chapter.

OBJECTIVES

8.1   Identify key structures of the male and female reproductive systems.

8.2   Discuss key functions of the male and female reproductive systems.

LEARNING THE LANGUAGE: TERMINOLOGY RELATED TO THE STRUCTURE AND FUNCTION OF THE REPRODUCTIVE SYSTEM

Match the hormones in Column A with the function in Column B.

Column A

1. _____ Corticotropin
2. _____ Estrogen
3. _____ Follicle-stimulating hormone (FSH)
4. _____ Gonadotropin-releasing hormone (Gn-RH)
5. _____ Luteinizing hormone (LH)
6. _____ Progesterone
7. _____ Prolactin
8. _____ Testosterone

Column B

A. Stimulates the pituitary to produce LH and FSH

B. Primary androgen responsible for the growth and division of the germinal cells that form sperm

C. In males, stimulates Leydig's cells to secrete testosterone; in females, stimulates estrogen production

D. Female sex hormones that produce cyclic changes in the uterine and vaginal endothelium

E. Helps prepare the endometrium for the fertilized ovum and promotes the development of the placenta

F. In males, stimulates Sertoli's cells and germinal cells to start and complete spermatogenesis; in females, stimulates the production of follicular cells

G. Helps prolactin maintain lactation

H. Initiates lactation

9. Identify the structures of the female pelvis.

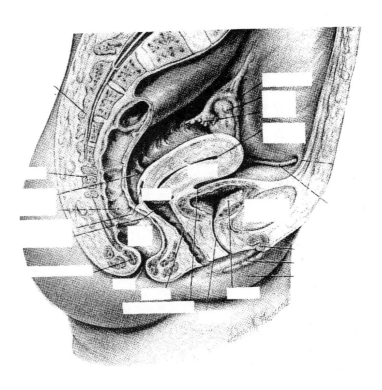

10. Identify the structures of the male pelvis and genitalia.

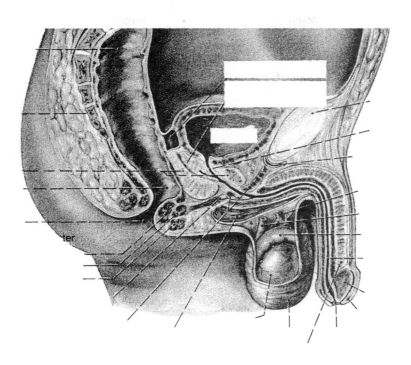

11. Label lymph nodes near the female breast.

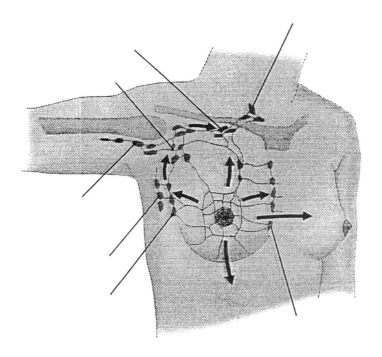

KNOWLEDGE BUILDING: FEMALE AND MALE REPRODUCTIVE STRUCTURE AND FUNCTION

12. In the female breast, the upper outer quadrant and tail of Spence is the location of most breast cancers. Why?

13. What is the function of Cooper's ligaments in the breast?

14. What is estrogen's effect on the breast?

15. What happens to breast tissue after menopause?

16. In the normal menstrual cycle, describe the roles of FSH, LH, estrogen, and progesterone.

17. What nonsexually related physiologic functions does estrogen influence?

18. What is the purpose of the prostate?

19. What is the primary purpose of the testes?

20. What are testosterone's three major functions?

Assessment of the Reproductive System

The process of assessing clients with gynecologic, reproductive, or urinary disorders needs to be completed with a great amount of sensitivity toward the client. Sometimes in the health care field, because we may work with clients every day who have a gynecologic, reproductive, or urinary problem, we forget that for the client this is not an everyday event and that these are very personal matters. The personal nature of the examination of the reproductive system necessitates an approach to the client that is supportive, sensitive, and maintains privacy and respect.

OBJECTIVES

37.1 Identify key elements of a comprehensive gynecologic assessment.

37.2 Describe diagnostic tests used for women with gynecologic disorders.

37.3 Examine key elements of a health assessment for men with reproductive disorders.

37.4 Describe diagnostic tests used for men with disorders of the reproductive system.

37.5 Discuss primary and secondary prevention related to reproductive disorders.

LEARNING THE LANGUAGE: TERMINOLOGY RELATED TO ASSESSMENT OF CLIENTS WITH REPRODUCTIVE DISORDERS

Match the terms in Column A with the correct definition/description in Column B.

Column A	Column B
1. _____ Bimanual examination	A. An enlargement of the breasts
2. _____ Cystocele	B. An examination in which one or two fingers are placed in the vagina and the other hand is placed on the abdomen to palpate the pelvic contents
3. _____ Epispadias	
4. _____ Gynecomastia	
5. _____ Hypospadias	C. Shine a flashlight through the scrotum
6. _____ Inframammary ridge	D. Opening to the penis is on the underside of the penile shaft
7. _____ Rectocele	E. Bulging of the rectum into the vagina
8. _____ Tail of Spence	F. Upper outer quadrant of the breast
9. _____ Transillumination of the scrotum	G. Opening to the penis is on the upper side of the penile shaft
	H. Curved ridge along the inferior breast
	I. Prolapse of the urinary bladder

Match the gynecologic tests and procedures in Column A with the correct definition in Column B.

Column A

10. _____ Cervical conization
11. _____ Colposcopy
12. _____ Endometrial smear
13. _____ Hysteroscopy
14. _____ Laparoscopy
15. _____ Mammography
16. _____ Papanicolaou (Pap) smear
17. _____ Pneumocystogram
18. _____ Schiller's test
19. _____ Wet smear

Column B

A. Swabbing the uterine lining to obtain cells and secretions for examination
B. Surgical removal of diseased part of cervix by cutting out a cone-shaped section of tissue
C. Visualization of the intrauterine cavity
D. Iodine is applied to the vagina and cervix to differentiate normal and abnormal tissue
E. Air is injected into a cyst and then a mammogram is taken
F. Used to detect *Candida albicans*
G. A telescope is inserted through a small incision on the abdomen to visualize abdominal and pelvic organs
H. Use of a magnifying instrument to examine the cervical epithelium, vagina, and vulva
I. Secretions are taken from the vaginal pool and the cervix for cytologic smear
J. Soft tissue radiographic examination

Match the diagnostic tests for male reproductive disorders in Column A with the correct definition/description in Column B.

Column A

20. _____ Alkaline phosphatase
21. _____ Prostate-specific antigen (PAS)
22. _____ Semen analysis
23. _____ Serum acid phosphatase
24. _____ Urodynamic assessment

Column B

A. Antigen found in the serum of men with prostate cancer
B. Enzyme found in the serum of men with advanced prostate cancer
C. Enzyme found in the serum of men whose prostate cancer has metastasized to the bone
D. Studies which measure pressure from bladder or urethra, urinary flow, and muscle activity
E. Analysis of sperm for fertility, the effectiveness of a vasectomy, to test DNA, or to establish paternity

THINKING CRITICALLY: UNDERSTANDING RATIONALES

Provide the rationales for the therapeutic nursing interventions listed.

Intervention   **Rationale**

Client Having a Gynecologic Examination

25. Assess for history of rubella.

26. Assess for history of alcohol and drug use.

27. Question about allergy to latex or rubber.

28. Delay examination of the breasts until after the assessment of lungs and heart.

29. Have the client press her hands firmly on her hips during the visual examination of the breasts.

30. Instruct clients not to douche, have intercourse, or take a tub bath immediately before a pelvic examination, or use vaginal products for 2–3 days before a pelvic examination.

Male Client Having an Assessment of the Reproductive and Urinary Tract

31. Assess for history of mumps.

32. Assess for taking antihypertensives.

33. Take client's sexual history.

CLIENT EDUCATION: KNOWING WHAT TO TEACH AND WHY

List rationale for the following teaching point.

34. Breast self-examination (BSE)
    Teaching: Teach premenopausal women to do a BSE 7–10 days after the onset of menses.
    Rationale:

THINKING CRITICALLY: KNOWING WHAT TO DO AND WHY

■ *Diagnostic Tests*

Test	Informed Consent	Pretest Nursing Care	Post-Test Nursing Care
35. Papanicolaou smear			
36. Ultrasound			
37. Endometrial biopsy			
38. Cervical biopsy			
39. Laparoscopy			
40. Mammography			
41. Prostatic biopsy			
42. Cystoscopy			

43. Describe normal and abnormal assessment findings of the prostate.

45. How often should a woman have a Pap smear, mammogram, and perform BSEs according to the American Cancer Society's recommendations?

44. What are the five sets of lymph nodes examined during the physical examination of the breast?

CHAPTER 38

Management of Men with Reproductive Disorders

The most common disorder of the reproductive/urinary tract in males is benign prostatic hypertrophy (BPH). By age 50 it is estimated that 50% of men have some degree of BPH. This figure increases to nearly 75% by age 80. Needless to say, nurses in many settings will come in contact with men with this disorder. Because this disorder involves an organ that has sexual, reproductive, and urinary functions, the nurse needs to be extra sensitive in his or her assessments and interventions with this client. Also, knowledge of the special needs of the older adult will be important to integrate into caring for many of these clients. Another additional set of needs and circumstances are involved when the client has cancer of the prostate.

While not the only other disorder of the reproductive and urinary system, care of the client with testicular cancer deserves special mention. This disorder most commonly occurs in men ages 15–35. Fortunately, the survival statistics for the disorder are improving; however, there are early detection guidelines that nurses need to know and teach to help further improve those figures.

OBJECTIVES

38.1 Identify assessment areas pertinent to males with reproductive disturbances.

38.2 Discuss disorders of infertility and impotence and their medical, surgical, and nursing management.

38.3 Discuss disorders of the prostate and their medical, surgical, and nursing management.

38.4 Discuss medical, surgical, and nursing management for the client with testicular disorders.

38.5 Define penile, scrotal, reproductive duct, and seminal vesical disorders.

LEARNING THE LANGUAGE: TERMINOLOGY RELATED TO CARE OF MEN WITH REPRODUCTIVE DISORDERS

Match the terms related to the male reproductive system in Column A with the correct definition in Column B.

Column A	Column B
1. _____ Azoospermia	A. Less than the normal number of sperm
2. _____ Balanitis	B. Penile foreskin (prepuce) is constricted at the opening
3. _____ Circumcision	C. Urethral meatus opens on top of the penis
4. _____ Epispadias	D. Surgical removal of the penile foreskin
5. _____ Eunuchoidism	E. Dilation and varicosity of the pampiniform plexus
6. _____ Hematocele	F. Absence of sperm
7. _____ Hydrocele	G. Rare, acute testicular inflammation
8. _____ Hypospadias	H. Twisted spermatic cord
9. _____ Oligozoospermia	I. Congenital condition in which puberty does not occur
10. _____ Orchitis	J. Collection of blood in the tunica vaginalis testis
11. _____ Paraphimosis	K. Prolonged, persistent erection
12. _____ Phimosis	L. Inflammation of the glans penis and mucous membranes beneath it
13. _____ Prostatitis	M. Collection of clear yellow fluid along the spermatic cord
14. _____ Priapism	N. Urethral meatus opens on the ventral side of the penis
15. _____ Testicular torsion	O. Tight foreskin that once retracted cannot be returned to its normal position
16. _____ Varicocele	P. Inflammation of the prostate

THINKING CRITICALLY: UNDERSTANDING RATIONALES

Provide the rationales for the therapeutic nursing interventions listed below.

Intervention	Rationale
Client with Benign Prostatic Hypertrophy	
17. Never force a urinary catheter.	
18. Measure and maintain urinary catheter output after prostatic surgery.	
19. Assess for use of antidepressants, decongestants, and anticholinergics.	
20. Assess for bladder spasms after transurethral prostatic resection (TURP).	

Client with a Potential Reproductive Disorder

21.   Assess for exposure to environmental and occupational chemicals.

22.   Assess for specific medication use.

23.   Ask about previous sexually transmitted diseases (STDs).

CLIENT EDUCATION: KNOWING WHAT TO TEACH AND WHY

List rationales for the following teaching recommendations.

Teaching Recommendation	**Rationale**
24. Avoid prolonged sitting after prostatic surgery.	
25. Avoid constipation and straining after prostatic surgery.	
26. Teach perineal exercises after prostatic surgery.	
27. Recommend annual rectal examinations for men over age 40.	

THINKING CRITICALLY: KNOWING WHAT TO DO AND WHY

28.   Describe the rationale for using estrogens with prostate cancer.

PUTTING IT ALL TOGETHER

■ *Case Study*

Mr. F. is a 65-year-old black male who comes to the clinic with a chief complaint of difficulty urinating. He reports getting up at least four times during the night to void and voiding small amounts with little force. With history, physical data, and the results of a diagnostic work-up, Mr. F. is diagnosed with BPH.

29.   BPH results from which of the following?
  A.   hypertrophy of periurethral glands that compresses the normal prostatic tissue
  B.   hyperplasia of periurethral glands that compresses the normal prostatic tissue
  C.   dysplasia of the prostatic cells that usually begins in the periphery of the posterior gland
  D.   inflammation of the prostatic gland that eventually compresses the urethra

Mr. F. is scheduled for a transurethral prostatectomy (TURP). Mr. F.'s wife misses the physician's explanation of the surgery and asks the nurse about the procedure.

30.   The nurse would explain to Mr. F. and his family that this procedure will involve which of the following?
  A.   a low abdominal incision to approach the prostate without entering the bladder
  B.   an incision into the area between the anus and the prostate
  C.   a transurethral incision of the prostate and a balloon dilation of the stricture
  D.   a lighted tube is placed in the urethra and excess prostatic tissue is removed

31.   Postoperatively the nurse identifies a nursing diagnosis of High risk for fluid volume deficit related to postoperative hemorrhage. Which of the following observations would the nurse expect to make in relation to the nursing diagnosis?
  A.   pink-tinged urine for several days postoperatively
  B.   multiple clots in the urine postoperatively
  C.   bright red blood in the urine postoperatively
  D.   clear, amber-colored urine postoperatively

32.   Another nursing diagnosis identified for Mr. F. notes the potential for pain postoperatively. The most likely cause of this pain would be which of the following?
  A.   lower abdominal incisional pain
  B.   pain from bladder spasms
  C.   pain from the urethral catheter
  D.   pain from bleeding in the bladder

Mr. F.'s output is 100 cc for the past 4 hours. Rank the following nursing actions in order of importance.

33.   _____ Notify physician.
34.   _____ Irrigate catheter as ordered.
35.   _____ Assess catheter patency.
36.   _____ Assess Mr. F.'s intake.

CHAPTER 39

Management of Women with Reproductive Disorders

Nursing care of the woman with a gynecologic disorder requires that the nurse understand various components of reproductive anatomy and the pathophysiology involved. It also requires accurate, sensitive history-taking and supportive assistance during the physical examination. Surgical therapies for several gynecologic disorders may involve removal of the uterus or ovaries, which results in sterilization. Women will exhibit a range of emotional responses to this type of surgery. The nurse's recognition of the trauma and support can help women begin coping with their sense of loss. Other women may be faced with gynecologic cancers. Nursing interventions for these women will fall into the psychosocial as well as the technical realm. Also, as in many areas previously discussed, there are instances for nurses to implement primary and secondary prevention so that in some cases women can avoid gynecologic disorders or at least seek early detection and treatment. Additionally, it is important for nurses to recognize and support variations in cultural and ethnic attitudes and practices toward female reproduction.

OBJECTIVES

39.1   Discuss menstrual disorders and menopause and their medical, surgical, and nursing management.

39.2   Discuss infectious and inflammatory uterine disorders and their medical, surgical, and nursing management.

39.3   Discuss malignant and nonmalignant tumors of the uterus and their medical, surgical, and nursing management.

39.4   Discuss other disorders of the uterus and their medical, surgical, and nursing management.

39.5   Discuss ovarian disorders and their medical, surgical, and nursing management.

39.6   Discuss vaginal disorders and their medical, surgical, and nursing management.

39.7   Discuss disorders of the vulva and their medical, surgical, and nursing management.

39.8   Define other gynecologic cancers.

LEARNING THE LANGUAGE: TERMINOLOGY RELATED TO NURSING CARE OF WOMEN WITH GYNECOLOGIC DISORDERS

Match the terms in Column A with the correct description/definition in Column B.

Column A

1. _____ Amenorrhea
2. _____ Atrophic vaginitis
3. _____ Bartholinitis
4. _____ Choriocarcinoma
5. _____ Cystocele
6. _____ Dysmenorrhea
7. _____ Dyspareunia
8. _____ Endometrial ablation
9. _____ Endometriosis
10. _____ Enterocele
11. _____ Hydatidiform mole
12. _____ Kraurosis
13. _____ Leiomyomas
14. _____ Leukoplakia vulvae
15. _____ Leukorrhea
16. _____ Menorrhagia
17. _____ Metrorrhagia
18. _____ Radical hysterectomy
19. _____ Radical vulvectomy
20. _____ Rectocele
21. _____ Uterine prolapse

Column B

A. Painful menstrual flow

B. Absence of menses

C. Excessive vaginal bleeding at normal intervals

D. Bleeding between periods, either spotting or outright bleeding

E. Thinning and drying of vaginal walls

F. Endometrial tissue located outside the uterus

G. Muscle and connective tissue tumors of the uterus

H. Protrusion of part of the urinary bladder through the vaginal wall

I. Protrusion of a portion of the rectum through the vaginal wall

J. Protrusion of a portion of the small intestine through the vaginal wall

K. Descent of the uterus into the vagina

L. Normal, nonbloody, asymptotic vaginal discharge

M. Thickened gray patches of epithelium scattered over the vulva and perineum

N. Excision of tissue from the anus to below the symphysis pubis (skin, labia majora and minora, and clitoris), and possibly groin lymph nodes

O. Inflammation of Bartholin's glands

P. Neoplasm of the chorion with grossly visible invasion of the uterine myometrium and, sometimes, adjacent tissue

Q. Painful intercourse

R. Lesion of the vulvae characterized by bright red, smooth, almost transparent epithelium

S. Laser fiber used to destroy endometrium by passing it through a hysteroscope

T. Removal of the uterus, cervix, ovaries, fallopian tubes, lymph nodes, upper third of the vagina, and parametrium

U. Rare trophoblastic disease in pregnancy with characteristic grapelike tissue

THINKING CRITICALLY: UNDERSTANDING RATIONALES

Provide the rationales for the therapeutic nursing interventions listed.

Intervention	Rationale

Client with Menopause

22. Use of hormone replacement therapy (HRT).

23. Do not recommend HRT for clients who have had breast or uterine cancer.

Client Postoperative Abdominal Hysterectomy

24. Assist client to ambulate and give an enema.

25. Insert Foley catheter during surgery.

Client Having History and Physical of Reproductive System

26. Assess for client's mother's use of diethylstilbestrol (DES) during pregnancy with client.

Provide the rationales for use of the following medications with the specified disorders.

Disorder	Rationale

Ibuprofen or indomethacin

27. Use with dysmenorrhea.

Spironolactone (Aldactone)

28. Use with premenstrual syndrome (PMS).

Oral contraceptives or progesterone

29. Use with endometriosis.

CLIENT EDUCATION: KNOWING WHAT TO TEACH AND WHY

Provide short answers to the following questions.

30. What would you teach in regard to risk factors for cervical cancer?

33. What would you teach the perimenopausal woman about prevention of osteoporosis?

31. What would you teach a group of women about the risk factors for endometrial cancer?

34. List teaching aspects of prevention for pelvic inflammatory disease (PID).

32. Why would you teach the woman with dysmenorrhea about exercise?

35. What would you teach about activity recommendations/restrictions postoperative hysterectomy?

THINKING CRITICALLY: KNOWING WHAT TO DO AND WHY

36. Provide interventions for women having hot flashes.

37. What would be your rationale for teaching women about the benefits of having regular Pap smears?

PUTTING IT ALL TOGETHER

■ *Case Study*

Ms. I., 28, comes to the gynecology clinic for a routine screening examination. She is gravida 2, para 2 with a history of Candidal infections but no other significant gynecologic history. Ms. I. receives a Pap smear and gynecologic examination. She is told that a report will be mailed to her within 2–3 weeks with the results of her Pap smear.

38. A Pap smear is the primary test to screen for
- A.   endometrial cancer.
- B.   vaginal cancer.
- C.   cervical cancer.
- D.   ovarian cancer.

39. In teaching Ms. I. about primary prevention of cervical cancer, it would be important to emphasize which of the following?
- A.   treat infections of the cervix early
- B.   use of oral contraceptives
- C.   daily use of commercial douches
- D.   assess her mother's use of DES

40. If Ms. I. were diagnosed with cervical cancer in situ, her prognosis would be
- A.   50% recovery.
- B.   60% recovery.
- C.   90% recovery.
- D.   100% recovery.

41. Ms. I. has cryosurgery with laser therapy for a positive Pap smear. In doing the discharge teaching, the nurse would include which of the following?
- A.   Avoid baths or sitz baths.
- B.   Call the physician if having malodorous discharge.
- C.   Call the physician if having clear, watery discharge.
- D.   No pain is expected postprocedure.

40

Management of Clients with Breast Disorders

The statistics on breast cancer incidence speak for themselves: one in eight women who live to be 85 years of age will get breast cancer; in 2000, 40,800 were estimated to die from breast cancer. Nurses do have a major role to play in teaching women about early detection methods and encouraging their use. When a woman is initially treated surgically for breast cancer, the actual physical nursing care may be fairly limited with the psychosocial and teaching role being paramount. If the woman has adjuvant therapy for breast cancer, in either the inpatient or outpatient setting, the complexity of both psychosocial and physical nursing interventions increases. Making referrals to community resources will be an additional way nurses can assist their clients in managing their own care. In almost any setting where nurses come in contact with women, there are teaching opportunities that can lead to early detection, which has the potential to decrease the extent of the disease, and therefore, the complexity of treatment. It is important that these opportunities are recognized and used.

OBJECTIVES

40.1 Discuss breast cancer and its medical, surgical, and nursing management.

40.2 Describe benign breast disorders and their medical and nursing management.

LEARNING THE LANGUAGE: TERMINOLOGY RELATED TO NURSING CARE OF CLIENTS WITH BREAST DISORDERS

Match the terms in Column A with the correct description or definition in Column B.

Column A

1. _____ Adjuvant therapy
2. _____ BRCA-1
3. _____ Carcinoembryonic antigen
4. _____ Estrogen receptor–positive
5. _____ Multicentric
6. _____ Neoadjuvant therapy
7. _____ Peau d'orange
8. _____ Tamoxifen

Column B

A. Indicates that the tumor is receptive to estrogen and may respond to anti-estrogen therapy

B. Therapy added to another treatment to enhance the effect; for example, with cancer therapy chemotherapy is given in addition to surgery and/or radiation to prolong disease-free survival

C. Radiation, hormonal therapy, or chemotherapy given before surgery

D. Gene on chromosome 17 which indicates a higher risk for breast, ovarian, and prostate cancer

E. Edema of the breast with an orange-peel appearance

F. Anti-estrogen used in treatment of estrogen receptor-positive breast cancer

G. Cancer is found in two or more locations

H. Tumor marker present in the serum of women with breast cancer that is used to follow the progress of the disease

Match the disorders in Column A with the correct description in Column B.

Column A

9. _____ Breast abscess
10. _____ Duct ectasia
11. _____ Fibroadenoma
12. _____ Fibrocystic breasts
13. _____ Fissure of the nipple
14. _____ Gynecomastia
15. _____ Hyperplasia and atypical hyperplasia
16. _____ Lactation mastitis
17. _____ Mastodynia and mastalgia
18. _____ Papillomas

Column B

A. Fluid-filled cysts that are round, well circumscribed, and movable

B. Cell changes that indicate an increased risk for breast cancer

C. Intraductal lesions in the terminal portion of the duct or throughout the ductal system

D. Disease of the ducts in the subareolar zone in aging breasts

E. Localized, indurated, painful area that may develop when bacteria enter the breast of a lactating woman

F. Subareolar, low-grade infection in nonlactating women or occurring during lactation when bacteria enter through a cracked nipple

G. A painful longitudinal ulcer in the nipple that occurs in nursing mothers

H. A common breast tumor, usually in younger women, that is a nontender, round, firm or rubbery mass

I. Breast pain

J. Hypertrophy in the male breast

Match the histopathologic types in Column A with the correct description in Column B.

Column A		**Column B**
19. _____ Infiltrating ductal carcinoma	A.	Arises from ductal epithelium, precancerous marker, indicates risk for invasive ductal breast cancer
20. _____ Infiltrating lobular carcinoma		
21. _____ Inflammatory breast cancer		
22. _____ Intraductal carcinoma	B.	Five to seven percent of breast cancers, reaches large size, better prognosis
23. _____ Lobular cancer in situ		
24. _____ Medullary carcinoma	C.	Occurs with other carcinomatous breast cancers, axillary metastasis uncommon
25. _____ Mucinous carcinoma		
26. _____ Paget's disease	D.	Ill-defined thickening rather than a lump, often involves both breasts
27. _____ Tubular carcinoma		
	E.	Seventy percent of breast cancers, stone-hard lump
	F.	Found with other breast cancers, slow growing, can become quite large
	G.	Crusting and scaling skin changes in the nipple with burning, itching, or bleeding
	H.	Skin redness, induration, edema, and warmth, often with lymph involvement
	I.	Arises in mammary lobules, is a precancerous marker, indicates higher risk for invasive cancer

Match the tumor characteristics in Column A with the type of tumor it most frequently describes in Column B.

Column A		**Column B**
28. _____ Usually fluid-filled	A.	Benign tumors
29. _____ Usually solitary	B.	Malignant tumors
30. _____ Usually bilateral		
31. _____ Skin dimpling		
32. _____ Mobile		
33. _____ Usually nontender		
34. _____ Irregular margins		
35. _____ Tend to be multiple		
36. _____ Borders well defined		

THINKING CRITICALLY: UNDERSTANDING RATIONALES

Provide the rationales for the therapeutic nursing interventions for postmastectomy clients listed below.

Intervention	**Rationale**
37. Take blood pressure readings on the nonoperated side.	
38. Have a Reach for Recovery volunteer visit the client.	

39.   What is the rationale for using Tamoxifen after a mastectomy?

CLIENT EDUCATION: KNOWING WHAT TO TEACH AND WHY

Discuss what you would teach and/or provide rationale for the intervention.

Teaching Point	**Rationale**

40.   Teaching arm exercises to women after a mastectomy.

41.   Advising a woman who has had a mastectomy with a lymph node resection to wear gloves when washing dishes or gardening.

42.   What would you teach a group of women about breast cancer risks?

43.   Teaching points about side effects from radiation.

44.   What are areas to include in teaching for the woman being discharged postmastectomy?

THINKING CRITICALLY: KNOWING WHAT TO DO AND WHY

45.   Identify nursing interventions to support a woman undergoing diagnostic work-up for breast cancer.

Putting It All Together

■ *Case Study*

Ms. J. is a 55-year-old postmenopausal female with a diagnosis of infiltrating ductal carcinoma of the right breast.

46. If Ms. J.'s symptoms were typical they would include which of the following?
    A. pain and edema
    B. a movable, round mass
    C. a fixed, irregular mass
    D. bilateral masses

After consulting with her physician about her options, Ms. J. decides to have a modified radical mastectomy. A lymph node dissection will also be done during the surgery.

47. The modified radical mastectomy includes removal of which of the following?
    A. cone of the breast
    B. lump and surrounding tissue
    C. cone of the breast and overlying skin
    D. quadrant of the breast and some underlying fascia

48. The nurse caring for her postmastectomy finds Ms. J. upset after a medical student explained that the pathology reports revealed her tumor to be estrogen receptor-positive. The nurse explains to Ms. J. that the estrogen receptor-positive (ER+) test gives the physician information about treatment options. The nurse further explains that ER+ makes Ms. J. a candidate for which of the following treatments?
    A. removal of her ovaries
    B. treatment with estrogen
    C. treatment with progesterone
    D. treatment with Tamoxifen

49. Within 24 hours after her mastectomy, Ms. J. should begin which of the following exercises?
    A. pendulum arm swings
    B. elbow flexion and extension
    C. shoulder abduction and external rotation
    D. hand wall climbing

50. Ms. J.'s mastectomy was performed on her right side. The rationale for not drawing blood from her right arm, and teaching Ms. J. to shave her underarm with an electric razor and to wear a glove on her right hand when working in the garden is
    A. increased risk for infection after lymph node removal.
    B. increased risk for edema after lymph node removal.
    C. decreased circulation after the lymph node removal.
    D. decreased lymph drainage after lymph node removal.

41

Management of Clients with Sexually Transmitted Diseases

Sexually transmitted diseases are the second most common communicable disease in the United States. In many cases the incidence of these diseases is on the increase. It is important for nurses to know about these disorders, such as how they can be prevented, how they are spread, how they are treated, and how to approach clients in a nonjudgmental manner, in order to do case finding and teaching.

OBJECTIVES

41.1   Examine the overall concept of sexually transmitted diseases (STDs) and medical and nursing management.

41.2   Discuss common sexually transmitted diseases and their medical and nursing management.

41.3   Describe the remaining, less common sexually transmitted diseases.

LEARNING THE LANGUAGE: TERMINOLOGY RELATED TO NURSING CARE OF CLIENTS WITH SEXUALLY TRANSMITTED DISEASES

Match the terms in Column A with the correct definition or description in Column B.

Column A

1. _____ Bacterial vaginosis
2. _____ Chancroid
3. _____ *Chlamydia trachomatis*
4. _____ Genital herpes
5. _____ Genital warts
6. _____ Gonorrhea
7. _____ Granuloma inguinale
8. _____ Hepatitis B
9. _____ Lymphogranuloma
10. _____ *Pediculosis pubis*
11. _____ Syphilis
12. _____ Trichomoniasis
13. _____ Vulvovaginal Candidiasis

Column B

A. A sexually transmitted infection caused by *Neisseria gonorrhoeae*, a gram-negative diplococcus, which affects the genitourinary tract

B. A sexually transmitted, recurrent, systemic infection caused by the herpes simplex virus type II that manifests as a genital ulceration

C. An infection of the vagina and vulva, which is occasionally transmitted sexually, caused by *Candida*, a fungal organism; it is not generally considered a sexually transmitted disease

D. A skin infestation with lice from either contaminated objects or close physical contact; it is sometimes considered a sexually transmitted disease

E. Highly contagious infection caused by the gram-negative *Haemophilus ducreyi* bacillus

F. Systemic infection common in the tropics caused by *Chlamydia trachomatis,* with a primary lesion that is a small, painless papule on the glans penis or vaginal mucosa

G. Chronic infection (rare in the United States) caused by *Calymmatobacterium granulomatis* characterized by genital and perianal papular lesions

H. Viral infection of the liver most frequently transmitted by sexual contact

I. Bacterial infection caused by an overgrowth of normal flora in the vagina

J. Most common STD; in men, can cause a stricture of the urethra or epididymis; in women, infections can extend to the endometrium and salpinx

K. Systemic, highly infectious disease caused by *Treponema pallidum* and characterized by stages

L. Benign growths that typically occur in multiple, painless clusters on the vulva, vagina, cervix, perineum, anorectal area, urethral meatus, or glans penis caused by the human papillomavirus (HPV)

M. Protozoal infection causing vulvovaginitis

THINKING CRITICALLY: UNDERSTANDING RATIONALES

14. What is the rationale for treating a client with gonorrhea for Chlamydia?

Listed below are specific medications and nursing implications associated with the medications. Provide the rationales for the nursing implications.

Implication	**Rationale**

Flagyl

15. Advise clients not to drink alcohol.

Doxycycline

16. Take 1–2 hours after meals and avoid iron, dairy products, and antacids.

CLIENT EDUCATION: KNOWING WHAT TO TEACH AND WHY

Discuss what you would teach and give rationales.

Teaching Point	**Rationale**

17. Teaching clients with human papillomavirus the importance of having an annual Papanicolaou (Pap) smear.

18. Teaching women about the risks of sterility with Chlamydial infections.

19. For the client with Chlamydia, syphilis, and gonorrhea, what would you teach about sexual contact during treatment?

20. What would you teach about immunity after a sexually transmitted disease?

THINKING CRITICALLY: KNOWING WHAT TO DO AND WHY

21. As a nursing student, you are assigned to do a teaching project on prevention of sexually transmitted diseases. If you wanted to target your teaching to people at highest risk, what age group(s) would you target?

22. Genital warts (*Condylomata acuminatum*) is associated with an increased incidence of
    A. sterility.
    B. pelvic inflammatory disease.
    C. hair loss.
    D. genital carcinoma.

23. The surest way to prevent sexually transmitted diseases is
    A. abstinence.
    B. education.
    C. condoms.
    D. single sex partner.

24. For the client newly diagnosed with gonorrhea, important teaching by the nurse would include which of the following?
    A. Penicillin will easily treat the disease.
    B Abstinence from sex for one month after treatment is necessary.
    C. All sexual partners must be identified.
    D. Towels and other personal items can carry the infection.

25. Teaching to a client receiving metronidazole (Flagyl) would include which of the following?
    A. Medication is usually taken for one week.
    B. Avoid consuming alcohol while taking medication.
    C. Medication is safe during pregnancy.
    D. Avoid taking medication with meals.

26. Teaching clients about the use of male condoms would include which of the following facts?
    A. Use natural membrane condoms.
    B. Use a new condom each time you have sex.
    C. Use petroleum jelly or baby oil for a lubricant.
    D. Pull the condom tight over the end of the penis.

UNIT 9

Metabolic Disorders

ANATOMY AND PHYSIOLOGY REVIEW: THE METABOLIC SYSTEMS

The endocrine system acts with the nervous system to control and integrate body function. The actions of the endocrine system may be localized to one area but can be generalized to all body cells.

A basic understanding of the structure and function of the endocrine system will facilitate an understanding of the pathophysiology of the disorders to be discussed in Chapters 42 through 45. It is suggested that you review the following definitions and study questions. If you have difficulty with the answers, spending some time with the review in Unit 9 in the textbook will be beneficial.

OBJECTIVES

9.1 Discuss regulation of endocrine activity by the two major endocrine glands, the hypothalamus and the pituitary.

9.2 Define negative feedback systems controlling blood levels of hormones.

9.3 Describe the role of the hypothalamus in endocrine function.

9.4 Identify the major functions of each endocrine gland by giving the action of each hormone produced by the gland.

9.5 Describe the normal structure of the liver, biliary tract, and exocrine pancreas.

9.6 Describe the normal function of the liver, biliary tract, and exocrine pancreas.

PUTTING IT ALL TOGETHER: REVIEW OF ENDOCRINE SYSTEM ANATOMY

1.   Label the diagram below with the name of each
      endocrine gland.

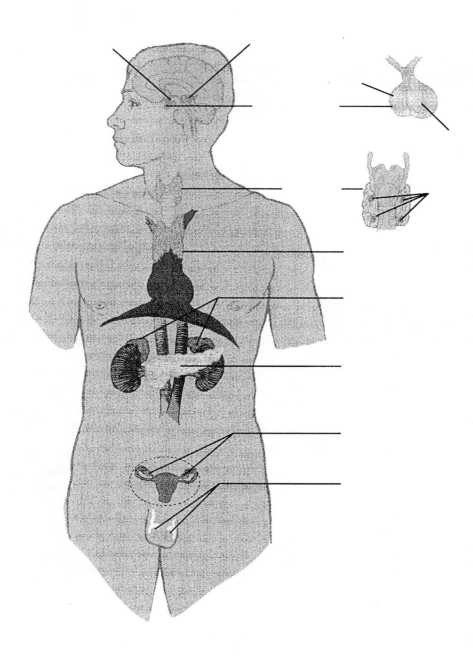

REVIEW OF ENDOCRINE SYSTEM PHYSIOLOGY

Match the hormones in Column A with the endocrine gland that secretes them in Column B. Some glands secrete more than one hormone.

Column A	**Column B**
2. _____ Thyroxine	A. Adrenal cortex
3. _____ Glucagon	B. Adrenal medulla
4. _____ Epinephrine	C. Ovaries
5. _____ Adrenocorticotropic hormone	D. Pancreas
6. _____ Parathormone	E. Thyroid
7. _____ Insulin	F. Parathyroid
8. _____ Antidiuretic hormone	G. Pituitary (anterior lobe)
9. _____ Melanocyte-stimulating hormone	H. Pituitary (posterior lobe)
10. _____ Mineralocorticoids	I. Testes
11. _____ Thyroid-stimulating hormone	
12. _____ Gonadotropic hormone	
13. _____ Thyrocalcitonin	
14. _____ Progesterone	
15. _____ Androgens	
16. _____ Prolactin	

Give the function of each of the following endocrine glands by filling in the information missing in the following descriptions.

17. **Adrenal (cortex)** influences fluid and electrolyte balance through the secretion of _____, which increases sodium retention and potassium excretion by the kidneys, raises blood glucose levels with the secretion of _____, and affects masculinization.

18. **Pancreas (islets of Langerhans)** regulates _____ of carbohydrates, fat, and protein, and controls glycogenolysis by mobilizing glycogen stores through the secretion of _____.

19. **Pituitary (anterior lobe)** stimulates thyroid and adrenocortical secretion, through the secretion of _____ and _____, respectively.

20. **Pituitary (posterior lobe)** promotes water _____, thus decreasing urine output.

21. **Thyroid** controls metabolic rate, and secretes a hormone whose effect is opposite that of the hormone from the _____ glands.

22. Synthesis of the two posterior pituitary hormones occurs within the _____.

LEARNING THE LANGUAGE: TERMINOLOGY RELATED TO STRUCTURE AND FUNCTION OF THE LIVER, BILIARY SYSTEM, AND EXOCRINE PANCREAS

Match the terms in Column A with the correct definition in Column B.

Column A	Column B
23. _____ Acinar cells	A. Supplies the liver with oxygenated blood
24. _____ Ampulla of Vater	B. Phagocytic macrophages that line the hepatic sinuses and serve as filters to remove bacteria and other debris from the blood as it enters the liver from the portal vein
25. _____ Bilirubin	
26. _____ Cholesterol	
27. _____ Cholecystokinin	C. The conversion of glucose to glycogen
28. _____ Deamination	D. Prevents intravascular fluid from leaking out of the blood vessels into the extravascular spaces where it produces ascites and edema
29. _____ Glycogenesis	
30. _____ Glycogenolysis	
31. _____ Gluconeogenesis	E. Carries nutrients, metabolites, and toxins from the digestive organs to the liver for processing, detoxification, or assimilation
32. _____ Hepatic artery	
33. _____ Hepatocyte	
34. _____ Kupffer's cells	F. A valve at the confluence of the common bile duct and the duodenum that opens to allow bile to flow into the intestinal tract
35. _____ Liver lobule	
36. _____ Portal vein	
37. _____ Plasma oncotic pressure	G. Site that connects the pancreas to the common bile duct
38. _____ Sphincter of Oddi	
	H. A yellow-greenish pigment in bile that is a product of hemoglobin breakdown
	I. A bile precursor
	J. Stimulates the contraction of the gallbladder in response to fatty foods in the small intestine
	K. The breakdown of glycogen to glucose
	L. The conversion of amino acids to glucose
	M. Cells in the pancreas that produce enzymes
	N. Functional unit of the liver
	O. Major cell in the liver
	P. The breakdown of amino acids

KNOWLEDGE BUILDING: THE STRUCTURE AND FUNCTION OF THE LIVER, BILIARY TRACT, AND EXOCRINE PANCREAS

39. What structures protect the liver?

41. If blood flow is impeded through the liver, what is the effect on the above listed veins?

40. The _____, _____, and _____ join to form the portal vein.

42. Blood returns to the inferior vena cava via the _____ vein.

43. What is the effect on the liver of any process affecting the blood flow through the right atrium?

44. What are the two major functions of bile salts?

45. What are the roles of the liver in fat metabolism?

46. The major processes of glucose production or breakdown that occur in the liver are _____, _____, and _____, _____, and _____.

47. As a part of the process of deamination, _____ waste product is left. The liver converts this waste product to _____ and it is excreted by the kidneys.

48. The liver synthesizes _____, _____, and clotting proteins _____, _____, _____, _____, and _____, and clotting factors.

49. The plasma protein essential for plasma oncotic pressure synthesized in the liver is _____.

50. The liver detoxifies _____, _____, and _____.

51. The liver functions as a reservoir for _____.

52. When the gallbladder is removed, what is the effect on fat digestion?

53. The major endocrine function of the pancreas is to secrete _____ and _____.

54. The major exocrine function of the pancreas involves secreting the digestive enzymes _____, _____, and _____.

55. What prevents the digestive enzymes produced by the pancreas from autodigesting the pancreas?

56. What is the purpose of the bicarbonate produced by the ducts and ductules leading from the acini?

42

Assessment of the Endocrine and Metabolic Systems

A thorough history and physical examination are important in assessing clients with endocrine disorders because the endocrine system affects every other body system. The client could present with a variety of manifestations. Understanding normal physiology of the endocrine system is essential to assessing endocrine dysfunction.

Assessment of the liver and biliary tract requires developing advanced psychomotor, observational, and communication skills. In addition to assessment skills, the nurse caring for clients with liver, biliary tract, and exocrine pancreatic disorders will have to interpret related laboratory tests. Additionally, the nurse will have to prepare clients for diagnostic tests and provide nursing care for them after the test.

OBJECTIVES

42.1   Discuss how the endocrine system affects every other body system and the resulting variety of manifestations that may occur with endocrine disorders.

42.2   Appreciate the importance of a thorough history and physical examination in the assessment of clients with endocrine disorders.

42.3   Demonstrate correct technique for palpation of the thyroid gland.

42.4   Identify common diagnostic tests for thyroid, adrenal, and posterior pituitary function.

42.5   Prepare a plan for complete assessment of an individual's liver, biliary tract, and pancreatic function.

42.6   Prepare a person with dysfunction of the liver, biliary tract, or pancreas for diagnostic tests.

42.7   Interpret results of laboratory and diagnostic tests.

LEARNING THE LANGUAGE: TERMINOLOGY RELATED TO ASSESSMENT OF CLIENTS WITH LIVER, BILIARY TRACT, AND EXOCRINE PANCREATIC DISORDERS

Match the terms in Column A with the correct definition in Column B.

Column A	**Column B**
1. _____ Acholic	A. Fluid accumulation in the peritoneal cavity
2. _____ Ascites	B. Bulky, foul-smelling, fatty stools
3. _____ Spider angiomas	C. Stools without bilirubin
4. _____ Steatorrhea	D. Dilated veins

Match the diagnostic studies in Column A with the correct description in Column B.

Column A

5. _____ Angiography
6. _____ Cholangiography
7. _____ Oral cholecystography
8. _____ Paracentesis
9. _____ Peritoneoscopy
10. _____ Radionuclide scan
11. _____ Ultrasonography

Column B

A.   X-ray of the gallbladder following oral intake of a radiopaque dye

B.   Injection of a contrast medium through the femoral artery in order to visualize the arteries of the spleen, biliary system, and pancreas

C.   Insertion of a long needle through the skin into the peritoneum to remove fluid

D.   Insertion of a lighted scope through a stab wound in the abdomen to permit visualization of the liver and peritoneum

E.   Following IV infusion of gamma-emitting isotopes, a scintillation detector is passed over the abdomen to investigate biliary tract patency, tumors, or abscesses

F.   High-frequency sound waves used to examine the interior of the body

G.   Following IV injection of an organic iodine dye, x-ray filming begins

Match the laboratory tests in Column A with the appropriate interpretation in Column B.

Column A

12. _____ Alkaline phosphatase
13. _____ Aspartate aminotransferase (SGOT)
14. _____ Direct (conjugated) bilirubin
15. _____ Globulin
16. _____ Mitochondrial antibody
17. _____ Serum γ-glutamyltransferase (GGI)
18. _____ Serum amylase
19. _____ Serum ammonia
20. _____ Total protein

Column B

A.   Enzyme elevated in biliary obstruction, also found in bone, intestine, and placenta

B.   Pancreatic digestive enzyme released with breakdown of acinar cells

C.   Enzyme released from damaged liver, heart, kidney, and muscle cells

D.   Elevated with impaired biliary excretion

E.   Elevated when severe liver damage reduces synthesis into urea

F.   Enzyme located in liver and kidney; an elevation indicates liver disorders

G.   Decreased with impaired protein synthesis caused by chronic liver disease

H.   May be increased with decreased removal of bacterial antigens from the portal blood or release of antigenic material from damaged liver cells

I.   Appears in 90% of people with primary biliary cirrhosis; an antibody directed against a component of the inner mitochondrial membrane

THINKING CRITICALLY: KNOWING WHAT TO DO AND WHY

Mr. W. is a 36-year-old male with suspected hepatitis. He has a percutaneous liver biopsy with local anesthesia. Questions 21–24 refer to Mr. W.

21.   Mr. W. is requested to hold his breath on exhalation for 5–10 seconds, during the insertion of the biopsy needle. State the reason for this request.

22.   Initially, after the biopsy, Mr. W. will be placed on his right side. What is the rationale for this order?

23.   Mr. W. is at risk for hemorrhage postbiopsy. Why?

24.   Describe nursing interventions that assess for and prevent post–liver biopsy hemorrhage.

25.   In completing a psychosocial history for a person with a suspected disorder of the liver or pancreas, why is assessment of alcohol intake important?

26.   Describe the procedure for percussing liver borders.

27.   If an enlarged spleen is percussed, what is the procedure for palpating the spleen? Why?

28.   What questions would you ask the client to determine if he/she had an iodine allergy?

29.   If a client has a hypersensitivity reaction to iodine, what symptoms might he/she exhibit?

30.   When taking the history of a client with a suspected or known liver disorder, what drugs and chemicals are particularly important to inquire about? Why?

■ Diagnostic Tests

Test	Informed Consent	Pretest Nursing Care	Post-Test Nursing Care
31. Ultrasonography			
32. Oral cholecystography			
33. Cholangiography			
34. Angiography			
35. Radionuclide scanning			
36. Paracentesis			
37. Peritoneoscopy			
38. Liver biopsy			

THINKING CRITICALLY: KNOWING WHAT TO DO AND WHY

Some manifestations are specific for certain endocrine disorders. Match the manifestations in Column A with the appropriate endocrine disorder in Column B.

Column A

39. _____ Tremors
40. _____ Tachycardia
41. _____ Kussmaul's respirations
42. _____ Weight gain
43. _____ Hirsutism (excessive body hair)
44. _____ Exophthalmos (bulging eyes)
45. _____ Buffalo hump and moon facies
46. _____ Constipation
47. _____ Diarrhea
48. _____ Dry, brittle hair

Column B

A. Hypothyroidism
B. Hyperthyroidism
C. Cushing's disease
D. Addison's disease
E. Diabetes mellitus

Answer Yes or No to the following questions regarding assessment of the endocrine system.

49. _____ Should you normally be able to palpate the thyroid gland?

50. _____ If the thyroid gland is enlarged, should you auscultate for bruits?

51. _____ Can Dilantin therapy decrease T_4 (thyroxin) levels?

52. _____ Do pregnancy and oral contraceptives increase T_4 (thyroxin) levels?

53. _____ Are cortisol levels normally higher in the morning than in the evening?

54. _____ Does the collection of a 24-hour urine specimen for ketosteroids (metabolites of the hormones produced by the adrenal cortex) require a bottle containing a preservative?

CHAPTER

43

Management of Clients with Thyroid and Parathyroid Disorders

The hormones secreted by the thyroid gland increase metabolic rate. Thus, hypofunction (hypothyroidism) will result in a sustained decrease in metabolic rate, whereas hyperfunction (hyperthyroidism) will result in a sustained increase in metabolic rate. Either of these conditions has significant ill effects on physiologic and psychologic functioning. The parathyroid glands regulate serum calcium levels. Hyperparathyroidism can elevate serum calcium, resulting in depressed neuromuscular functioning and damage to the renal system. Hypoparathyroidism can decrease serum calcium, resulting in increased neuromuscular irritability producing tetany and causing convulsions.

OBJECTIVES

43.1   Describe three types of thyroid enlargement (goiter, thyroiditis, and thyroid tumors), giving definition, assessment and methods of diagnosis, and interventions.

43.2   Identify two major forms of hypothyroidism.

43.3   Discuss the etiology of hypothyroidism in adults.

43.4   Discuss the etiology of Graves' disease as an autoimmune disorder.

43.5   Compare and contrast the signs and symptoms of hypo- and hyperthyroidism.

43.6   Describe the complications of hypo- and hyperthyroidism.

43.7   Discuss the usual medical treatments for hypo- and hyperthyroidism.

43.8   Discuss nursing responsibilities regarding thyroid function tests.

43.9   Describe the needs of clients experiencing hypo- and hyperthyroid function.

43.10   Plan nursing care interventions to meet the needs of clients experiencing hypo- and hyperthyroid function.

43.11   Recognize the signs of under- and overdose of thyroid hormones.

43.12   Give the action and toxic or side effects of antithyroid medications.

43.13   Discuss nursing care for a person receiving radioactive iodine (^{131}I) therapy.

OBJECTIVES (CONTINUED)

43.14 Discuss types of thyroid cancer as to incidence, characteristics, intervention, and prognosis.

43.15 Discuss nursing care needed to help assure that the client scheduled for a thyroidectomy is euthyroid, relaxed, well-nourished, and has no uncontrolled cardiac problems.

43.16 Describe nursing assessment needed to recognize early signs and symptoms of the major complications that may follow a thyroidectomy.

43.17 Plan postoperative nursing care to decrease strain on the suture line, relieve discomfort from sore throat and tracheal irritation, prevent pooling of respiratory secretions, and prevent or relieve the complications of thyroidectomy.

43.18 Describe hypo- and hyperparathyroidism as to etiology, assessment and methods of diagnosis, and interventions.

43.19 Discuss specifically the treatment of hypercalcemia.

43.20 List nursing diagnoses that may apply to clients experiencing parathyroid disorders.

43.21 Plan nursing interventions based on the list of nursing diagnoses.

43.22 Discuss nursing care needed to meet the goals of preoperative care for a client having a parathyroidectomy.

43.23 Describe nursing assessments needed to recognize early signs and symptoms of the major complications that may follow parathyroid resection.

43.24 Plan postoperative nursing care for clients undergoing parathyroid gland resection.

THINKING CRITICALLY: KNOWING WHAT TO DO AND WHY

■ *Comparison of Hypo- and Hyperthyroidism*

Indicate whether each of the following signs or symptoms is more closely associated with hypo- *or* hyper*thyroidism. Check your answers by referring to Table 43-1, "Manifestations of Hypothyroidism and Hyperthyroidism" in the text.*

1. _____ Lethargy and apathy
2. _____ Exophthalmos
3. _____ Mood swings
4. _____ Hand tremor at rest
5. _____ Weight loss
6. _____ Warm, smooth skin
7. _____ Profuse diaphoresis

8. _____ Generalized nonpitting edema
9. _____ Dry hair and skin
10. _____ Intolerance to cold
11. _____ Loose bowel movements
12. _____ Good appetite
13. _____ Tachycardia
14. _____ Incoordination

■ *Study Questions*

15. Explain why a goiter may be a sign of hypo- or hyperthyroidism.

16. Explain why both hypo- and hyperthyroidism can result in diminished cardiac output and cardiac damage.

17. Give two nursing diagnoses and an appropriate intervention for each for a client with hypothyroidism.

18. Give two nursing diagnoses and an appropriate intervention for each for a client with hyperthyroidism.

19. What type of IV fluid is preferred to treat hypercalcemia and which diuretic is preferred to promote urinary calcium excretion?

■ *Case Study*

Ms. W., 35, has trouble sleeping, a fine hand tremor, tachycardia, and weight loss in spite of an increased appetite. Laboratory test results show elevated T_3, T_4, and ^{131}I uptake values. She is diagnosed as having Graves' disease with mild exophthalmos, and is admitted to the hospital for a subtotal thyroidectomy.

20. Which of the following environments would be best for her?
    A. warm, quiet private room with extra blankets on her bed
    B. warm room with increased sensory stimulation
    C. restful physical environment with low levels of sensory stimulation
    D. lower temperature and increased physical activities

21. What is the best intervention for Ms. W. since she has exophthalmos?
    A. Keep the head of her bed flat.
    B. Give her artificial tears and dark glasses.
    C. Instill ophthalmic antibiotic ointment.
    D. Patch both of her eyes.

22. What is the most likely reason she has sustained tachycardia and a bounding pulse?
    A. Her metabolic rate has increased her heart rate.
    B. She is anxious about the upcoming surgery.
    C. The lower thyroxin level has decreased her blood pressure (B/P).
    D. Her water intake has decreased significantly.

23. She received saturated solution of potassium iodide (SSKI) before being admitted for surgery to
    A. establish a diagnosis with the ^{131}I uptake.
    B. prevent the formation of a corneal ulcer.
    C. relieve her anxiety.
    D. decrease the thyroid gland's vascularity.

24. Which of the following symptoms and signs would she most likely have on admission?
    A. constipation
    B. dry skin
    C. mood swings
    D. cold intolerance

25. What would you need to have available when she returned from surgery?
    A. nasogastric tube with suction
    B. oral suction
    C. cervical collar
    D. tracheostomy care kit

26. Which of the following medications would you need to have available for her?
    A. calcium gluconate
    B. levothyroxine sodium (Synthroid)
    C. propranolol (Inderal)
    D. SSKI

44

Management of Clients with Adrenal and Pituitary Disorders

Adrenal and pituitary disorders can affect many body systems and thus lead to a wide variety of problems. Providing client education is an essential part of nursing care so that clients with these disorders can maintain healthy lives. In order to teach clients, nurses need to gain an understanding of the pathophysiology which underlies these disorders. A review of normal physiology will greatly facilitate this process.

OBJECTIVES

44.1   Compare and contrast the signs and symptoms of adrenocortical insufficiency and adrenocortical hyperfunction.

44.2   Relate the signs and symptoms of Addison's disease to a decrease in production of each of the three groups of adrenocortical hormones.

44.3   Identify four conditions that may cause secondary adrenocortical insufficiency.

44.4   Discuss the danger of acute adrenal insufficiency (Addisonian crisis).

44.5   Describe two types of adrenocortical hyperfunction (Cushing's syndrome and Conn's syndrome) as to definition, etiology, assessment and methods of diagnosis, and interventions.

44.6   Describe the adrenomedullary disorder of pheochromocytoma as to pathophysiology, usual signs and symptoms, methods of diagnosis, and interventions.

44.7   Discuss nursing responsibilities regarding laboratory diagnostic tests to detect specific dysfunctions of the adrenal glands.

44.8   Identify nursing diagnoses based on the needs of clients experiencing dysfunction of the adrenal glands.

44.9   Plan nursing interventions that will decrease the risk of acute paroxysmal hypertension preoperatively and profound shock postoperatively for a person undergoing surgical excision of a pheochromocytoma.

Objectives (Continued)

44.10 Recognize the signs of under- and overdosage of corticosteroids.

44.11 Develop a teaching plan for helping a person learn self-administration of steroids.

44.12 List nursing interventions, with rationale for each action, necessary for a person experiencing Addisonian crisis.

44.13 Summarize the pre- and postoperative nursing care of clients undergoing unilateral or bilateral adrenalectomy.

44.14 Describe hyperpituitarism and hypopituitarism as to etiology, assessment and diagnostic methods, and interventions.

44.15 Compare and contrast the signs and symptoms of diabetes insipidus with the syndrome of inappropriate antidiuretic hormone (SIADH).

44.16 Describe diabetes insipidus and SIADH as to etiology, assessment and diagnostic methods, and interventions.

44.17 Discuss teaching needed by the person who is to undergo surgical removal of the pituitary gland.

44.18 Describe a focused but thorough nurse's assessment of the person prior to surgical removal of the pituitary gland.

44.19 Differentiate between nursing assessment and intervention following hypophysectomy via a craniotomy and via the transsphenoidal approach.

Putting It All Together: Care Plan for a Client with Addison's Disease

Ms. B. is a 58-year-old widow who lives alone on her family farm. She has Addison's disease and has been maintained on hydrocortisone 30 mg orally (PO) daily. Now, she is admitted to the hospital with weakness, dizziness, and weight loss. She appears thin and anxious and says she needs to be back on the farm to gather the vegetables from her garden and tend to the chickens and dogs. Her hands, forearms, and face have a deep tan. Her orders include serum electrolytes and glucose, adrenocorticotropic hormone (ACTH) stimulation test, 24-hour urine for 17 OH and ketosteroids, hydrocortisone 30 mg PO daily, fluid intake over 1500 cc/24 hours, and a liberal sodium diet.

1. Develop a care plan for Ms. B. Include nursing actions to meet the following desired goal. No development of adrenal crisis as evidenced by: normal mental status, normal skin turgor, normal serum sodium and potassium, stable vital signs, and no nausea, vomiting, or abdominal pain.

CLIENT EDUCATION: KNOWING WHAT TO TEACH AND WHY

■ Discharge Teaching for a Client Posthypophysectomy

The following items should be included as the important things to report to the health care professional when teaching a client posthypophysectomy:

excessive thirst	constant swallowing	double or blurred vision	fatigue
stiff neck	persistent headache	increased nasal congestion	impotence
weight gain	sensitivity to cold	decreased sex drive	loss of appetite

Which of the signs or symptoms listed above could indicate:

2. the need for thyroid replacement?

3. the need for gonadotropin replacement therapy?

4. the need for ADH replacement?

5. that there may be a leak in the cerebrospinal fluid (CSF)?

6. that meningitis may be present?

Management of Clients with Diabetes Mellitus

Diabetes mellitus is the most common endocrine disorder, and complications from this disorder make it the third leading cause of death by disease in the United States. Complications from diabetes mellitus make it the leading cause of new blindness in adults, the leading cause of new cases of renal failure, and the leading cause of amputations of the lower extremities. It is also responsible for increased risk of coronary artery disease and strokes. As a nurse you will probably work with clients who have diabetes mellitus because you will encounter them in any field of nursing you choose. The primary responsibility of the nurse is to teach the client self-care for management of this lifelong condition.

OBJECTIVES

45.1   Discuss current knowledge regarding the etiology of diabetes mellitus.

45.2   Describe the effect of diabetes mellitus on carbohydrate, fat, and protein metabolism.

45.3   List the cardinal symptoms of diabetes mellitus and give the pathophysiologic basis for each.

45.4   Compare and contrast two common types of diabetes mellitus: type I and type II.

45.5   Discuss methods of early detection and assessment factors used in screening and diagnosis of diabetes mellitus.

45.6   Discuss the goal of care for clients with diabetes mellitus and include the criteria for "good control."

45.7   Teach the client the importance of balancing diet, exercise, and rest in order to control or regulate blood glucose levels.

45.8   State the action, side effects, and nursing implications for insulin and oral hypoglycemic agents.

45.9   List the nursing diagnoses, with rationale and intervention, commonly indicated with diabetes mellitus.

45.10   Differentiate between the pathophysiologies of diabetic ketoacidosis and hyperglycemic, hyperosmolar, nonketotic coma.

45.11   Describe clinical manifestations, diagnostic findings, and management for each of the acute complications listed in Objective 45.10.

OBJECTIVES (CONTINUED)

45.12 Differentiate among the long-term complications of diabetes mellitus regarding reversible and irreversible changes.

45.13 Identify the nurse's role in preventing long-term complications for a client with diabetes mellitus.

45.14 Explain the need for the special perioperative care necessary for a client with diabetes mellitus.

PUTTING IT ALL TOGETHER: MEAL PLANNING

1. Use the Dietary Guidelines for Americans (Food Guide Pyramid) issued by the U.S. Department of Agriculture (USDA) and Health and Human Services in 1992 to develop a menu plan for yourself for one day. In the table, write in the specific food serving to be used for each meal. Use foods which give 65% CHO, 15% protein, and 20% fat and 25 calories/kg to maintain your present weight.

MENU PLAN

Breakfast	Snack	Lunch	Snack	Dinner	Snack
Milk					
Vegetable					
Fruit					
Bread					
Meat					
Fat					

■ Review of Foot Care

Foot care is essential for the client with diabetes mellitus. Neglect or improper care could result in an amputation. Use the following questions as guidelines when providing care.

2. What type of shoes is the client wearing? Are they in good condition? Do they fit well?

3. What type of socks or stockings is the client wearing? Are they clean? Do they fit?

4. What is the color and temperature of the feet compared to that of the hands and forearms?

5. Is there any edema? If so, how much?

6. What is the skin condition? Dry or moist? Cuts or ulcers?

7. Does hair grow on the toes?

8. What is the condition of the toenails? Any in-grown? How are they cut?

9. Are there bunions, corns, calluses, or pressure points?

10. Are the peripheral pulses strong and equal bilaterally?

11. How is the sensation?

Include the following questions when interviewing the client to obtain data about foot care.

12. How often do you check your feet?

13. How often do you wash your feet? Do you check the water temperature? If so, how?

14. How do you dry your feet?

15. Do you put anything on your feet like lotions, powders, medicines? If so, what?

16. How do you trim your toenails?

17. If you get a cut or sore, what do you do about it?

18. Do your feet get cold? How do you keep them warm?

19. Do you ever go barefoot? What do you wear on your feet in the house?

20. Do your feet ever feel numb? Do they burn or hurt?

21. Have you ever had a nurse teach you how to care for your feet?

When teaching foot care, try to use the person's own foot care tools and have the client give a return demonstration. Use the "Bridge to Home Care" and the "Care Plan" on foot care in Chapter 45 of the text.

REVIEW OF INSULIN AND ORAL HYPOGLYCEMICS

Answer the following questions regarding medications given to control diabetes mellitus.

22. Why can't insulin be administered by mouth?

23. Which type of insulin can be administered intravenously?

24. How does exercise affect the body's need for insulin?

25. Does the level of stress a person is experiencing affect their insulin requirements? How?

26. If regular insulin is given subcutaneously before breakfast, when is a hypoglycemic reaction most likely to occur?

27. If regular and NPH insulins are given together before breakfast, when is a hypoglycemic reaction likely to occur?

28. How should insulin be stored?

29. Should the routine order of regular insulin before breakfast be given if the client is nothing by mouth (NPO) for a procedure such as a colonoscopy? Why or why not?

30. What type of syringes should be used to administer U-100 insulin and U-500 insulin?

31. How should glucagon be administered?

32. What is the reason for giving glucagon to a person with diabetes mellitus?

33. What are the actions of the oral hypoglycemics?

34. Draw the time-action curves of the two types of insulin, regular and NPH, given at 7:30 am. Pay particular attention to the peak action of each type of insulin, as this is the time when a hypoglycemic reaction is most likely to occur. Check your drawing by referring to Figure 45-2 in Chapter 45 of the text.

7 am   **1 pm**   **7 pm**   **1 am**   **7 am**

46

Management of Clients with Exocrine Pancreatic and Biliary Disorders

Nursing care of clients with disorders of the biliary system, particularly gallbladder disorders, is a relatively common experience. However, the medical therapy for these disorders is changing and these changes will require nursing care to refocus from care and teaching in the hospital setting to the outpatient and home care setting. For example, when caring for clients with pancreatic disorders, the frequency will not be as great but the complexity will still be present. One example is pain management for clients with both acute and chronic pancreatitis. Another example of challenging nursing care is maintaining nutrition for the client who initially cannot eat and, in later stages of the disease, has difficulty with digestion because of damage to the exocrine function of the pancreas. The complexity of the disorders and the rapidly changing technology require an understanding of the pathophysiology and medical therapy and nursing care that is carefully planned, flexible to changing client situations, and scientifically sound.

OBJECTIVES

46.1 Discuss clinical problems most frequently associated with the gallbladder and biliary tract and their medical, surgical, and nursing management.

46.2 Discuss clinical problems most frequently associated with the exocrine function of the pancreas and their medical, surgical, and nursing management.

LEARNING THE LANGUAGE: TERMINOLOGY RELATED TO NURSING CARE OF CLIENTS WITH BILIARY TRACT AND EXOCRINE PANCREATIC DISORDERS

Match the terms in Column A with the correct definition in Column B.

Column A

1. _____ Acalculous cholecystitis
2. _____ Cholangiography
3. _____ Cholecystectomy
4. _____ Cholecystitis
5. _____ Cholecystography
6. _____ Cholecystostomy
7. _____ Choledocholithiasis
8. _____ Choledochostomy
9. _____ Cholelithiasis
10. _____ ERCP
11. _____ Lithotripsy
12. _____ Murphy's Sign
13. _____ Ursodeoxycholic acid
14. _____ Whipple's disease

Column B

A. X-ray of bile ducts
B. Presence of gallstones
C. Inflammation of gallbladder without stones
D. X-ray of gallbladder
E. Incision and drainage of gallbladder
F. Endoscopic retrograde cholangiopancreatography
G. Exploration of common bile duct
H. Oral agent that dissolves stones
I. Stones in common bile duct
J. Cessation of breathing on inspiration and extreme pain
K. Removal of the gallbladder
L. Inflammation of the gallbladder
M. Pancreaticoduodenal resection
N. Shock waves used to crush gallbladder stones

THINKING CRITICALLY: UNDERSTANDING RATIONALES

Provide the rationales for the therapeutic nursing interventions listed below.

Intervention	**Rationale**

Client Postoperative Cholecystectomy

15. Use meticulous lung hygiene measures.

16. Pay attention to oral hygiene.

Client with Cholelithiasis

17. Insert nasogastric (NG) tube.

18. Assess for gag reflex after retrograde endoscopy.

19. Teach about low-fat meals.

Client with Pancreatitis

20. Assess for epigastric or umbilical pain that may extend to the back and flank.

21.   Assess for hypovolemic shock.

22.   Nothing by mouth (NPO) and/or gastric suctioning.

23.   Carefully assess lungs.

24.   Teach about restriction of alcohol, tea, coffee, spices, and heavy meals.

25.   Encourage clients to seek counseling as appropriate about alcohol problem.

Client with Chronic Pancreatitis
26.   Assess for hyperglycemia.

27.   Teach about use of pancreatic enzymes.

28.   What is the rationale for assessing for pregnancy before administering Chenodiol (chenodeoxycholic acid)?

Putting It All Together

■ Case Study

Ms. D. is a 45-year-old African-American female who is admitted to the hospital with a diagnosis of acute cholelithiasis. Past history includes four pregnancies with four live births, history of hypertension, a hysterectomy, oophorectomy, and salpingectomy 3 years ago. She is taking hormone replacement and antihypertensive medication. Assessment data include: height 6' 2", weight 165 lbs., B/P 140/84, P 88 reg, T 99.6° F. Her chief complaint is of pain starting in the upper abdominal area which worsens after meals with fried foods. She rates her pain a 7 on a scale of 10. Laboratory values include white blood cell count (WBC) of 10,000/mm³ and total bilirubin of 1.0 mg/dl.

29.   Based on the information listed above, what data would be considered risk factors for gallbladder disease?
A.   race, gender, and number of pregnancies
B.   age, hormone replacement, and weight
C.   hypertension, gender, and race
D.   hysterectomy, number of pregnancies, and weight

Ms. D. is scheduled for a cholecystectomy and common bile duct exploration.

30. In completing preoperative teaching, the nurse would include which of the following explanations?
    A. information about a midabdomen vertical incision
    B. information on extracorporeal shock wave therapy to break up the gallstones
    C. a description of a T-tube
    D. information about taking insulin postoperatively

31. If Ms. D. had an elevated bilirubin level, the most likely explanation would be a stone blocking the
    A. common bile duct.
    B. gallbladder.
    C. ampulla of vater.
    D. cystic duct.

32. Preoperatively, the physician will more likely order meperidine (Demerol) than morphine to treat Ms. D.'s pain because
    A. Demerol is a stronger narcotic.
    B. morphine has more respiratory effects.
    C. morphine can increase spasms of the sphincter of Oddi.
    D. only Demerol can be given intravenously.

33. Postoperatively, if Ms. D. were to have a T-tube, nursing care plans would include which of the following?
    A. Hang drainage bag below the bed.
    B. Report first day's output of 500 cc to physician.
    C. Irrigate the T-tube every 4 hours.
    D. Record volume and color of drainage every 8 hours.

CHAPTER 47

Management of Clients with Hepatic Disorders

Clients with disorders of the hepatic system present multiple challenges for nursing care. It is particularly important with these disorders to understand the underlying pathophysiology as this understanding will help the nurse develop plans of care that include assessment for important complications of hepatic disorders—complications that can be life-threatening. With hepatitis it is critical for nurses to understand the need for and use of safety precautions to protect themselves. There may also be situations that necessitate a nonjudgmental approach to nursing care, such as when the client's disorder is caused by alcohol intake. Additionally, there are some aspects of primary prevention that nurses can teach clients in order to prevent some of the hepatitis disorders.

OBJECTIVES

47.1   Discuss the liver disorder jaundice and related medical and nursing management.

47.2   Describe the clinical problems associated with hepatitis and related medical and nursing management.

47.3   Discuss the liver disorder cirrhosis and its medical, surgical, and nursing management.

47.4   Define other hepatic disorders.

47.5   Describe surgical, medical, nursing, and long-term management of the client with a liver transplant.

LEARNING THE LANGUAGE: TERMINOLOGY RELATED TO LIVER DISORDERS

Match the terms in Column A with the correct definition in Column B.

Column A

1. _____ Active immunization
2. _____ Ascites
3. _____ Asterixis
4. _____ Bilirubin
5. _____ Esophageal varices
6. _____ Hepatitis
7. _____ Hepatic encephalopathy
8. _____ Icterus
9. _____ Passive immunity
10. _____ Portal hypertension
11. _____ Sengstaken-Blakemore
12. _____ Sclerotherapy

Column B

A. Yellow pigmentation of the skin; jaundice
B. Bile pigment, product of red blood cell breakdown
C. Inflammation of the liver
D. Abnormal muscle tremors; liver flap
E. Fluid accumulation in the peritoneum
F. Increase in pressure in the portal vein resulting from obstruction of blood flow through the liver
G. Nasogastric tube used in the treatment of esophageal varices through inflation of balloons that provide tamponade on the bleeding varices
H. Injection with a killed virus vaccine to produce immunity
I. Immune globulin given after exposure to hepatitis
J. Enlarged esophageal veins resulting from portal hypertension
K. CNS disturbances caused by a buildup of ammonia in the blood
L. Treatment for esophageal varices involving injection of sclerosing agent

Match the liver disorders in Column A with the correct description in Column B.

Column A

13. _____ Amyloidosis
14. _____ Caroli's syndrome
15. _____ Congenital hepatic fibrosis
16. _____ Hemochromatosis
17. _____ Wilson's disease

Column B

A. Congenital disorder of the liver characterized by portal fibrosis
B. Congenital disorder that leads to accumulation of copper in the liver, brain, and kidney
C. Congenital disorder of the liver characterized by dilated bile ducts and cyst formation
D. Proteinaceous, starch-like substance that infiltrates the liver and other organs causing the tissue to cease functioning
E. A recessive inherited metabolic defect that causes increased iron absorption from the gastrointestinal tract

Match the descriptions in Column A with the appropriate laboratory test in Column B. (More than one answer may apply.)

Column A		Column B
18. _____ Indicates previous exposure and immunity to hepatitis A	A.	HAV–Ab/IgM
	B.	HAV–Ab/IgG
19. _____ Indicates progression from active hepatitis to chronic hepatitis B	C.	HBsAg
	D.	HBsAb
20. _____ Indicates past infection with hepatitis B	E.	HBgAb
21. _____ Indicates acute stage of hepatitis A	F.	HBeAg
22. _____ Indicates previous exposure to hepatitis B, a continuous chronic infection, or immunization with hepatitis B vaccine		
23. _____ Indicates resolution of acute stage of hepatitis B		
24. _____ Indicates that the person is infectious		

Match the descriptions in Column A with the type of hepatitis in Column B. (More than one answer may apply.)

Column A		Column B
25. _____ Always found with hepatitis B	A.	Hepatitis A
26. _____ Also known as infectious hepatitis	B.	Hepatitis B
27. _____ Spread by carriers	C.	Hepatitis C
28. _____ Spread by blood	D.	Hepatitis D
29. _____ Primary prevention by careful hand-washing	E.	Hepatitis E
30. _____ Primary prevention by active immunity	F.	Toxic hepatitis
31. _____ Caused by benzene and chloroform		
32. _____ Health care workers at risk		
33. _____ Spread by contaminated shellfish, water, and milk		
34. _____ Contracted through travel in high-incidence areas		

Match the types of jaundice in Column A with the correct description in Column B and which bilirubin test will be elevated with the disorder in Column C. (More than one answer may apply.)

Column A		Column B		Column C
35. _____ Hemolytic jaundice	A.	Defective uptake, conjugation, or transport of bilirubin by the liver	a.	Conjugated (direct bilirubin)
36. _____ Hepatocellular jaundice			b.	Unconjugated (indirect bilirubin)
37. _____ Obstructive jaundice	B.	Impaired bilirubin transport and excretion in the biliary system	c.	Total bilirubin
	C.	Results from excessive blood cell destruction		

THINKING CRITICALLY: KNOWING WHAT TO DO AND WHY

Provide short answers to the following questions.

38. The client has an elevated bilirubin and severe pruritus. Identify appropriate nursing interventions.

39. Describe the cause and outcome of portal hypertension with cirrhosis.

40. Identify nursing interventions for the following nursing diagnosis: Potential for decreased cardiac output related to blood volume loss secondary to rupture of esophageal varices and resultant secondary bleeding.

41. Identify the three main causes of ascites and the pathophysiologic bases for these.

42. List four measures used to assess ascites.

43. Describe the causes of hepatic encephalopathy.

44. List nursing measures to assess a person at risk for developing hepatic encephalopathy.

45. Explain the rationale and methods for reducing protein and bacteria in the gastrointestinal tract as a treatment for hepatic encephalopathy.

46. Your client with cirrhosis and ascites has a nursing diagnosis of Ineffective breathing pattern. What nursing interventions would you implement? Why?

47. Your client is post-op for a liver transplant and at risk for rejection of the donor tissue. What key assessments would you need to make?

PUTTING IT ALL TOGETHER

■ Case Study

Mr. G., 36, is admitted to the medicine unit with symptoms of jaundice, lethargy, loss of appetite, nausea, and aching joints. He states that he has had these symptoms for about one week. His preliminary diagnosis is hepatitis. The physician orders laboratory tests to confirm the diagnosis.

48. If Mr. G. has hepatitis B, which of the following laboratory studies would be positive?
    A. HBsAb
    B. HBsAg
    C. HBcAb
    D. HBV–Ab/IgM

Mr. G.'s diagnosis of hepatitis B is confirmed.

49. Precautions to use when caring for Mr. G. include
    A. wearing a mask while giving direct care.
    B. wearing gloves when entering the room.
    C. ordering meals on disposable dishes.
    D. marking the patient's serum with special labels.

50. When Mr. G.'s appetite returns, the usual diet recommendations include
    A. low protein and carbohydrates, with moderate fat.
    B. normal protein, high carbohydrates, and low fat.
    C. moderate protein, high carbohydrates, and low fat.
    D. high protein and carbohydrates, with moderate fat.

51. Mr. G.'s nurse has identified a nursing diagnosis of Activity intolerance related to fatigue. Which of the following interventions would be most appropriate to include under this diagnosis?
    A. Encourage ambulation three times daily.
    B. Ambulate as tolerated without fatigue.
    C. Encourage total bed rest.
    D. Encourage active range of motion three times a day.

52. Mr. G. has an order for prochlorperazine maleate (Compazine) 10 mg IM q 4–6 hours p.r.n. for nausea. The nurse would
    A. give the Compazine as ordered.
    B. verify the order with the physician.
    C. give Compazine 5 mg.
    D. give Compazine 10 mg suppository.

53. Mr. G.'s discharge plans would most likely include which of the following?
    A. Resume usual activity level.
    B. Limit total calories to 2000 daily.
    C. Avoid alcohol and aspirin.
    D. Get passive immunization vaccine.

Integumentary Disorders

ANATOMY AND PHYSIOLOGY REVIEW: THE INTEGUMENTARY SYSTEM

Skin, the largest body organ, acts as a thermoregulator to help maintain a normal body temperature and serves as a protector between the body's internal and external environments. Skin is also the most visible body organ and is important to one's body image. It is necessary for a sense of touch, which is an important means of communication.

OBJECTIVES

10.1   Describe the structure and function of the following three layers of the skin: (1) epidermal (epidermis), (2) dermal (dermis), and (3) subcutaneous (subcutaneous fat).

10.2   Describe the structure and function of the following epidermal appendages: eccrine and apocrine sweat units, sebaceous glands, hair, and nails.

10.3   Discuss the effects of normal aging on the skin.

PUTTING IT ALL TOGETHER

■ *Review of Skin Structure and Function*

Label the specific parts of the three layers of the skin in the following diagram.

1.   5.

2.   6.

3.   7.

4.   8.

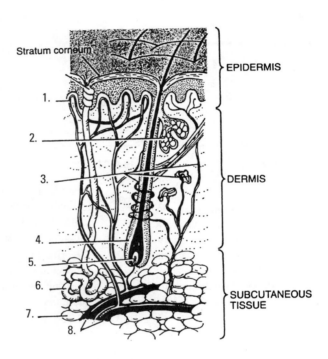

Give the function of each of the specific parts identified above (in the same order).

9.   13.

10.   14.

11.   15.

12.   16.

CHAPTER

48

Assessment of the Integumentary System

Thorough assessment is needed for accurate diagnosis of skin disorders and the nurse is often given the opportunity to assess the client's skin. A well-lit, private room is conducive to obtaining a thorough assessment because inspection is so important. Symptoms of systemic disorders are often observed in the skin. Knowledge of biocultural differences is essential for accurately assessing integumentary disorders in clients of all races and cultures.

OBJECTIVES

48.1   Obtain a thorough health history, including pertinent past history as well as current abnormalities or problems related to an integumentary assessment.

48.2   Use observation and palpation to obtain an accurate physical integumentary assessment.

48.3   Explain in layman's terminology commonly used diagnostic skin procedures.

48.4   Identify biocultural variations in assessing the integumentary system.

LEARNING THE LANGUAGE: TERMINOLOGY RELATED TO ASSESSMENT OF SKIN LESIONS

Match the definitions of types of skin lesions in Column A with the correct term in Column B.

Column A	Column B
1. _____ Irregularly shaped, exudative, depressed lesion in which entire epidermis and upper layer of dermis are lost; results from trauma or tissue destruction	A. Atrophy
2. _____ Wasting of epidermis; skin appears thin and transparent	B. Bulla
3. _____ Dried serum, blood, or pus on skin surface	C. Crust
4. _____ Elevated lesion that is larger than a nodule; may be benign or malignant	D. Cyst
5. _____ Elevated thick-walled lesion containing fluid or semisolid matter	E. Excoriation
6. _____ Elevated lesion containing serous fluid; usually less than 1 cm	F. Fissure
7. _____ Skin color change without elevation; less than 1 cm	G. Lichenification
8. _____ Elevated, solid lesion; less than 1 cm; varies in color	H. Macule
9. _____ Dried fragments of sloughed epidermal cells	I. Papule
10. _____ Fleeting skin elevation; irregularly shaped due to edema	J. Plaque
11. _____ Superficial linear abrasion of epidermis	K. Pustule
12. _____ Epidermal thickening resulting in elevated plaque with skin markings	L. Scale
13. _____ Raised, flat lesion formed from merging papules or nodules	M. Tumor
14. _____ Deep linear split through epidermis into dermis	N. Ulcer
15. _____ Elevated lesion containing purulent material; less than 1 cm	O. Vesicle
16. _____ Large, elevated, fluid-filled lesion; greater than 1 cm	P. Wheal

DIAGNOSTIC TESTS: KNOWING WHAT TO DO AND WHY

Explain in layman's terms the following diagnostic tests related to the integumentary system.

17.   Wood's light exam

18.   Excision biopsy

49

Management of Clients with Integumentary Disorders

Nurses need to know how to use topical medications and therapies because nurses frequently manage skin care and disorders. Since the client is often responsible for self-care for dermatologic disorders, the nurse needs to be able to teach self-care information. Prejudice against clients with skin diseases must be avoided. The client with skin problems may withdraw from social situations and it is important that health care professionals be accepting and available to help.

Successful plastic surgery requires a high degree of client participation. Many plastic surgery procedures are done on an outpatient basis; therefore, important aspects of nursing care for these clients are postoperative teaching and discharge planning. Nursing care of all clients having plastic surgery, whether as an outpatient or inpatient, includes physiologic and psychological aspects.

OBJECTIVES

49.1 Discuss common dermatologic topical therapies as to action and nursing interventions.

49.2 Describe the purpose and possible complications of ultraviolet light treatment.

49.3 Discuss the psychosocial aspects of skin disorders and associated nursing implications.

49.4 Describe inflammatory skin conditions, in general, as to pathophysiology and etiology, and appropriate nursing and medical interventions.

49.5 Give examples of inflammatory skin conditions (pruritus, eczema/dermatitis, psoriasis, acne, and pemphigus).

49.6 Describe the risk factors, pathophysiology, and four stages of pressure ulcers.

49.7 Discuss medical and nursing interventions for the client with pressure ulcers.

49.8 Describe skin infections and infestations, in general, as to pathophysiology and etiology, and appropriate nursing and medical interventions.

49.9 Give some examples of skin infections (bacterial, fungal, viral, parasitic).

49.10 Describe common nail disorders, in general, as to pathophysiology and etiology, and appropriate nursing and medical interventions.

OBJECTIVES (CONTINUED)

49.11   Discuss the following specific premalignant and malignant skin conditions as to pathophysiology and etiology, and appropriate nursing and medical interventions: actinic keratosis, basal cell carcinoma, squamous cell carcinoma, malignant melanoma, mycosis fungoides, and Kaposi's sarcoma.

49.12   Outline specific ways to protect the skin from sunlight.

49.13   Teach the client skin self-examination.

49.14   Differentiate between the purposes of aesthetic plastic surgery and reconstructive surgery.

49.15   Differentiate between expectations of clients having aesthetic plastic surgery and those having reconstructive surgery.

49.16   List the basic principles of plastic surgery.

49.17   Discuss how body image is an important consideration when providing care for clients undergoing plastic surgery.

49.18   Outline the following common plastic surgical procedures by including the purpose, brief description of the procedure, and potential complications: rhytidectomy, blepharoplasty, rhinoplasty, and lipectomy.

49.19   Differentiate among the types of grafts used in reconstructive surgery.

49.20   Discuss nursing assessment and interventions for a client with a recent skin graft or tissue transfer that focus on promoting capillary formation.

49.21   Describe laser treatment used in plastic surgery.

49.22   Describe assessment findings characteristic of facial fractures.

49.23   Discuss types of facial fractures and stabilization procedures.

49.24   Discuss general nursing intervention for the client with facial fractures.

49.25   Discuss general nursing intervention for the client with facial lacerations.

49.26   Discuss immediate care of a client following traumatic amputation.

49.27   Describe, in general terms, replantation surgery.

49.28   Discuss nursing intervention for the client following replantation.

THINKING CRITICALLY: UNDERSTANDING RATIONALES

■ Topical Medications

Listed below are some important considerations of medications administered topically for treating integumentary disorders. List the rationales for these considerations.

Consideration	**Rationale**

Antipruritic

1.   Apply frequently if the drug contains no anesthetic.

2.   Assess for contact sensitivity.

Antiviral

3.   Apply with a gloved hand.

4.   Start treatment early during prodromal stage.

Keratolytic

5.   Apply carefully only to lesion.

6.   Cover with dressing.

Corticosteroids

7.   Apply in thin, even amounts.

8.   Monitor length of treatment.

Emollients

9.   Avoid applying petrolatum-based products to intertriginous sites.

10.   Reapply when product has worn off or been absorbed.

Tars

11.   Advise person how to restrict sun exposure.

12.   Advise person to wear old, easily washed clothing.

Scabicides/Pediculicides

13.   Advise person to contact physician or nurse if pruritus occurs following treatment.

14.   Discourage repeated and unnecessary use.

THINKING CRITICALLY: KNOWING WHAT TO DO AND WHY

■ *Dermatologic Disorders*

Provide short answers to the following questions.

Who is at high risk for developing the following disorders?

15.   Skin cancer

16.   Decubitus ulcers

17.   Stasis dermatitis

18.   Systemic infection from a local skin disorder

19.   Yeast and fungal infections

20. What are appropriate nursing interventions to relieve pruritus due to dry skin?

21. What is the most effective medical treatment for acne?

22. What is the most common skin lesion in the elderly?

23. Why does a potential for self-concept alteration often accompany psoriasis?

24. What is the etiology of herpes zoster and what is the recommended treatment?

25. Which stage of pressure ulcers is a full-thickness skin loss involving damage or necrosis of subcutaneous tissue but not the underlying fascia?

26. How often should the client with a pressure ulcer be repositioned?

27. What is the causative organism in cellulitis?

28. What are potential complications from cellulitis?

29. Which skin cancer has the greatest metastatic potential? Which has the least?

Thinking Critically: Understanding Rationales

■ Clients Undergoing Plastic Surgery

Provide the rationales for the following nursing interventions.

Intervention	Rationale
30. Preoperatively, ask open-ended questions about postsurgical expectations.	
31. Postoperatively, report to the surgeon the presence of blisters in the area of a skin graft.	
32. Gently assist the client in looking at and touching the healed surgical site.	
33. Teach clients who are discharged following rhytidectomy to sleep with the head of their bed elevated for one week following surgery.	
34. Position a client who has a flap so that the flap can be assessed at all times.	
35. Instruct a woman not to raise her arms above her head for three weeks following breast reconstructive surgery with implants.	
36. Administer mannitol intravenously, as ordered, to the client following a blepharoplasty.	
37. Administer adequate analgesia to the client following an abdominoplasty.	
38. Following blepharoplasty, teach the client to use eye drops during the day and eye ointment at night for a few days.	
39. Preoperatively, assess near and distant vision of a client who is having a blepharoplasty.	
40. Administer a test dose of collagen in the client's forearm prior to collagen injections.	

■ *Clients Undergoing Plastic Surgery* **(Continued)**

Intervention	Rationale
41. Use the pulse oximeter to monitor for viability of reimplanted digits.	
42. Assess for excessive swallowing in the client following a rhinoplasty.	
43. Instruct individuals with nasal fractures to sneeze through the mouth and not to blow the nose.	
44. Keep suction equipment and a wire cutter easily available at the bedside of a client whose jaws are wired shut.	
45. Teach the client with facial incision lines to keep the incision lines clean by applying a topical antibiotic and not to allow the incision lines to get wet.	
46. Give aspirin as prescribed following replantation.	
47. Instruct a woman with a subpectoral implant not to wear a bra immediately postoperatively.	
48. Administer oral care following repair of facial fractures.	
49. Report a decrease in temperature of 2° C or more in an hour or a decline to 32° C (89.6° F) as measured by the temperature probe placed on the replanted extremity.	

Management of Clients with Burn Injury

The American Burn Association has developed an injury severity grading system that categorizes burns as major, moderate, and minor (see Table 50-2 in Chapter 50 of the text). Clients with minor burns are often treated in the clinic or emergency department. Clients with moderate burns usually require hospitalization. It is preferable that clients with major burns be treated in a burn center or facility with expertise in burn care. A major burn injury is a traumatic event requiring a long recovery period. Psychological rehabilitation is as important as physical rehabilitation in the overall recovery process.

OBJECTIVES

50.1   Discuss the etiology of burns by describing four categories of burn injuries.

50.2   Identify specific areas to address when planning strategies to prevent burns.

50.3   Describe the systemic effects of burns.

50.4   Describe the effects of carbon monoxide and smoke poisoning.

50.5   List the factors determining burn severity.

50.6   Describe the major categories of burn depth.

50.7   Assess burn size by the "Rule of Nines" technique.

50.8   Describe the Berkow method of determining burn size.

50.9   Discuss how burn location, the medical history and age of the client, and mechanism of injury affect burn severity.

50.10   Discuss appropriate interventions during the emergent phase for the following types of burns: thermal, chemical, and electrical.

50.11   Identify nursing diagnoses common for burned clients.

50.12   Discuss specific nursing interventions, including assessment, appropriate for each of the above nursing diagnoses.

50.13   Describe airway management and oxygen therapy for the client with burns.

50.14   Discuss fluid resuscitation in the first 24 hours and second 24 hours following burn injury.

OBJECTIVES (CONTINUED)

50.15   Describe management of the client with a circumferential burn.

50.16   Identify basic principles of infection control.

50.17   Discuss hydrotherapy as to purpose, advantages and disadvantages, and nursing considerations.

50.18   Describe the major methods of debridement as to purpose, and advantages and disadvantages.

50.19   Discuss topical therapy as to purpose, advantages and disadvantages, and nursing considerations of specific examples.

50.20   Differentiate between the two methods of burn wound management: (1) open and (2) closed.

50.21   Discuss care of the skin graft and the donor site.

50.22   Differentiate among the main types of biologic dressings and synthetic dressings.

50.23   Describe the aggressive nutritional support necessary for the client with burns.

50.24   Discuss pharmacologic and nonpharmacologic methods of pain management.

50.25   Describe the psychosocial reactions typical of burned clients.

50.26   Demonstrate correct methods of positioning to prevent contractures.

THINKING CRITICALLY: KNOWING WHAT TO DO AND WHY

■ Care of the Client with Burn Injuries

1.   What are the four causes of burns?

2.   How can nurses help in the prevention of burn injuries?

3.   What six factors determine the severity of a burn?

4.   What is the appearance of each category of burn depth?

5.   What is the sensation of each category of burn depth?

6.   What is the course of each category of burn depth (time and factors associated with healing)?

7. Why would the nurse assess capillary refill following a burn injury? How?

8. Burns in which location are associated with pulmonary complications?

9. Burns in which location are highly prone to infection?

10. Which age groups have a higher mortality with similar burns?

11. Why are electrical burns so dangerous?

12. What are the major goals of first aid for a burned person?

13. Why should information be obtained from a burned person as soon as possible after the injury?

14. What assessment findings are associated with burn shock?

15. What is the appropriate intervention to prevent burn shock?

16. What is an escharotomy and why is it done?

17. How can localized infection after a burn injury be controlled?

18. How should medications to control pain be administered to the burned person?

19. Why are there special nutritional needs for the burned person?

20. How long are pressure garments worn?

21. Given the following situation, compute the size of body surface area burned by first using the "Rule of Nines" without a chart (see Figure 50-8 in Chapter 50 of the text), and then using the Lund and Browder formula (similar to the Berkow formula), with the chart provided below.

On physical exam, a 33-year-old male has large, thick-walled blisters over deep red, wet, and shiny tissue over all his upper extremities and half of his face. The upper half of his face is red with small, thin blisters. His hands appear dry and deep red with some brown tissue.

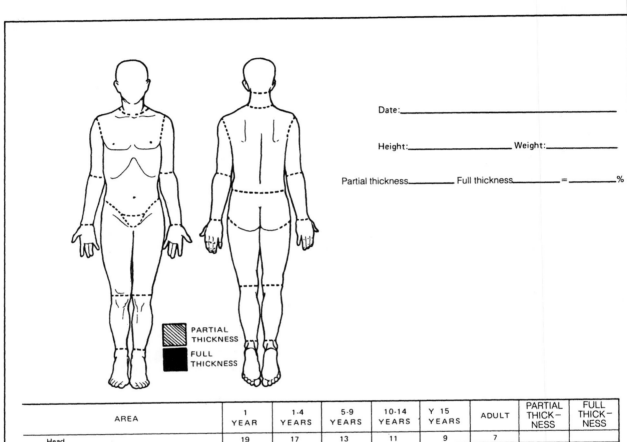

Date:_____

Height:_____ Weight:_____

Partial thickness_____ Full thickness_____ = _____%

AREA	1 YEAR	1-4 YEARS	5-9 YEARS	10-14 YEARS	Y 15 YEARS	ADULT	PARTIAL THICK- NESS	FULL THICK- NESS
Head	19	17	13	11	9	7		
Neck	2	2	2	2	2	2		
Ant. Trunk	13	13	13	13	13	13		
Post.Trunk	13	13	13	13	13	13		
R. Buttock	2½	2½	2½	2½	2½	2½		
L. Buttock	2½	2½	2½	2½	2½	2½		
Genitalia	1	1	1	1	1	1		
R. U. Arm	4	4	4	4	4	4		
L. U. Arm	4	4	4	4	4	4		
R. L. Arm	3	3	3	3	3	3		
L. L. Arm	3	3	3	3	3	3		
R. Hand	2½	2½	2½	2½	2½	2½		
L. Hand	2½	2½	2½	2½	2½	2½		
R. Thigh	5½	6½	8	8½	9	9½		
L. Thigh	5½	6½	8	8½	9	9½		
R. Leg	5	5	5½	6	6½	7		
L. Leg	5	5	5½	6	6½	7		
R. Foot	3½	3½	3½	3½	3½	3½		
L. Foot	3½	3½	3½	3½	3½	3½		
TOTAL								

HOSP. NO.	NAME	ROOM

22. What is the primary goal during the emergent phase following a burn injury?
    A. prevent infection
    B. maintain organ perfusion
    C. control pain
    D. promote healing

23. How thick should a topical antimicrobial agent be applied to a burned area?
    A. 1/16"
    B. 1/4"
    C. 1/2"
    D. 1"

24. Which of the following actions is appropriate for donor site care?
    A. Change dressing daily.
    B. Use normal saline wet-to-dry dressings.
    C. Keep fine-mesh gauze dressing dry.
    D. Apply topical antimicrobial ointment b.i.d.

25. Which of the following lab values will be decreased in the acute phase of a major burn injury?
    A. hematocrit
    B. hemoglobin
    C. serum potassium
    D. blood urea nitrogen (BUN)

26. When should a p.r.n. pain medication be given in relation to a dressing change?
    A. 1 hour before
    B. 30 minutes before
    C. during
    D. immediately after

Circulatory Disorders

ANATOMY AND PHYSIOLOGY REVIEW: THE CIRCULATORY SYSTEM

The peripheral vascular system is the vascular system outside of the heart and aorta. It is composed of arteries, arterioles, capillaries, venules, veins, and lymphatic channels. Overall, the main purpose of the peripheral vascular system is to deliver oxygen and nutrients to the cells and to carry carbon dioxide and other metabolic waste to excretory organs. In addition, hormones and vasoactive substances are transported through the peripheral vascular system.

Blood flow in the peripheral vascular system depends on the efficiency of the heart as a pump and patency of the blood vessels. Circulation is influenced by blood viscosity (thickness), hydration, mechanisms affecting coagulation and fibrinolysis of the blood, and local changes in the size of the vessels.

OBJECTIVES

11.1 Discuss the major terms related to the peripheral vascular system.

11.2 Identify the major structures of the peripheral vascular system.

11.3 Discuss the functions of the peripheral vascular system.

11.4 Explain the mechanisms that maintain arterial blood pressure.

11.5 Discuss blood flow through the tissues.

11.6 Discuss the effect of aging on the peripheral vascular system.

LEARNING THE LANGUAGE: TERMINOLOGY RELATED TO ANATOMY AND PHYSIOLOGY OF THE CIRCULATORY SYSTEM

Fill in the blanks.

1. Arteries carry oxygenated blood _____ the heart.

2. The _____ layer provides a smooth passageway for blood. It is the layer that atherosclerosis begins.

3. Approximately 75% of the total blood volume at any given time is found in the _____ _____ system.

4. The functional units of the peripheral vascular systems are the _____.

5. The lymphatic system returns _____ fluid to the general circulation and assists with immune reactions and _____ digestion.

6. The spleen, thymus, and _____ are all lymph organs.

7. Ultimately all lymphatics converge and empty into the junction of the internal jugular and right subclavian veins at two main ducts: the _____ duct and the right lymphatic duct.

■ Blood Flow Through the Large Arteries

Match the terms in Column A with the descriptions in Column B.

Column A **Column B**

8. _____ The veins' ability to stretch
9. _____ Regulates the diameter of blood vessels
10. _____ Constricts and dilates to maintain peripheral vascular resistance
11. _____ Regulates blood pressure by sensing pressure changes in the aortic arch, carotid sinus, and right atrium
12. _____ Developed by excess venous pressure
13. _____ Senses arterial oxygen, carbon dioxide, and hydrogen ion pressures
14. _____ Small oval bodies that lymph flows through
15. _____ Pressure within the large systemic arteries

A. Arterial blood pressure
B. Vasomotor nerve fibers
C. Arterioles
D. Baroreceptors
E. Aortic and carotid bodies
F. Lymph nodes
G. Incompetent valves
H. Capacitance vessels

THINKING CRITICALLY

■ Effects of Chemicals and Hormones

Match the chemicals or hormones in Column A with the effect in Column B.

Column A **Column B**

16. _____ Bradykinin
17. _____ Norepinephrine
18. _____ Acetylcholine
19. _____ Renin
20. _____ Vasopressin
21. _____ Histamine
22. _____ Epinephrine
23. _____ Serotonin
24. _____ Angiotensin II

A. Constriction
B. Vasodilation

■ *Factors that Influence Venous Return*

Indicate how the following factors affect venous return. Mark (I) for increase or (D) for decrease.

25. _____ Person in sitting position
26. _____ Legs elevated
27. _____ Prolonged standing
28. _____ Flexing calf muscles
29. _____ Bed rest

30. _____ Walking
31. _____ Inhalation
32. _____ Valsalva's maneuver
33. _____ Vasodilator medications

THINKING CRITICALLY: SHORT ANSWER QUESTIONS

34. What is the difference between arteriosclerosis and atherosclerosis?

35. Why are arteriosclerosis and atherosclerosis commonly diagnosed in the older population?

36. How do vasodilators and vasoconstrictors affect the arterial blood pressure?

51

Assessment of the Vascular System

A thorough health history provides the basis for a peripheral vascular assessment. The nurse needs to have a good understanding of the structure and function of the peripheral vascular system and the risk factors and etiology of peripheral vascular disorders. Demographic and biographical data, family history, current medications, diet and exercise, and a review of systems can help the nurse identify those clients who have, or are at risk for, peripheral vascular disorders.

The physical examination follows the health history. The mnemonic "8 Ps of peripheral vascular assessment" can guide the nurse in gathering pertinent physical assessment data. Diagnostic tests and procedures supplement the assessment data. Nurses must prepare the client physically and psychologically for these tests. In addition, they must monitor the client after tests and anticipate and plan for possible complications.

OBJECTIVES

51.1   Describe important assessment data to obtain during the peripheral vascular nursing history.

51.2   Discuss signs and symptoms associated with peripheral vascular disorders.

51.3   Perform basic physical assessment of the peripheral vascular system.

51.4   Describe pathophysiologic bases for selected assessment data.

51.5   Describe pre- and postprocedure nursing care of selected noninvasive and invasive diagnostic techniques.

LEARNING THE LANGUAGE: TERMINOLOGY RELATED TO ASSESSMENT OF PERIPHERAL VASCULAR DISORDER

Match the statements in Column A with the correct term in Column B.

Column A

1. _____ Caused by turbulent blood flow
2. _____ Indicates possible phlebothrombosis
3. _____ Assesses patency of radial and ulnar artery
4. _____ Caused by long-standing lymphatic obstruction
5. _____ Fluid accumulation in the tissue
6. _____ Assesses venous disorders
7. _____ Assesses arterial disorders
8. _____ Cramping leg pain upon walking
9. _____ Pain and paresthesia during rest
10. _____ The distance the client is able to walk without pain

Column B

A. Intermittent claudication
B. Rest pain
C. Homans' sign
D. Allen's test
E. Pitting edema
F. Brawny edema
G. Trendelenburg's test
H. Claudication distance
I. Elevation pallor
J. Bruits

THINKING CRITICALLY

Match the signs or symptoms in Column A with the appropriate peripheral insufficiency in Column B.

Column A

11. _____ Decreased peripheral pulses
12. _____ Muscular atrophy
13. _____ Dependent cyanosis
14. _____ Thin, shiny, hairless skin
15. _____ Brown skin discolorations
16. _____ Cool skin temperature
17. _____ Pale color
18. _____ Pain with elevation
19. _____ Exercise decreases pain

Column B

A. Venous
B. Arterial

THINKING CRITICALLY: KNOWING WHAT TO DO AND WHY

■ Diagnostic Tests

Discuss the purpose of each test. Complete the grid.

	Test Purpose	Informed Consent	Pretest Nursing Care	Post-Test Nursing Care
20.	Impedance Plethysmography (IPG)	No		None
21.	Contrast Angiography			• Peripheral vascular checks and vital signs q15min X 1h then q2h • Assess puncture site • Bed rest 6–8 hours • IV and fluid hydration • Intake and output • Monitor blood urea nitrogen (BUN) and creatinine
22.	Contrast Venography	Yes	• Baseline peripheral vascular checks • Teaching • Allergies • Clear liquids before test	

List the pertinent assessment data related to peripheral vascular disorders in the following table.

Functional Health Pattern-Focused Health History

23. Health Perception–Health Management	24. Nutrition–Metabolic	25. Elimination	26. Activity–Exercise
27. Sleep–Rest	28. Cognitive–Perceptual	29. Self-Perception–Self-Concept	30. Role–Relationship
31. Sexuality–Reproductive	32. Coping–Stress Tolerance	33. Values–Beliefs	

The "8 Ps" of the peripheral vascular assessment: briefly discuss below why it is important to assess each "P" indication.

Mnemonic "8 Ps"	Assessment	Rationale
34. **Pain**	Symptom analysis Health History	Different peripheral vascular disorders have specific pain patterns.
35. **Pulses**	Quality, circulation	
36. **Pallor**	Color	
37. **Poikilothermy**	Temperature	
38. **Paresthesia**	Sensations, numbness, tingling	
39. **Paralysis**	Movement, muscle strength	
40. **Puffiness**	Edema	
41. **Pinkies**	Capillary refill, nails, trauma	

Clients with Hypertensive Disorders: Promoting Positive Outcomes

The prevention, detection, evaluation, and treatment of hypertension has improved in the last decade. However, according to the JNC-VI (Joint National Committee of Health's sixth report) and *Healthy People 2000,* the incidence of hypertension is again on the rise. One in four Americans have arterial hypertension. The highest occurrence is among the elderly, the less educated and poorer populations, and African Americans. The JNC-VI guidelines are prevention-focused and recommend the use of nonpharmaceutical as well as pharmaceutical measures to prevent and treat hypertension. Nurses who are knowledgeable and committed to prevention, detection, evaluation, and treatment of hypertension provide a pivotal force in decreasing the incidence of hypertension.

OBJECTIVES

52.1   Identify and describe the major classifications of hypertension.

52.2   Identify primary and secondary prevention measures for primary hypertension.

52.3   Discuss incidence, risk factors, etiology, clinical manifestations, and pathophysiology of primary hypertension.

52.4   Describe possible complications of hypertension.

52.5   Describe nonpharmaceutical medical management of primary hypertension.

52.6   Describe the classification, action, expected response, side effects, and nursing considerations of drugs used to treat hypertension: diuretics, sympatholytic agents, vasodilators, angiotensin-converting enzyme inhibitors, and calcium channel blockers.

LEARNING THE LANGUAGE: TERMINOLOGY RELATED TO HYPERTENSION

■ Classification of Hypertension

Match the descriptive statements in Column A with the appropriate classification in Column B.

<table>
<tr><td align="center">**Column A**</td><td align="center">**Column B**</td></tr>
</table>

1. _____ Has an identifiable cause
2. _____ Develops with arteriosclerosis
3. _____ Most common in elderly
4. _____ Idiopathic hypertension
5. _____ Results from increased blood viscosity
6. _____ Most common type of hypertension
7. _____ Essential hypertension
8. _____ Normotensive except when blood pressure is measured by a health care professional

A. "White coat" hypertension
B. Isolated systolic hypertension
C. Primary hypertension
D. Secondary hypertension

THINKING CRITICALLY: UNDERSTANDING RATIONALES

■ Medications for Hypertension

Listed below are medications and nursing implications associated with the medications. Provide the rationale for the nursing implications.

Implications	**Rationale**

Diuretics

9. Daily weights

10. Assess for dehydration

11. Avoid taking drug prior to bedtime

12. Monitor electrolytes

Adrenergic-Inhibiting Agents: Beta Blockers

13. Instruct client on taking own pulse

14. Contraindicated for clients with bronchial asthma

15. Warn diabetic clients that these medications may mask signs of hypoglycemia

16. Warn about orthostatic hypotension

17. Do not stop abruptly

Angiotensin-Converting Enzyme (ACE) Inhibitors
18. Monthly urine protein analysis and leukocyte count

19. Taste loss is a frequent side effect

Calcium Antagonist (Calcium Channel Blockers)
20. Monitor for sudden hypotension

Centrally Acting Alpha₂ Agonists—Clonidine
21. Avoid alcohol

22. Diabetics monitor blood sugar

PUTTING IT ALL TOGETHER

■ *Case Study: Hypertension*

Mr. Y., a 72-year-old black male, came to the clinic with complaints of fatigue. The physical examination revealed the following information: blood pressure 190/88 mm Hg, pulse 86, height 5' 6", weight 210 pounds.

23. Identify the classification of hypertension demonstrated by this client.

24. Using Table 52-2 in the text, identify the classification of severity assessed in Mr. Y.

25. List risk factors contributing to Mr. Y.'s hypertensive state.

26. Using Table 52-1 of the text, identify the appropriate follow-up criteria for Mr. Y.

27. Using Box 52-4, describe *step 1* of the stepped care approach to management for hypertension.

CHAPTER

53

Management of Clients with Vascular Disorders

Chapter 53 focuses on disorders of arteries, veins, and the lymphatic system. The chapter includes the etiologies, risk factors, pathophysiology, clinical manifestations, and medical and nursing management of many disorders. In addition, the chapter discusses the perioperative care of clients with vascular disorders.

As with other chapters encompassing numerous similar conditions, you may have difficulty pinpointing the essential information. Again, try not to memorize. Instead, concentrate on the pathophysiology of each disorder. Recall the normal physiology and determine how this condition alters the normal function of the artery, vein, or lymphatic system. It also helps to organize the arterial and venous disorders as acute or chronic.

In contrast, nursing care of clients with arterial disorders emphasizes promoting circulation and adequate tissue perfusion, while nursing care of clients with venous disorders centers on monitoring thrombolytic therapy and controlling and preventing thrombus formation. Infectious lymphatic processes require nursing care directed at the primary infection, and nursing care for lymphedema is palliative. Thus, these disorders require a broad range of nursing knowledge and skill.

OBJECTIVES

53.1 Differentiate between acute and chronic arterial disorders and acute and chronic venous disorders.

53.2 Summarize the etiology, risk factors, pathophysiology, complications, and medical and surgical treatment of peripheral vascular disorders.

53.3 Discuss the nursing management of the client with peripheral vascular disorders.

53.4 Discuss the nursing management of the surgical client undergoing percutaneous transluminal angioplasty, arterial bypass, amputation, and abdominal aortic aneurysm surgery.

53.5 Differentiate between primary and secondary lymphedema.

53.6 Discuss the outcome management of lymphedema.

THINKING CRITICALLY: ASSESSMENT DATA AND ASSOCIATED PATHOPHYSIOLOGY OF ARTERIAL AND VENOUS DISORDERS

Match the assessment data in Column A with the appropriate pathophysiologic bases in Column B.

Column A	Column B
1. _____ Cellulitis	A. Severe and prolonged ischemia
2. _____ Dryness, scaling of skin, brittle toenails	B. Increased metabolic needs; arteries unable to dilate to supply oxygen
3. _____ Death of tissues of extremities	C. Vessels no longer able to constrict; remain dilated
4. _____ Cyanosis of tissues	D. Stagnant blood pooling in tissues of extremities
5. _____ Reddish-blue tissue color	E. Presence of abnormal amounts of deoxygenated hemoglobin
6. _____ Pain in calf muscles accompanying exercise	F. Venous insufficiency
	G. Prolonged ischemia; malnutrition of tissues

NURSING INTERVENTIONS FOR PERIPHERAL VASCULAR DISORDERS

Match the interventions in Column A with the appropriate rationale in Column B.

Column A	Column B
7. _____ Wash feet with tepid water	A. Reduces venous congestion
8. _____ Use foot cradle on bed	B. Allows ulcers to drain more easily
9. _____ Use sheepskin under heels	C. Embolus can occur quickly
10. _____ Use coarse mesh gauze dressings	D. Prevents friction and allows air to circulate
11. _____ Avoid extended periods of knee flexion	E. Gravity increases blood flow
12. _____ Legs should be dependent with arterial disease	F. Prevents popliteal compression
13. _____ Monitor peripheral pulses	G. Minimizes foot trauma
14. _____ Wear supportive, closed-toe shoes	H. Absorbs excess moisture

Match the interventions in Column A with the correct nursing diagnosis in Column B.

Column A	Column B
15. _____ Encourage range of motion (ROM) and progressive ambulation.	A. Altered tissue perfusion
16. _____ Monitor vital signs for increase in pulse and decrease in blood pressure.	B. Risk for impaired skin integrity
17. _____ Check dressings for excessive drainage.	C. Fluid volume deficit
18. _____ Monitor albumin levels.	D. Impaired physical mobility
19. _____ Assess color, temperature, movement, sensation.	
20. _____ Use bed cradle and heel protector p.r.n.	
21. _____ Instruct client to avoid crossing legs.	
22. _____ Monitor hemoglobin and hematocrit levels.	
23. _____ Use lanolin-based lotion.	

Provide rationales for the following interventions associated with deep vein thrombosis (DVT), postphlebitic syndrome (PPS), and venous stasis ulcers.

Intervention	**Rationale**

Deep Vein Thrombosis (DVT)

24.   Bed rest for 5–7 days after onset of thrombus formation.

25.   Elevate legs.

26.   Apply continuous warm, moist packs.

27.   Administer heparin intravenously.

Venous Stasis Ulcers

28.   Apply wet-to-dry dressings.

29.   Apply Unna boot.

Match the statements in Column A with the correct medication in Column B.

Column A	**Column B**
30. _____ Avoid aspirin	A. Heparin
31. _____ Fast-acting	B. Coumadin (Warfarin)
32. _____ Slow-acting	
33. _____ Prevents clotting factor IX	
34. _____ Antidote: Mephyton	
35. _____ Avoid green leafy vegetables	
36. _____ Administered intravenously	
37. _____ Administered orally	
38. _____ Inhibits synthesis of vitamin K-dependent clotting factors	
39. _____ Prothrombin time (PT)	
40. _____ Antidote: protamine sulfate	
41. _____ Partial prothrombin time (PTT)	

Indicate which of the following factors will increase (I) or decrease (D) prothrombin time.

42. _____ Alcohol

43. _____ Diet high in vitamin K

44. _____ Aspirin

45. _____ Antihistamines

46. _____ Barbiturates

47. _____ Vitamin K deficiency

Provide rationales for the following interventions used in the nursing management of a client with an amputation.

Intervention	Rationale

48. Keep a large tourniquet at the bedside.

49. Elevate stump on pillow for 24–48 hours.

50. Do not elevate stump for more than 48 hours.

51. Perform ROM exercises three times a day.

52. Place client in a prone position several hours each day.

53. Teach client about phantom limb pain.

54. Assess for erythema along the surgical incision.

Provide rationales for the following stump and prosthesis care.

Intervention	Rationale

55. Inspect the stump daily.

56. Do not apply alcohol or creams to the stump.

57. Put the prosthesis on immediately upon arising.

58. Dry prosthesis socket thoroughly after removing from stump.

59. Differentiate between arterial insufficiency and venous insufficiency.

60. What is Raynaud's syndrome?

61. Describe the physiologic action of fibrinolytic medications.

62. Differentiate between primary and secondary lymphedema.

■ *Case Study: Deep Vein Thrombosis (DVT)*

Ms. N., a 32-year-old white female, was admitted to the hospital for knee surgery. She was placed on nothing by mouth at 10 PM the evening before surgery. During the surgery, a leg cuff was placed on her thigh to decrease blood flow and increase visibility in the surgical site. Following the surgery, she was placed in a cast that extended from her right ankle to mid-thigh. Within 36 hours after the surgery, the client experienced pain in the calf of her right leg when attempting to stand. When the pain persisted, the surgeon removed the cast to facilitate assessment of the extremity. The right leg was edematous; deep indentations (more than 1 cm) were created by thumb pressure. The circumference of the thigh was 2 inches more than the circumference of the left thigh. Ms. N. was diagnosed with deep vein thrombosis and anticoagulant therapy was started.

63.   Based on the data in the case study, what factors contributed to the development of DVT in this client?

64.   Ms. N.'s pitting edema would be classified as
   A.   1+.
   B.   2+.
   C.   3+.
   D.   4+.

65.   Initially, Ms. N. received 5000 units of heparin by intravenous (IV) bolus followed by an intravenous infusion of heparin at 750 units per hour. Which of the following diagnostic studies would be used to measure the effectiveness of the heparin?
   A.   prothrombin time
   B.   bleeding time
   C.   partial thromboplastin time
   D.   clotting time

66.   The IV heparin is supplied premixed: heparin 50,000 units/500 mL D_5W. How many mL will she receive per hour?

67.   The physician wants the PTT to be two times the control. Ms. N.'s PTT is 45 seconds. The control is 30 seconds. Is Ms. N.'s PTT in the physician's desired PTT range?

68.   Based on the PTT results the infusion rate is increased to 800 units per hour. How many mL/hour will you give?

69.   After approximately 48 hours, the physician added sodium warfarin (Coumadin) to the regimen. Which one of the following is correct about sodium warfarin?
   A.   Protamine sulfate is the antidote for sodium warfarin.
   B.   A prothrombin time of 1 1/2 to 2 times the normal is desired.
   C.   Coumadin derivatives are fast-acting.
   D.   Anticoagulant therapy is usually discontinued after a few days.

70.   The nurse caring for Ms. N. would consider which one of the following as an appropriate nursing intervention?
   A.   Perform active range of motion to the right leg.
   B.   Position a pillow under the right leg.
   C.   Apply continuous cold, moist packs.
   D.   Elevate legs above the level of the heart.

■ *Case Study: Abdominal Aortic Aneurysm*

Mr. B. is a 67-year-old male with a history of hypertension and coronary artery disease. He is seen in the emergency room complaining of a sudden onset of severe, excruciating, abdominal pain and back pain. The physical assessment reveals a pulsating abdominal mass. Vital signs are: B/P 100/70; HR 100. Femoral and dorsalis pedis pulses are strong. He is alert and oriented. He tells the nurse that he feels like he is dying. A computed tomography scan reveals a 7-cm dissecting abdominal aortic aneurysm. He undergoes an emergency repair of the abdominal aortic aneurysm (AAA) with a Dacron graft.

71.   What is a 7-cm dissecting abdominal aortic aneurysm?

72. What factors probably contributed to the development of an abdominal aortic aneurysm ?

73. What is the reason for emergency surgery?

■ *Postoperative Nursing Management*

74. How will you know that hemorrhage has not occurred?

75. How will you know that he is not experiencing impaired gas exchange?

76. How will you know that he is not experiencing altered tissue perfusion?

77. How will you know that he is not experiencing ischemia of the bowel?

78. How will you know that the pain related to the surgical incision is improving?

79. What is the major reason for maintaining the postoperative systolic blood pressure below 130 mm Hg?

U N I T 12

Cardiac Disorders

ANATOMY AND PHYSIOLOGY REVIEW: THE HEART

The cardiovascular system consists of the heart, arteries, capillaries, veins, and lymphatics. The heart works continuously. It beats approximately 72 times per minute and pumps approximately 5 quarts of blood each minute and 75 gallons of blood per hour. The heart pumps oxygenated blood into the arterial system. The arterial system transports the oxygenated blood to the cells. The venous system collects deoxygenated blood and delivers it to the right side of the heart where it is pumped to the lungs for reoxygenation. The function of the arteries, capillaries, veins, and lymphatics is to carry blood to and from the tissues and cells throughout the body.

OBJECTIVES

12.1   Discuss normal cardiac structure and function.

12.2   State the two primary functions of the heart.

12.3   Diagram normal blood flow through the heart chambers and valves.

12.4   Explain the factors that influence the mechanical properties of the heart, including preload, afterload, and contractile state.

12.5   List factors that will cause variations in heart rate.

12.6   Discuss the effects of aging on the cardiovascular system.

LEARNING THE LANGUAGE: TERMINOLOGY RELATED TO ANATOMY AND PHYSIOLOGY OF THE HEART

Match the prefixes in Column A with the correct definition in Column B.

Column A

1. _____ Epi-
2. _____ Myo-
3. _____ Endo-

Column B

A.   Within, inner
B.   Upon or over
C.   Relating to muscle

Fill in the blanks.

4.   The _____ layer covers the outer surface of the heart.

5.   The _____ layer is the middle layer of the heart that consists of striated muscle fibers.

6. The _____ layer lines the inner chambers and heart valves.

7. The _____ is a loose-fitting covering that protects the heart from trauma and infection.

8. The left atrium receives _____ blood from the _____ and pumps it out through the aorta to _____ circulation.

9. The right atrium receives _____ blood from the _____ and pumps it to the _____ via the _____.

10. The _____ valves open during systole and close during diastole.

11. The _____ valves open during diastole and close during systole.

12. _____ is the working phase of the cardiac cycle and _____ is the resting phase.

Match the definitions in Column A with the correct term in Column B.

Column A	**Column B**
13. _____ The amount of resistance to left ventricular ejection	A. Cardiac output
14. _____ The amount of stretch in the left ventricle at the end of diastole	B. Stroke volume
15. _____ The amount of blood ejected from the ventricles each minute	C. Preload
	D. Pulse pressure
16. _____ The volume of blood ejected with each contraction	E. Cardiac cycle
	F. Ventricular diastole
17. _____ The difference between systolic and diastolic pressure	G. Ventricular systole
18. _____ One complete heartbeat	H. Afterload
19. _____ Pressure in the ventricles exceeds the aortic and pulmonic pressure	
20. _____ Resting/filling phase of the cardiac cycle	

Match the definitions in Column A with the correct term in Column B.

Column A	**Column B**
21. _____ Adrenergic receptors located in the heart	A. Baroreceptors
22. _____ Adrenergic receptors located in arteries and veins	B. Stretch receptors
	C. Chemoreceptors
23. _____ Adrenergic receptors located in the lungs	D. Sympathetic nervous system
24. _____ Decreases the heart rate	E. Parasympathetic nervous system
25. _____ Increases the heart rate	F. Norepinephrine and epinephrine
26. _____ Affected by changes in arterial pressure	G. Acetylcholine
27. _____ Sensitive to changes in oxygen content and arterial pH	H. Beta$_1$ receptors
28. _____ Sensitive to pressure changes in vena cava and right atrium	I. Beta$_2$ receptors
	J. Alpha receptors
29. _____ Increases heart rate, respirations, and blood pressure	
30. _____ Decreases heart rate and blood pressure	

Indicate the effect of the following on the blood pressure: (I) increase or (D) decrease.

31. _____ Antidiuretic hormone (ADH)
32. _____ Renin-angiotensin
33. _____ Aldosterone
34. _____ Histamine

35. _____ Bradykinin
36. _____ Serotonin
37. _____ Acetylcholine
38. _____ Epinephrine

THINKING CRITICALLY: SHORT ANSWER QUESTIONS

39. Describe the primary function of the circulatory system.

41. Demonstrate your knowledge of Starling's law by describing the phenomenon in your own words.

40. Describe two factors that determine cardiac output.

42. Discuss the effects of aging on the cardiac system.

43. Using the Figure U12-2 on p. 1436 of the textbook, trace the flow of blood through the heart systemic circulation. Color the oxygenated blood red and the deoxygenated blood blue. Label the great vessels, chambers, and valves.

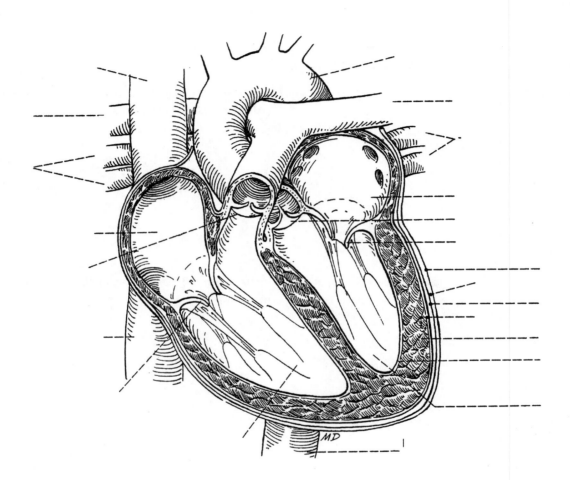

54

Assessment of the Cardiac System

Cardiovascular disease remains the number one cause of death in the United States. To care for a client with a cardiovascular disorder, the nurse must know how to assess the cardiovascular system. Assessment of the cardiovascular system incorporates data from the health history, including the past medical history, family medical history, psychosocial history, and lifestyle analysis. Assessment also includes the performance of a basic cardiovascular examination. In addition to the health history and physical examination, noninvasive and invasive diagnostic tests are ordered. The nurse must prepare the client physically and psychologically for these tests. In addition, they must monitor the client after tests and anticipate and plan for possible complications.

OBJECTIVES

54.1   Obtain a health history that focuses on the client's cardiovascular (CV) status.

54.2   Analyze risk factors for cardiovascular disease.

54.3   Perform a basic CV physical examination.

54.4   Prepare the client both physically and psychologically for diagnostic studies.

54.5   Describe nursing responsibilities for selected diagnostic procedures used to evaluate CV function.

LEARNING THE LANGUAGE: TERMINOLOGY RELATED TO ASSESSMENT OF CARDIOVASCULAR DISORDERS

Use Functional Health Patterns Framework to list the pertinent assessment data for cardiovascular disorders in the following table.

Functional Health Pattern-Focused Health History for Cardiovascular Disorders

1. Health Perception–Health Management	2. Nutrition–Metabolic	3. Elimination	4. Activity–Exercise
5. Sleep–Rest	6. Cognitive–Perceptual	7. Self-Perception–Self-Concept	8. Role–Relationship
9. Sexuality–Reproductive	10. Coping–Stress Tolerance	11. Values–Beliefs	

■ *Physical Examination*

Give the rationale for examining the following.

Focus of Physical Examination	**Rationale**
12. General appearance	
13. Blood pressure (B/P)	
14. Pulse	
15. Respirations	
16. Edema	
17. Neck vein distention	
18. Palpation of point of maximal impulse (PMI)	
19. Auscultation of heart sounds	
20. Auscultation of lungs	
21. Inspection and palpation of abdomen	

THINKING CRITICALLY: KNOWING WHAT TO DO AND WHY

■ *Laboratory Tests*

Laboratory Test	**Rationale**
22. Complete blood count (CBC)	
23. Cardiac enzymes: CK and CK-MB, LDH_1 and LDH_2, Troponin	
24. Blood coagulation	
25. Serum lipids	
26. Serum electrolytes	
27. Blood glucose	

Mark Yes or No if an informed consent is required for the following tests. Give the rationale for the interventions listed.

■ **Diagnostic Tests**

Test	Informed Consent	Pretest Nursing Care	Post-Test Nursing Care
28. Electrocardiogram (ECG)			Remove electrode patches.
29. Holter Monitoring		Explain the procedure. Instruct the client to keep a diary of activity and any symptoms that occur.	
30. Exercise Electrocardiogram (Stress Test)		Obtain a baseline resting ECG immediately prior to test.	During the test: monitor constantly for changes in ECG, chest pain.
31. Electrophysiologic Studies (EPS)			Keep extremity straight. Encourage fluids.
32. Cardiac Catheterization		Assess for allergies. Mark peripheral pulses.	Assess for rash, nausea, and vomiting.
33. Magnetic Resonance Imaging (MRI)		Assess for any metal objects. Remove glasses, clothing with zippers or metal snaps.	

■ *Postural Blood Pressure*

Indicate the expected changes: (I) increase or (D) decrease.

34. **Supine**   **Sitting**   **Standing**

    B/P _____   B/P _____   B/P _____

    Pulse _____   Pulse _____   Pulse _____

35. List the parameters for postural hypotension.

LEARNING THE LANGUAGE: TERMINOLOGY RELATED TO CARDIAC DISORDERS

Match the definitions in Column A with the correct term in Column B.

Column A	**Column B**
36. _____ Shortness of breath	A. Orthopnea
37. _____ Difficulty breathing in supine position	B. Neck vein distention (NVD)
38. _____ Sudden respiratory distress at rest	C. Paroxysmal nocturnal dyspnea (PND)
39. _____ Chest pain	D. Water-hammer pulse
40. _____ Strong heartbeats/weak heartbeats	E. Palpitations
41. _____ Sensation of rapid heartbeats	F. Pulsus alternans
42. _____ Associated with increased stroke volume	G. Angina
43. _____ Increased central venous pressure (CVP)	H. Dyspnea

Match the statements in Column A with the normal heart sound in Column B.

Column A	**Column B**
44. _____ Closure of pulmonic and aortic valves	A. First heart sound (S_1)
45. _____ Best heard at apex of heart	B. Second heart sound (S_2)
46. _____ Closure of mitral and tricuspid valves	
47. _____ Signifies the end of systole and onset of diastole	
48. _____ Marks onset of systole	
49. _____ Best heard at base of heart	

THINKING CRITICALLY

50. Describe four major symptoms that are commonly associated with CV disorders.

53. Explain the significance of engorged external jugular veins.

51. Discuss what descriptive data associated with chest pain should be gathered in the CV history.

54. Identify what characteristics of a murmur should be assessed in order to classify the murmur as to type.

52. Describe three lifestyle areas that can affect an individual's potential for developing CV disorders.

Indicate if the following conditions would cause an increased (I) or decreased (D) CVP.

55. _____ Right-sided heart failure

58. _____ Valvular stenosis

56. _____ Decreased circulating blood volume

59. _____ Hypertension

57. _____ Vasodilation

Indicate if the following conditions would cause an increased (I) or decreased (D) pulmonary artery pressure (PAP).

60. _____ Heart failure or volume overload

61. _____ Hypovolemia

62. _____ Pulmonary hypertension

Management of Clients with Structural Cardiac Disorders

Disorders of cardiac structure include the heart muscle (cardiomyopathies), infection and inflammatory disorders of the heart, and valvular heart disease. The chapter includes the etiologies, risk factors, pathophysiology, clinical manifestations, diagnostic tests, complications, and medical and nursing management of a variety of disorders. In addition, the perioperative care of clients having cardiac surgery is presented.

When numerous similar conditions are studied, it sometimes becomes difficult for students to determine what is essential information. Try not to memorize. Instead, focus your efforts on the pathophysiology that is involved with each cardiac disorder. Recall the normal physiology and determine how this condition alters the normal function of the heart. Also, remember that regardless of the cardiac disorder being discussed, the result will probably be decreased oxygenated blood to the tissues of the body and diminished ability to remove metabolic end products from the tissues.

OBJECTIVES

55.1 Describe the predisposing factors, pathophysiology, etiology, clinical manifestations, and complications for the disorders that are the result of an inflammatory response.

55.2 Describe the predisposing factors, pathophysiology, etiology, clinical manifestations, and complications for selected structural abnormalities of the heart.

55.3 Describe the pathophysiologic changes that occur with cardiac tamponade.

55.4 Describe medical management and nursing care of clients with cardiac conditions.

55.5 Describe the surgical management and nursing care for selected cardiac disorders.

55.6 Identify postoperative collaborative problems that may occur with cardiac surgery.

LEARNING THE LANGUAGE: TERMINOLOGY RELATED TO THE STRUCTURE OF THE HEART

■ *Pathophysiology of Inflammatory Cardiovascular Disorders*

Match the characteristic lesions in Column A with the appropriate cardiac disorder in Column B.

Column A

1. _____ Chorea
2. _____ Osler's nodes
3. _____ Small, firm, painless nodules
4. _____ Tiny vegetations along line of closure of valve leaflets
5. _____ Aschoff's bodies
6. _____ Rapidly progressing or insidious onset infection
7. _____ Four to six weeks antibiotic therapy
8. _____ Symptoms: heart murmurs, embolic pneumonia, high fever
9. _____ Roth's spots
10. _____ Symptoms: erythema marginatum, weakness, malaise, weight loss
11. _____ Splinter hemorrhages
12. _____ Caused by a streptococcal infection

Column B

A. Rheumatic fever
B. Infective endocarditis

■ *Pathophysiology of Idiopathic Cardiomyopathies*

Match the statements in Column A with the appropriate type of idiopathic cardiomyopathy in Column B.

Column A

13. _____ Signs of congestive heart failure (CHF) exist
14. _____ May be genetically transmitted
15. _____ Enlargement of all four heart chambers
16. _____ Least common of the three classes of cardiomyopathies
17. _____ Appears most often in young adults
18. _____ Often asymptomatic
19. _____ Associated with amyloidosis
20. _____ CHF without cardiac enlargement occurs
21. _____ Small, elongated left ventricular chamber occurs

Column B

A. Dilated
B. Restrictive
C. Hypertrophic

■ *Pathophysiology of Valvular Heart Disease*

Match the statements in Column A with the appropriate valvular heart disease in Column B.

Column A		**Column B**	
22. _____	Most common among women	A.	Mitral stenosis
23. _____	Most common cause is rheumatic valvulitis	B.	Mitral regurgitation
24. _____	Systemic emboli common	C.	Mitral valve prolapse
25. _____	Heightened awareness of own heartbeat	D.	Aortic stenosis
26. _____	Mitral valve fails to close completely	E.	Aortic regurgitation
27. _____	Loud first heart sound; low-pitched, rumbling, diastolic murmur		
28. _____	Blowing, high-pitched systolic murmur		
29. _____	Syncope is frequent symptom		
30. _____	Prevents passage of blood from left atrium to left ventricle		
31. _____	Soft, high-pitched blowing decrescendo diastolic murmur		
32. _____	Chest pain common manifestation		

MANAGEMENT OF THE CLIENT DURING CARDIAC SURGERY

Match the rationales in Column A with the appropriate intervention in Column B.

Column A		**Column B**	
33. _____	Performs gas exchange functions for the body	A.	Hypothermia
34. _____	Circulates oxygenated, filtered blood	B.	Extracorporeal circulation
35. _____	Decreases the client's metabolic needs		
36. _____	Filters, rewarms, or cools the blood		
37. _____	Reduces the client's need for oxygen		

THINKING CRITICALLY: KNOWING WHAT TO DO AND WHY

■ *Nursing Management of Clients Having Cardiac Surgery*

Provide the rationale for the following nursing interventions.

Interventions	Rationale
38. Check for pedal pulses.	
39. Measure urine volume hourly for first 8–10 hours after surgery.	
40. Obtain daily weights.	
41. First 24 hours: administer Demerol judiciously.	
42. Place a calendar and clock at the bedside.	
43. Perform passive exercises and leg flexion every 2 hours.	
44. Wash hands before and after dressing changes.	
45. Teach the person to check own pulse daily for rate and regularity.	
46. Maintain blood pressure (B/P) with 20 mm Hg of baseline.	
47. First 48 hours: assess heart sounds every 2 hours.	
48. Observe and measure chest tube drainage.	

Place a check mark by the client who should have the highest priority for your immediate nursing care.

49. _____ A. Client with nursing diagnosis: Ineffective breathing pattern related to increased pulmonary secretions.

_____ B. Client with nursing diagnosis: High risk for infection related to thoracic incision.

50. _____ A. Client with nursing diagnosis: Activity intolerance related to dyspnea.

_____ B. Client with nursing diagnosis: Ineffective individual coping related to change in health status.

EVALUATION: HOW WILL YOU KNOW IF THE CLIENT IS GETTING BETTER?

Briefly describe how you would evaluate each of the following nursing diagnoses or collaborative problems for a client having cardiac surgery.

Nursing Diagnosis/ Collaborative Problem	Expected Outcome
51. Risk for decreased cardiac output	
52. Risk for cardiac tamponade	
53. Risk for paralytic ileus	
54. Pain	

PUTTING IT ALL TOGETHER

■ Case Study

J.K., an 8-year-old girl who lives in a crowded urban slum, is brought to the clinic. She complains of joint pain and her right knee is swollen and red. Her mother indicates that during the last few days J.K. has been "moping around the house" instead of playing with other children. In addition, she isn't eating as much as usual. The physical examination reveals small, painless nodules around the left elbow, a temperature of 38° C, and leukocytosis. J.K. is admitted to the hospital and placed on bed rest. The physician prescribes antibiotics and steroids to reduce her symptoms.

55. From the assessed data, identify the existing predisposing factors for rheumatic fever.

56. Using Jones' criteria (Box 55-1), determine which of J.K.'s symptoms are major manifestations and which are minor manifestations of rheumatic fever.

57. Explain why bed rest is ordered for a client with rheumatic fever.

58. Discuss how the nurse can help an 8-year-old adjust to imposed activity restriction.

59. Describe the criteria that must be considered before J.K.'s activities are increased.

60. Explain why antibiotics and steroids are prescribed for the client with rheumatic fever.

61. State one nursing diagnosis based on the assessed data in the above situation.

62. List the main complications of rheumatic fever.

CHAPTER

56

Management of Clients with Functional Cardiac Disorders

Chapter 56 focuses on coronary artery disease and congestive heart failure. The chapter discusses etiologies, risk factors, pathophysiology, clinical manifestations, and medical and nursing management of these disorders.

Although each of the cardiac disorders in this chapter has many causes, the nurse can view them as stemming from coronary artery disease. The presence of atherosclerosis can contribute to angina pectoris, myocardial infarction, (covered in Chapter 58) and congestive heart failure. Therefore, the nurse must have a clear understanding of coronary artery disease: its etiology, risk factors, clinical manifestations, diagnostic tests, complications, and related medical and nursing management.

OBJECTIVES

56.1   Describe the pathogenesis of atherosclerosis.

56.2   Discuss risk factors associated with coronary artery disease.

56.3   Describe the etiology and clinical manifestations of coronary artery disease and congestive heart failure.

56.4   Describe diagnostic studies used to assess clients with coronary artery disease and congestive heart failure.

56.5   Describe medical management and nursing management for clients with coronary artery disease and congestive heart failure.

56.6   Explain the rationales for selected nursing interventions.

56.7   Discuss the goals of cardiac rehabilitation after CABG (coronary artery bypass grafting surgery).

THINKING CRITICALLY: CORONARY ARTERY DISEASE

Indicate if the following are nonmodifiable (N), modifiable (M), or contributing factors (CF) to CAD.

1. _____ Age
2. _____ Sex
3. _____ Race
4. _____ Obesity
5. _____ Sedentary lifestyle
6. _____ Heredity

7. _____ Smoking
8. _____ Environment
9. _____ High cholesterol
10. _____ Diabetes
11. _____ Response to stress

Number the sequence of events in the development of atherosclerotic plaque.

12. _____ Lipid entry and accumulation
13. _____ Endothelial injury
14. _____ Thrombus formation
15. _____ Smooth muscle cell proliferation

16. _____ Platelet–fibrin interaction
17. _____ Ulceration and calcification
18. _____ Fibrosis

Ms. C. is a 53-year-old secretary who has been diagnosed as having atherosclerotic heart disease. Recently, she had to resign from her place of employment because of fatigue, weakness, and inability to climb the stairs to her second-floor office without experiencing chest pain. At home, Ms. C. is able to perform only light housework.

19. Classify this client's heart disease according to the New York Heart Association's guidelines (Box 56-2).

SIGNS, SYMPTOMS, AND TREATMENT OF CONGESTIVE HEART FAILURE

Match the objective and subjective findings in Column A with the causative factor in Column B.

Column A	**Column B**
20. _____ Cough	A. Left ventricular failure
21. _____ Weight gain	B. Right ventricular failure
22. _____ Fatigue	
23. _____ Orthopnea	
24. _____ Hepatomegaly	
25. _____ Dependent edema	
26. _____ Dyspnea	
27. _____ Ascites	

Listed below are some important implications associated with drugs used to treat heart failure. Write the rationales for each implication.

Implications	Rationale

Digoxin (Lanoxin)

28. Take the client's pulse for one full minute apically before giving the drug.

29. Check most recent digoxin levels and potassium levels.

30. Ask the client if he or she is seeing flickering flashes of light.

31. Ask the client if he or she has experienced nausea and vomiting.

Furosemide (Lasix)

32. Monitor laboratory results for potassium levels.

33. Weigh the client daily.

INTERVENTIONS FOR CLIENTS WITH CONGESTIVE HEART FAILURE

Match the interventions in Column A with the appropriate goal in Column B.

Column A

34. _____ Reduce physical stress performance
35. _____ Administer oxygen therapy
36. _____ Administer diuretics
37. _____ Place client in upright position
38. _____ Administer vasodilators
39. _____ Administer inotropic agents
40. _____ Restrict fluid intake
41. _____ Restrict sodium intake

Column B

A. Improve ventricular pump
B. Reduce preload
C. Reduce afterload

■ Case Study

Ms. L., 61 years old, is admitted to the emergency department in acute respiratory distress. Her color is ashen, blood pressure 190/100, respirations 32, and apical pulse 120. She is extremely anxious and complains of chest pain and nausea. She tells you that 10 days ago she stopped taking all of her medications because she thought that they were no longer helping her. She is diagnosed with congestive heart failure, complicated by pulmonary edema.

42. You administer intravenous morphine sulfate as ordered. You should assess Ms. L.'s response to the drug by noting its effect on which of the following?
    A. nausea
    B. blood pressure
    C. ashen appearance
    D. pain

43. When auscultating the client's lungs, you would most likely hear
    A. wheezing.
    B. crackling.
    C. metallic ringing.
    D. crepitation.

44. In which of the following positions will Ms. L. be the most comfortable?
    A. low Fowler's
    B. Trendelenburg's
    C. Sims'
    D. high Fowler's

45. The client is to receive intravenous digoxin. One of the actions of the drug is to
    A. decrease cardiac dysrhythmias.
    B. dilate atherosclerotic coronary arteries.
    C. increase ventricular contractility.
    D. decrease cardiac output.

46. The client needs to be assessed carefully for digitalis toxicity. Which one of the following findings could indicate toxicity?
    A. anorexia
    B. constipation
    C. slow respiratory rate
    D. decreased blood pressure

47. Ms. L. is to be discharged with a prescription for furosemide. To help her evaluate the effectiveness of the drug, you instruct her to
    A. check her pulse daily.
    B. weigh herself daily.
    C. check her blood pressure daily.
    D. monitor her urinary output.

48. Ms. L. is to follow a low-sodium diet. Which of the following foods should she avoid?
    A. oranges
    B. broiled chicken
    C. catsup
    D. skim milk

CHAPTER 57

Management of Clients with Dysrhythmias

The heart has its own intrinsic conduction system that has the ability to conduct electrical impulses spontaneously and continuously in a regular sequence and rhythm. Once stimulated the whole heart muscle contracts and pumps blood into systemic circulation.

Dysrhythmias, also called arrhythmias, are disorders of the heart's conduction system. They result from disturbances in three major mechanisms: automaticity, conduction, and problems with reentry impulses. *Automaticity* is the normal heart rate produced by various pacemaker cells in the myocardium. *Conduction* is the speed at which the impulse travels through the conduction system. Problems with reentry impulses occur when pacemaker cells other than the sinoatrial (SA) node generate impulses. Dysrhythmias can decrease the pumping effectiveness of the heart. They vary from minor changes in the heart's rate and rhythm to life-threatening dysrhythmias. The dysrhythmias and their management are presented as problems arising from the atria, then the atrioventricular (AV) junction, and finally the ventricles.

OBJECTIVES

57.1 Define the terms related to disorders of cardiac rhythm.

57.2 Trace the cardiac conduction system.

57.3 Identify the components of the electrocardiogram (ECG) pattern.

57.4 Interpret selected rhythm strips.

57.5 Discuss the medical management of selected dysrhythmias.

57.6 Describe the management of life-threatening dysrhythmias.

57.7 Discuss the surgical management of dysrhythmias.

57.8 Discuss the major nursing interventions related to disorders of the cardiac rhythm.

LEARNING THE LANGUAGE: TERMINOLOGY RELATED TO DISORDERS OF CARDIAC RHYTHM

Trace and label the normal electrical conduction pathway in the cardiac muscle. Refer to Figure U12-6A in the textbook.

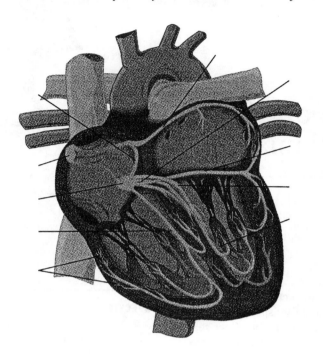

■ Normal ECG Pattern

Label the following components of this normal ECG pattern: P wave, P-R interval, QRS Complex, T wave, ST segment, U wave.

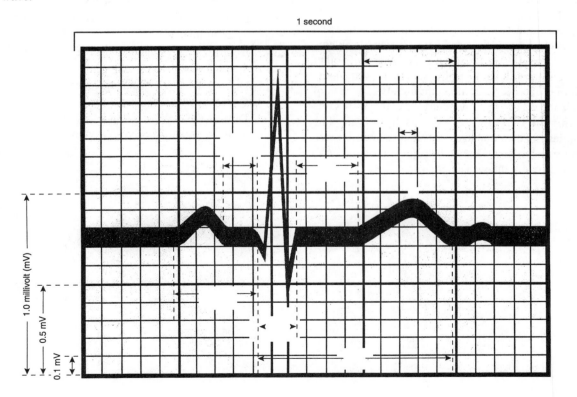

■ *Intrinsic Heart Rates*

Complete the following.

1. Sinoatrial Node (SA) _____ BPM (beats per minute)
2. AV Node _____ BPM
3. Ventricles _____ BPM

■ *Dysrhythmia Interpretation Guide*

Use Box 57-1 to rank the basic steps of dysrhythmia interpretation.

4. _____ Name the rhythm
5. _____ Measure the regularity (atrial and ventricular rhythms)
6. _____ Calculate the heart rate
7. _____ Measure the P-R interval

8. _____ Examine the P waves
9. _____ Examine the ST segment
10. _____ Measure the QRS complex and Q-T interval
11. _____ Examine the T wave

Match the definitions in Column A with the correct term in Column B (refer to Chapter 57 as needed).

Column A

12. _____ The ability of the cardiac muscle to depolarize in response to a stimulus
13. _____ The cell returns to its resting stage
14. _____ The ability of a cardiac cell to initiate an impulse
15. _____ The heart's inability to respond to a stimulus
16. _____ The ability of the heart muscle to move an impulse over the entire muscle mass
17. _____ The ability of the heart to contract

Column B

A. Excitability
B. Repolarization
C. Automaticity
D. Conductivity
E. Contractility
F. Refractoriness

THINKING CRITICALLY

■ *ECG Waveforms/Cardiac Electrical Events*

Match the ECG waveforms in Column A to the electrical event in Column B.

Column A

18. _____ P wave
19. _____ QRS complex
20. _____ T wave

Column B

A. Ventricular repolarization
B. Atrial depolarization
C. Ventricular depolarization
D. Atrial repolarization

Match each of the ECG intervals in Column A with its normal duration in Column B.

Column A	Column B
21. _____ P-R interval	A. < 0.44 seconds
22. _____ QRS complex	B. 0.12–0.20 seconds
23. _____ Q-T interval	C. 0.04–0.10 seconds

■ Defining Characteristics (Signs) of Dysrhythmias

Match the objective findings in Column A with the appropriate dysrhythmia in Column B.

Column A	Column B
24. _____ Heart rate less than 60 per minute	A. Paroxysmal atrial tachycardia
25. _____ P waves appear early; short P - P intervals	B. Sinus bradycardia
26. _____ Rapid, repetitive rhythm; rate of 160–230 per minute	C. Atrial flutter
	D. Premature ventricular contractions
27. _____ P waves inverted, producing "saw-toothed" pattern	E. Junctional rhythms
	F. Premature atrial contractions
28. _____ Abnormal upward direction of impulse spread	G. Atrial fibrillation
	H. Sinus tachycardia
29. _____ Rapid, regular rhythm; rate of 100–180 per minute	
30. _____ Chaotic atrial depolarization; more than 500 per minute	
31. _____ Wide, bizarre QRS	

■ Disturbances in Conduction

Match the types of heart block in Column A with the appropriate identifying information in Column B.

Column A	Column B
32. _____ First-degree heart block	A. All impulses from atria blocked
33. _____ Wenckebach or Mobitz I	B. Conduction in AV node slows; P-R interval longer than 0.20 seconds
34. _____ Mobitz II	
35. _____ Third-degree heart block	C. Recurrent cycle; P-R interval prolonged; QRS complex intermittently dropped
	D. P-R intervals constant; intermittently dropped QRS complex

■ Treatment for Dysrhythmias

Match the dysrhythmias in Column A to the appropriate intervention in Column B.

Column A	Column B
36. _____ Paroxysmal atrial tachycardia	A. Automatic Implantable Cardioverter Defibrillator (AICD)
37. _____ Sinus bradycardia	
38. _____ Complete heart block	B. Insertion of a pacemaker
39. _____ Premature ventricular contraction	C. Lidocaine HCl
40. _____ Sudden death	D. Carotid sinus massage
41. _____ Atrial fibrillation	E. Digoxin
42. _____ Ventricular fibrillation	F. Defibrillate
	G. Atropine

CLIENT EDUCATION: KNOWING WHAT TO TEACH AND WHY

■ Pacemakers

Intervention	Rationale
43. Report any signs of inflammation.	
44. Take pulse daily.	
45. Carry identification card.	
46. Avoid metal detectors.	
47. Do not lift more than 10 lbs the first 6 weeks.	
48. Avoid firing a rifle with butt end against affected shoulder.	

COMMUNITY AND SELF-CARE

■ How Will You Evaluate the Following Discharge Criteria?

Discharge Criteria	Evaluation
49. Vital signs stable	
50. Stable cardiac rhythm with dysrhythmias controlled	
51. Absence of fever, pulmonary, or cardiovascular complications	
52. Laboratory values within expected levels	
53. Ability to tolerate adequate nutritional intake	
54. Absence of urinary and bowel dysfunction	
55. Ability to perform activities of daily living	
56. Mental status within normal limits for client	
57. Referral to community support group for cardiac conditions	
58. Response of client and family to teaching/discharge planning	
59. Family response to illness and support	

■ *Rhythm Strip Interpretation*

Using the information provided in Box 57-1 of the text, interpret the following ECG tracings.

60.

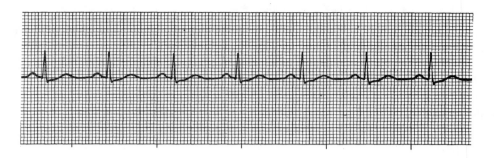

61.

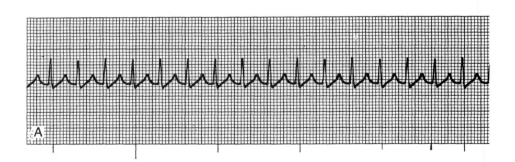

62.

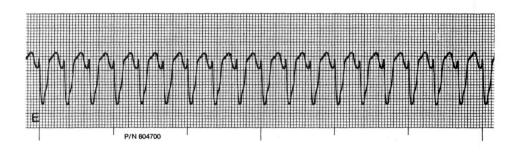

63.

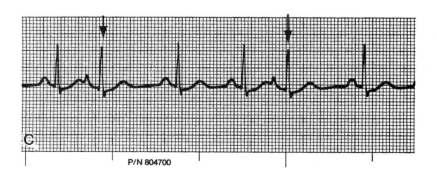

64.

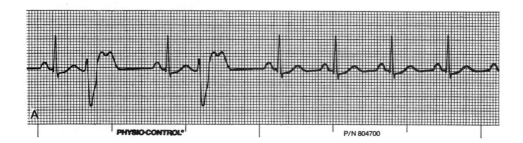

65.

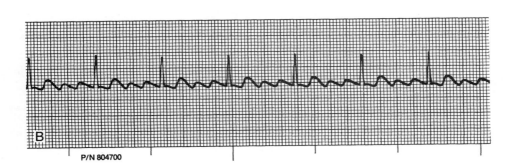

66.

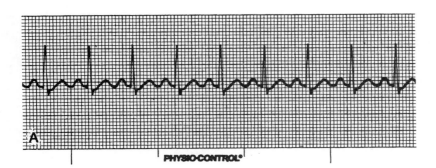

58

Management of Clients with Myocardial Infarction

Myocardial infarction is the leading cause of death in America. There are approximately 500,000 deaths annually. The presence of atherosclerosis and subsequent coronary artery disease is the major cause of angina pectoris and myocardial infarction. Therefore, nurse must have a clear understanding of coronary artery disease: its etiology, risk factors, clinical manifestations, diagnostic tests, complications, and related medical and nursing management. This chapter discusses etiologies, risk factors, pathophysiology, clinical manifestations, and medical and nursing management of angina pectoris and myocardial infarction.

OBJECTIVES

58.1   Describe the relationship between coronary artery disease, angina pectoris, and myocardial infarction.

58.2   Discuss risk factors associated with angina and myocardial infarction.

58.3   Describe the etiology and clinical manifestations of angina pectoris and myocardial infarction.

58.4   Describe diagnostic studies used to assess clients with angina pectoris and myocardial infarction.

58.5   Describe medical management and nursing management for clients with angina pectoris and myocardial infarction.

58.6   Explain rationale for selected nursing interventions for nursing management of clients with angina pectoris and myocardial infarction.

LEARNING THE LANGUAGE: TERMINOLOGY RELATED TO MYOCARDIAL INFARCTION

Match the description listed in Column A with the type of angina pectoris in Column B.

Column A

1. _____ Similar to classic angina but lasts longer; may result from coronary artery spasm
2. _____ Associated with REM sleep
3. _____ Occurs when client reclines and improves with sitting or standing
4. _____ Chronic pain unresponsive to interventions
5. _____ Occurs after an MI when the heart muscle is ischemic
6. _____ Anticipated or predictable pain following exertion or emotion
7. _____ Unpredictable pain that may occur at any time. Signals a high degree of blockage.

Column B

A. Stable angina
B. Unstable angina
C. Variant (Prinzmetal's) angina
D. Nocturnal angina
E. Angina decubitus
F. Intractable angina
G. Postinfarction angina

Listed below are some important implications associated with drugs used to treat angina pectoris. Write the rationale for each implication.

Implication   **Rationale**

Nitroglycerin (NTG)

8. Place sublingual tablet under the tongue at the first indication of an attack.

9. Store tablets in a dark bottle and in a dry place.

10. Monitor blood pressure.

Propranolol (Inderal)

11. Do not administer to people with bronchial asthma.

Nifedipine (Procardia)

12. Monitor client's heart rate.

KNOW THE DIFFERENCE: SIGNS, SYMPTOMS, AND TREATMENT OF ANGINA AND MYOCARDIAL INFARCTION

Match the manifestations listed in Column A with the appropriate cardiac disorder in Column B.

Column A	Column B
13. _____ Pain relieved by nitroglycerin	A. Angina pectoris
14. _____ Muscle hypoxia	B. Myocardial infarction
15. _____ Elevated serum level of CPK-MB	
16. _____ Irreversible	
17. _____ Intense, crushing, substernal pain	
18. _____ Pathologic Q waves	

Number in correct order the following changes that occur after an acute MI.

19. _____ Necrotic tissue replaced by gray, fibrous scar tissue.

20. _____ Infarcted area looks anemic and grayish-brown.

21. _____ Necrotic area becomes sharply defined.

22. _____ Central tissue of necrotic tissue is soft.

LABORATORY STUDIES USED TO DIAGNOSE A MYOCARDIAL INFARCTION

23. Based on your understanding of the laboratory findings specific for an MI, identify which line on the following diagram represents (A) Lactate dehydrogenase (LDH) serum level, (B) CPK-MB serum level, and (C) AST serum level.

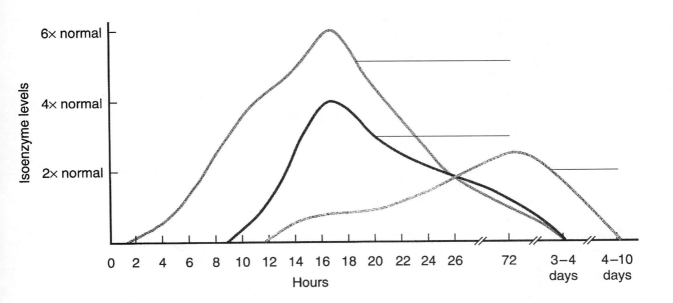

24. Which blood test is the most reliable indicator of an MI?

THINKING CRITICALLY: UNDERSTANING TREATMENT FOR MYOCARDIAL INFARCTION

25. What is the rationale for an increase in the white blood cell count following an MI?

What is the rationale for administering the following treatments?

28. Morphine

26. What is the rationale for taking an aspirin at the onset of chest pain?

29. Heparin

30. IV Nitroglycerin

27. What is the priority of treatment of a client with chest pain?

31. Oxygen

32. Thrombolytic therapy

Oxygenation Disorders

ANATOMY AND PHYSIOLOGY REVIEW: THE RESPIRATORY SYSTEM

The primary function of the respiratory system is to conduct air into the lungs, deliver oxygen via capillary membranes to the blood, and remove carbon dioxide. The respiratory system is divided into two anatomic areas, which are called the upper and lower airways. The upper airway (nasal cavities, pharynx, and larynx) conducts the air to the lower airway. As the inspired air passes through these structures, it is warmed, filtered, and humidified. The lower airway consists of the trachea, main bronchi, segmental bronchi, subsegmental bronchi, terminal bronchioles, and alveoli. It is in the alveoli that exchange of oxygen and carbon dioxide occurs.

The term *pulmonary ventilation* refers to the process of inspiration and expiration. The movement of air into and out of the lungs is aided by the muscles used in ventilation. The basic rate of ventilation is 14–18 respirations per minute. Regulation is accomplished by the respiratory center in the medullar oblongata and pons, peripherally and centrally located chemoreceptors, and autonomic nervous system.

OBJECTIVES

13.1 Explain the structure and function of the upper and lower airways.

13.2 Explain the process of ventilation, perfusion, and gas exchange.

13.3 Describe the process of gas exchange that occurs in the alveolar-capillary system.

13.4 Describe the mechanical, neural, and chemical stimuli that can affect ventilation.

13.5 Discuss the defense mechanisms that protect the integrity of the respiratory system.

13.6 Describe the effects of aging on the lungs.

LEARNING THE LANGUAGE: TERMINOLOGY RELATED TO STRUCTURE AND FUNCTION OF THE RESPIRATORY SYSTEM

Match the description in Column A with the structure in Column B.

Column A   **Column B**

1. _____ Voice box   A.   Nasal cavity
2. _____ Receives air   B.   Pharynx
3. _____ Serves both respiratory and digestion   C.   Larynx
4. _____ Connects upper pharynx with lower trachea
5. _____ Esophagus lies posterior
6. _____ Eustachian tube opens in this area
7. _____ Palatine and lingual tonsils

■ Function of Upper Airway and Lower Airway

Match the functions in Column A with the correct structure in Column B.

Column A   **Column B**

8. _____ Air conduction   A.   Upper airway
9. _____ Warms, filters, humidifies   B.   Lower airway
10. _____ Gas exchange
11. _____ Sneeze reflex
12. _____ Cough reflex
13. _____ Immunologic responses
14. _____ Primary clearance mechanism

■ Structure and Function of the Thorax, Diaphragm, and Pleura

Match the description in Column A with the correct structure in Column B.

Column A   **Column B**

15. _____ Dome-shaped   A.   Thorax
16. _____ Visceral and parietal membranes   B.   Diaphragm
17. _____ Maintains expansion of the lungs   C.   Pleura
18. _____ Protects the lungs
19. _____ Forced expiration and coughing
20. _____ Lower boundary
21. _____ Pneumothorax
22. _____ Nerve supply: phrenic nerve
23. _____ Flattens and lifts rib cage
24. _____ Maintains shape and diameter

■ *Structure and Function of the Lungs*

Match the descriptions in Column A with the correct structure in Column B.

Column A		Column B
25. _____ Contains two lobes	A.	Right lobe
26. _____ Working part of the lung	B.	Bronchopulmonary segments
27. _____ Gas exchange	C.	Terminal bronchus
28. _____ Self-contained; can be surgically removed	D.	Alveoli
29. _____ Anatomic dead space	E.	Lung parenchyma
30. _____ Contains three lobes	F.	Bronchioles
31. _____ Propels debris from the lungs to the mouth	G.	Left lobe
32. _____ Contain no cartilage, can collapse and trap air	H.	Mucociliary system

■ *Oxygen Transport and Gas Exchange*

Match the descriptions in Column A with the correct process in Column B.

Column A		Column B
33. _____ Blood flow	A.	Ventilation
34. _____ Atelectasis	B.	Perfusion
35. _____ Diffusion	C.	Gas exchange
36. _____ Carries oxygen and carbon dioxide		
37. _____ Occurs in the alveolar-capillary bed		
38. _____ Movement of air in and out of the lungs		
39. _____ Pulmonary embolism		
40. _____ Air flow		

■ *The Effects of Aging*

Fill in the blanks.

41. The majority of changes that occur with aging are seen in the _____ airway.

42. The movement of _____ in the _____ airway slows and becomes less effective. This change predisposes the older client to increased respiratory _____.

43. Changes in lung structure occur. The lungs become _____. Enlargement of _____ occur, which is not referred to as emphysema because it is not a result of disease.

44. There is an increased frequency of true _____ and a greater prevalence of chronic cough and sputum production. These changes predispose the elderly client to decreased lung _____ and respiratory _____.

■ *Short Answer*

45. What is the purpose of the pleural fluid?

46. Explain the role of diffusion in gas exchange.

47. What is the relationship between intrathoracic and atmospheric pressure during inspiration? During exhalation?

48. Compare and contrast the sneeze reflex and the cough reflex.

49. List the defense mechanisms that protect the integrity of the respiratory system.

50. List two things that affect ventilation and one thing that affects perfusion.

51. You are at the movies eating popcorn and drinking a cola. You aspirate a piece of popcorn. How long does it take the mucociliary system to propel the popcorn from the large bronchi, bronchial tree, and peripheral airway?

CHAPTER 59

Assessment of the Respiratory System

A thorough health history is the basis for a respiratory assessment. The history collects information about the client's present condition and previous respiratory problems. Information concerning common symptoms of respiratory disorders (cough, sputum production, dyspnea, hemoptysis, wheezing, and chest pain) is gathered, as well as a past medical history and family history. The physical examination or assessment follows the health history. The techniques of inspection, palpation, percussion, and auscultation are used to collect data. Diagnostic procedures are used to augment the assessment data. Common diagnostic procedures are chest x-ray, arterial blood gas analysis, pulmonary function tests, sputum tests, and bronchoscopy. Nurses must prepare the client physically and psychologically for these procedures. In addition, they must monitor the client after tests and anticipate and plan for possible complications.

OBJECTIVES

59.1 Give rationale for a focused respiratory assessment, including history-taking and physical examination.

59.2 Perform a basic respiratory health history and physical examination.

59.3 Prepare clients and significant others, both physically and psychologically, for various diagnostic procedures.

59.4 Discuss nursing responsibilities related to selected diagnostic procedures used to evaluate respiratory function.

LEARNING THE LANGUAGE: TERMINOLOGY RELATED TO ASSESSMENT OF CLIENTS WITH RESPIRATORY DISORDERS

Match the descriptions in Column A with the chest percussion sound in Column B.

Column A	Column B
1. _____ Increased air in lungs or pleural space	A. Resonant
2. _____ Thud-like sound; dense tipsier	B. Hyperresonant
3. _____ Drum-like; large air-filled chambers	C. Tympanic
4. _____ Airless tissue such as bone or muscle	D. Dull
5. _____ Normal lung sounds	E. Flat

Match the descriptions in Column A with the term used to describe normal or adventitious breath sounds in Column B.

Column A	Column B
6. _____ Consolidation	A. Bronchial
7. _____ Inflammation	B. Bronchovesicular
8. _____ High-pitched, crowing heard over trachea	C. Vesicular
9. _____ Constricted or narrowed airway	D. Fine crackles (rales)
10. _____ Pulmonary edema	E. Coarse crackles (coarse rales)
11. _____ Medium-pitched, heard over central airways	F. Atelectatic crackles
12. _____ Short crackling during inspiration	G. Wheeze
13. _____ Loud, low-pitched bubbling sound	H. Stridor
14. _____ Previously deflated airway, pops open	I. Pleural friction rub
15. _____ High-pitched, heard anteriorly over large tracheal airways	J. Voice sounds
16. _____ Inhaled air collides with secretions in trachea and large bronchi	
17. _____ Disappears after first few breaths, heard over dependent lungs	
18. _____ Low-pitched, heard over peripheral lung fields	
19. _____ Restrictive disease	
20. _____ Obstructive disease	
21. _____ Elderly clients, bedridden, first awakening	

Match the definitions in Column A with the appropriate pattern of respiration in Column B.

Column A	Column B
22. _____ Faster than normal rate of respiration	A. Cheyne-Stokes
23. _____ Normal respirations followed by periods of apnea	B. Hyperventilation
24. _____ Normal respiration: 12–16 breaths per minute	C. Tachypnea
25. _____ Periods of hyperpnea alternating with periods of apnea	D. Biot's breathing
	E. Eupnea

The following terms describe the appearance of sputum. Match the descriptions in Column A with the appropriate term in Column B.

Column A	Column B
26. _____ Yellow or green	A. Purulent
27. _____ Clear and white	B. Hemoptysis
28. _____ Mucus contains blood	C. Mucoid
29. _____ Contains more mucus than pus	D. Mucopurulent

Match the assessment findings in Column A with the correct term in Column B.

Column A	Column B
30. _____ S-shaped spinal curve	A. Clubbing
31. _____ Markedly sunken sternum	B. Barrel chest
32. _____ One side of chest moves more than the other	C. Pectus excavatum—funnel chest
33. _____ Concave spinal curve	D. Pectus carinatum—pigeon chest
34. _____ Enlarged angle of digital nailbed inward	E. Scoliosis
35. _____ Anteroposterior-transverse ratio 1:1	F. Lordosis
36. _____ Forward protrusion of sternum	G. Kyphosis
37. _____ Exaggerated posterior curvature, humpback	H. Paradoxical movement

■ Functional Health Pattern: Focused Health History for Clients with Respiratory Disorders

List pertinent assessment data for respiratory disorders in the following table.

38. **Health Perception–Health Management** Family history Past medical history Allergies Smoking Alcohol Immunizations Medications	39. **Nutrition–Metabolic** 24-hour diet recall Weight loss Energy to buy and prepare food	**Elimination**	40. **Activity–Exercise** Dyspnea Cough Sputum Hemoptysis Chest pain Exercise
41. **Sleep–Rest** Position of sleep	42. **Cognitive–Perceptual** LOC/orientation	**Self-Perception–Self-Concept**	43. **Role–Relationship** Occupation Home environment
Sexuality–Reproductive	**Coping–Stress Tolerance**	**Values–Beliefs**	

THINKING CRITICALLY: STUDY QUESTIONS RELATED TO ASSESSMENT OF CLIENTS WITH RESPIRATORY DISORDERS

■ *Short Answer*

Provide the rationales for the focused physical exam of clients with respiratory disorders.

44.   Respirations

45.   Skin color

46.   Cranial nerve I—olfactory

47.   Chest-wall configuration

48.   Fingers and toes

49.   Palpation: sinuses, trachea, and chest wall

50.   Chest percussion

51.   Chest palpation

52.   Chest auscultation

Indicate the reason for the test, whether an informed consent is required, and provide the rationale for the selected diagnostic tests for clients with respiratory disorders.

■ Diagnostic Tests

Test Purpose	Informed Consent	Pretest Nursing Care	Post-Test Nursing Care
53. Arterial blood gases (ABGs)		• Allen's test	• Hold pressure at site for 5 minutes
54. Pulmonary function tests (PFTs)		• Explicit instructions for each maneuver • No smoking or bronchodilators for 6 hours before test	
55. Chest x-ray		• Remove bra and any metal	
56. Pulse oximeter		• Do not place sensor distal to blood pressure cuff, pressure dressing, or arterial line	
57. Lung scan		• Explain procedure and assure client that sitting up during the test is possible • Assessment for iodine allergies *not required*	
58. Bronchoscopy		• NPO 6 hours prior to test • Assess cranial nerves IX and X	• Do not give anything to eat or drink until gag reflex returns. • Keep head of bed elevated. • Observe for respiratory distress. • Expect blood-tinged secretions.
59. Sputum		• Oral care prior to test • Collect prior to antimicrobials • May use direct or indirect method	
60. Thoracentesis		• Position upright, leaning over bedside table • Insertion of needle will be painful • Instruct against sudden movement during the test	• Position on unaffected side for 1 hour. • Vital signs and respiratory assessment • Amount of fluid withdrawn recorded on output record

CHAPTER

60

Management of Clients with Upper Airway Disorders

Tumors, polyps, a deviated nasal septum, or nasal fractures can cause disorders of the upper airway. Hemorrhagic, infectious, and inflammatory conditions also can affect the upper airway. Regardless of the etiology of the respiratory disorder, you must collect a complete assessment. These data will be the basis of your nursing care.

OBJECTIVES

60.1 Discuss etiology, incidence, risk factors, clinical manifestations, complications, diagnostic tests, and medical-surgical treatment of selected disorders of the upper airway.

60.2 Describe nursing management of the client with selected disorders of the upper airway.

60.3 Discuss respiratory disorders that produce chronic airway obstruction.

60.4 Plan care for a client with a tracheostomy.

LEARNING THE LANGUAGE: TERMINOLOGY ASSOCIATED WITH THE NOSE AND SINUSES

Match the definitions in Column A with the appropriate term in Column B.

Column A

1. _____ Nosebleed
2. _____ Loss of the sense of smell
3. _____ Common cold
4. _____ Procedure to straighten septum
5. _____ Offensive-smelling nasal discharge
6. _____ Abuse or overuse of topical nasal sprays or intranasal cocaine

Column B

A. Anosmia
B. Ozena
C. Rhinitis medicamentosa
D. Epistaxis
E. Rhinoplasty
F. Acute rhinitis

■ *Short Answer*

Give the rationale for the following interventions.

Intervention	**Rationale**

Tonsillectomy

7.   Teach client to expect tar-like stools.

8.   Place tonsillectomy client in side-lying position.

9.   Monitor vital signs closely.

10.   Give soft, bland food.

Rhinitis

11.   Give antihistamines to treat allergic rhinitis.

12.   Avoid overuse of topical nasal sprays.

13.   Consult physician if clear drainage becomes green or yellow.

Laryngitis

14.   Assess for heartburn, changes in sleep pattern.

15.   Implement voice rest.

16.   Refer to specialist for voice retraining.

Sinusitis

17.   Give decongestants to treat sinusitis.

Sinus Surgery

18.   Maintain drip pad for first 2 days.

19.   Avoid blowing the nose.

20.   Instruct client to sneeze with mouth open.

21.   Instruct client to increase fluids.

■ Clients with a Tracheostomy

Fill in the blanks.

22. A _____ is a surgical opening made into the trachea for airway management. It can be temporary or permanent. Indications for a temporary one include prolonged _____ and upper airway obstruction. Indications for a permanent one include _____, _____, and _____.

23. A universal tracheostomy tube consists of three parts. The outer cannula with cuff, _____, and _____. The outer cannula fits in the stoma to keep it _____. The flange has holes on each side to attach and secure tapes or ties. The secured flange keeps the tracheostomy tube from being dislodged.

24. The inner cannula can be removed for cleaning or replacement. The _____ facilitates insertion of the tracheostomy tube into the stoma.

25. Potential problems associated with tracheostomy tubes and cuffs include _____, _____, and _____.

26. With accidental extubation, if the stoma is less than 4 days old, it may close because a _____ is not formed. If extubation occurs, call for help and maintain _____ and _____ by bag and mask. Reinsert the tube if possible.

27. Weaning from a temporary tracheostomy tube is accomplished by _____ the cuff, and _____ the tube. The weaning process will vary from 2–5 days, depending on the person's ability to _____.

28. Tracheostomy suctioning is indicated when the client is unable to _____ and remove secretions. Extra hydration is needed because the hydrating mechanisms of the upper airway are _____. A room humidifier, humidified oxygen, and extra fluids help to liquefy secretions.

29. When securing the tracheostomy ties avoid placing the knot over the client's carotid artery because it can alter the _____ and erode the _____.

30. A person with a tracheostomy is at risk for constipation because he cannot perform the _____.

31. A person with a tracheostomy should always have some type of emergency call system and a prior agreed-upon form of communication because the tracheostomy prevents _____.

Match the descriptions in Column A with the risk factors and levels of prevention for laryngeal cancer in Column B.

Column A	Column B
32. _____ Educate the public on the hazards of smoking	A. Risk factor
33. _____ Refer clients to smoking cessation programs	B. Primary prevention
34. _____ Voice abuse	C. Secondary prevention
35. _____ Reduce the risk of progression of malignancy	D. Tertiary prevention
36. _____ Teach warning signs	
37. _____ Smoking	
38. _____ Alcohol abuse	

Match the signs or symptoms in Column A with the type of laryngeal cancer in Column B.

Column A	Column B
39. _____ No early symptoms	A. Glottic tumor
40. _____ Early hoarseness	B. Supraglottic tumor
41. _____ Early aspiration on swallowing	C. Subglottic tumor
42. _____ Carcinoma of false cord	
43. _____ Metastasis through regional lymph nodes	
44. _____ Early weight loss	

Select the best answer for the following questions.

45. Which type of tumor most commonly affects the larynx?
    A. basal cell carcinoma
    B. squamous cell carcinoma
    C. adenocarcinoma
    D. melanomas

46. Laryngeal carcinoma often metastasizes to the
    A. brain.
    B. breast tissue.
    C. lungs.
    D. uterus.

47. Following a nasal polypectomy, the client is placed in the
    A. Trendelenburg position.
    B. left side-lying position.
    C. Sims' position.
    D. semi- to high-Fowler's position.

48. The initial treatment of epistaxis is
    A. pressure on the anterior portion of the nose.
    B. application of warm compresses to the nose.
    C. insertion of nasal packing.
    D. cauterization of the bleeding vessel.

49. If the client is having posterior epistaxis, nasal packing and posterior plugs may be inserted. Nursing care for this client would include
    A. application of warm compresses to the nose.
    B. close monitoring for hypoxia.
    C. close monitoring for indications of anemia.
    D. application of cold compresses to the back of the neck.

50. Medical management of sinusitis includes
    A. use of steroid nasal sprays
    B. administration of dehumidified oxygen.
    C. use of diuretics.
    D. restriction of oral fluids.

PUTTING IT ALL TOGETHER

■ *Case Study*

Mr. F. is a 65-year-old man who retired from a chemical plant 5 years ago. Smoking history is 2 packs per day for approximately 50 years. Since retirement he drinks a six-pack of beer daily. He enjoys water-skiing, yard work, and gardening. Two weeks ago he began experiencing hoarseness and a sensation that something was caught in his throat. He is being evaluated for laryngeal cancer.

51. What are the risk factors for laryngeal cancer?

52. What are the common clinical manifestations of laryngeal cancer?

Mr. F. undergoes a laryngoscopy and biopsy. He is diagnosed with a subglottic tumor.

53. The physician orders ABGs, a chest x-ray, complete blood count (CBC), serum electrolytes, kidney and liver function tests, and a bone scan. Mr. F. is upset and wants to know why the physician is wasting time and spending his money on tests when he knows that he has cancer. How should the nurse respond?

54. Mr. F.'s tumor is classified and staged as a $T_3, N_2 M_0$. Explain what this means.

Mr. F. undergoes a total laryngectomy and radical neck dissection.

55. Explain why a radical neck dissection was performed.

56. List the complications of laryngeal surgery.

Identify the major nursing interventions for the following nursing diagnoses.

57. Risk for aspiration

58. Ineffective airway clearance

59. Risk for impaired gas exchange

60. Altered nutrition: less than body requirements

61. Impaired verbal communication

62. Potential for enhanced community coping

Explain why the following functions are altered in the client with a total laryngectomy. Use the picture below (Figure 60-8) to facilitate understanding.

63. Sense of smell

64. Ability to perform Valsalva's maneuver

65. Ability to blow his or her nose

66. Ability to gargle or whistle

67. Ability to breathe in normal manner

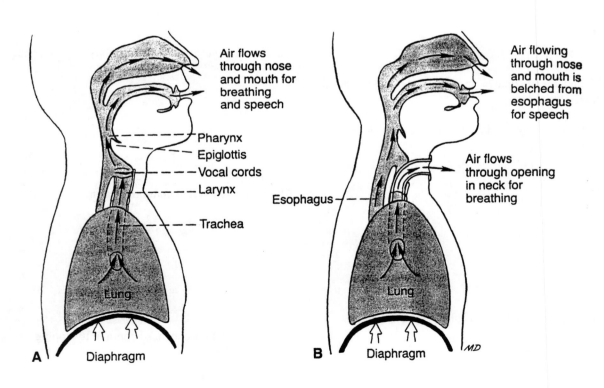

CHAPTER

61

Management of Clients with Lower Airway and Pulmonary Vessel Disorders

Common disorders of the lower respiratory tract include disorders of the lower airways and pulmonary vessels. Some disorders of the lower airways are asthma, chronic obstructive lung disease (COPD), and pulmonary embolism. The etiology and risk factors associated with these disorders are varied. Nursing care must be based on a complete assessment of each client. Teaching and post-hospital care of these clients are important and, therefore, must be included in the plan of care for these clients.

OBJECTIVES

61.1   Describe the incidence, etiology, risk factors, clinical manifestations, diagnostic tests, and complications associated with disorders of the lower airways and pulmonary vessels.

61.2   Summarize the medical/surgical management of selected disorders of the lower airways and pulmonary vessels.

61.3   Discuss the nursing management of disorders of the lower airways and pulmonary vessels.

61.4   Discuss the physical and psychosocial adjustments required of clients with chronic lower respiratory disorders.

Match the clinical manifestations in Column A with the appropriate disorder in Column B.

Column A	**Column B**
1. _____ Inspiratory and expiratory wheeze	A. Chronic bronchitis
2. _____ Enlarged anteroposterior chest diameter	B. Emphysema
3. _____ Wheezing; productive cough	C. Asthma
4. _____ Nonproductive coughing	D. Bronchiectasis
5. _____ Cough is uncommon	
6. _____ Elevated hematocrit	
7. _____ Hyperreactive airways	
8. _____ Purulent sputum production	
9. _____ Fever	
10. _____ Cachectic appearance, pink skin color	
11. _____ Barrel chest, cyanosis, dependent edema	

Match the descriptions in Column A with the appropriate disorder in Column B.

Column A	**Column B**
12. _____ Develops from thrombi in the extremities	A. Pulmonary embolus
13. _____ Occlusion of a pulmonary blood vessel	B. Pulmonary hypertension
14. _____ Occurs in young adults age 30–40 years	
15. _____ Acute chest pain aggravated by breathing	
16. _____ Cardiac catheterization	
17. _____ Give anticoagulants and thrombolytics	
18. _____ Give morphine for pain	
19. _____ Prolonged elevation of pulmonary artery pressure	
20. _____ Tachypnea, dyspnea, hemoptysis	
21. _____ Ventilation-perfusion lung scan	
22. _____ Heart-lung transplant	

THINKING CRITICALLY: KNOWING WHAT TO DO AND WHY

Provide the rationale for the following nursing interventions for the client with asthma, chronic obstructive pulmonary disease, and tracheobronchitis.

Intervention	**Rationales**

Client with Asthma

23.   Assess lung sounds every hour

24.   Monitor color and consistency of sputum

25.   Encourage fluids

26. Frequent oral hygiene

27. Beta-blockers contraindicated

28. Assess for triggering events

29. Teach step care program/action plan

Client with COPD
30. Administer chest physiotherapy

31. Teach diaphragmatic breathing

32. Offer frequent small meals

33. Encourage a diet high in fiber and bulk

34. Teach the client pursed-lip breathing

35. Teach the importance of low-dose oxygen therapy

36. Encourage client and family to vent feelings about living with a chronic progressive disease

37. Encourage relaxation techniques at bedtime

38. Suggest measures that may facilitate sexual activity

Client with Tracheobronchitis
39. Increase inspired humidity

40. Avoid cold environment air

41. Teach signs and symptoms of sinusitis

THINKING CRITICALLY: UNDERSTANDING RATIONALES

■ *Medications*

Listed below are medications used to treat respiratory disorders and nursing implications associated with these medications. Provide rationales for medication and the nursing implications.

Medication and Implications	**Rationale**
42. *Cephalexin (Keflex)*	
43. Check for allergy to penicillins before administering	
44. *Gentamicin (Garamycin)*	
45. Assess client for auditory and vestibular damage before beginning the drug	
46. *Theophylline (Theobid Duracaps)*	
47. Monitor blood pressure; use with caution in clients with hypertension	
48. Monitor theophylline levels	
49. *Prednisone*	
50. Administer with food	
51. Assess carefully for signs of infections	
52. *Diphenhydramine hydrochloride (Benadryl)*	
53. Monitor for dry mucous membranes	
54. Warn client about sedation	
55. *Metaproterenol (Alupent)*	
56. Teach client how to use inhaler	
57. *Heparin*	
58. Monitor partial thromboplastin time (PTT)	

Match the type of oxygen delivery systems in Column A with the appropriate oxygen concentration in Column B.

Column A		Column B	
59. _____	Nasal cannula	A.	95–100%
60. _____	Simple face mask	B.	24–44%
61. _____	Nonrebreathing mask	C.	40–60%
62. _____	Venturi mask	D.	Precise to within 1%; 24%–50%

PUTTING IT ALL TOGETHER

63. Which one of the following is an appropriate primary preventive measure for asthma?
    A. reducing air pollution
    B. monitoring peak airflow volumes
    C. teaching breath-retraining exercises
    D. administering pneumococcal pneumonia vaccine

64. Which one of the following is a cause of intrinsic asthma?
    A. mold spores
    B. smoke
    C. upper respiratory infections
    D. dust

65. During chronic bronchitis, airways collapse and air is trapped in the distal portion of the lung. This obstruction causes
    A. increased alveolar ventilation.
    B. alkalosis.
    C. hypoxia.
    D. increased tissue perfusion.

66. Low-flow oxygen therapy (1–3 L/minute) is ordered for clients with COPD because high flow rates
    A. dry mucous membranes.
    B. increase respiratory drive.
    C. increase carbon dioxide retention.
    D. constrict bronchial smooth muscles.

■ Case Study

Ms. P., a 77-year-old white female, has been experiencing shortness of breath during the last few years. She also experiences a mild cough when arising in the morning. Recently, Ms. P. has noticed that she has difficulty climbing stairs and walking any distance, even to her mailbox. She indicates that she must stop at intervals to catch her breath. In addition, she complains of excessive fatigue and loss of appetite.

She makes an appointment and is seen by her internist. The physician notes that she is using pursed-lip breathing. In addition, he notes a slight increase in the anteroposterior diameter of her chest. Although she does not smoke at present, she has a history of smoking 1 to 1 1/2 packs of cigarettes a day for a 50-year period. After a series of diagnostic studies, the physician tells Ms. P. that she has emphysema.

67. Which of the following is the most likely cause of Ms. P.'s shortness of breath?
    A. increased lung compliance
    B. increased elastic recoil
    C. obstruction of air passages
    D. excessive secretions

68. The increased diameter of her chest is caused by
    A. hypoventilation.
    B. hyperinflation of the lungs.
    C. dilation of the bronchial tree.
    D. hypoxemia.

69. Which of the following might improve Ms. P.'s appetite?
    A. increased amounts of milk and milk products
    B. a bedtime snack
    C. frequent small meals
    D. increased amounts of fluids containing caffeine

70. Which of the following should be included in Ms. P.'s teaching plan?
    A. signs and symptoms of left-side heart failure
    B. ways to increase social activities
    C. need to avoid outdoor activities
    D. need for immunization against influenza

CHAPTER

62

Management of Clients with Parenchymal and Pleural Disorders

Nursing care of clients with disorders of the lung parenchyma and pleura includes a wide range of disorders. The lung parenchyma is the essential working part or tissue of the lung. Disorders of the parenchyma include pneumonia, cancer of the lung, and adult respiratory distress syndrome (ARDS). Disorders of the pleura include pleural effusion. The etiology, risk factors, clinical manifestations, and treatment associated with disorders of the lung parenchyma and pleura are varied. Nurses play a major role in the care of clients with respiratory disorders. Therefore, it is essential to have an understanding of normal structure and function of lung parenchyma and pleura and the pathophysiology of each disorder. In addition, care of clients having thoracic surgery and being mechanically ventilated is presented.

OBJECTIVES

62.1 Describe the incidence, etiology, risk factors, clinical manifestations, diagnostic tests, and complications associated with disorders of the lung parenchyma and pleura.

62.2 Summarize the medical and surgical management of selected disorders of the lung parenchyma and pleura.

62.3 Discuss the nursing management of disorders of the lung parenchyma and pleura.

62.4 Discuss the nursing management of clients with chest tubes or those being mechanically ventilated.

LEARNING THE LANGUAGE: TERMINOLOGY RELATED TO CLIENTS WITH DISORDERS OF THE LUNG PARENCHYMA AND PLEURA

Match the clinical manifestations in Column A with the appropriate form of pneumonia in Column B.

Column A

1. _____ Sudden onset with single shaking chill
2. _____ Prodrome of 24–48 hours with fever, headache, and malaise
3. _____ Insidious onset; slowly rising fever
4. _____ Sudden onset with fever; multiple chills

Column B

A. Pneumococcal
B. Staphylococcal
C. *Legionella pneumophilia*
D. Mycoplasmal
E. Viral

Match the descriptions in Column A with the type of lung cancer in Column B.

Column A	**Column B**
5. _____ Rapid growth	A. Epidermoid (squamous cell)
6. _____ Responds well to chemotherapy	B. Adenocarcinoma
7. _____ Slow growth, metastasis uncommon	C. Large cell
8. _____ Secondary infections	D. Small cell (oat cell)
9. _____ Strongly linked with smoking	
10. _____ Slow growth, large tumor mass	
11. _____ Hilar or central mass	
12. _____ Pleural effusions	
13. _____ Arises from glandular tissue	
14. _____ Most common occurrence	

THINKING CRITICALLY: KNOWING WHAT TO DO AND WHY

Provide the rationale for the following nursing interventions for the client with pneumonia, pulmonary tuberculosis, fungal pulmonary disease, and cystic fibrosis.

Intervention	**Rationale**
Client with pneumonia	
15. Turn client frequently.	
16. Routinely auscultate the chest.	
17. Space activities.	
18. Splint chest wall with pillow.	
Client with pulmonary tuberculosis	
19. Instruct client to cough into paper tissues.	
20. Administer daily dose of INH at bedtime.	

Client with fungal pulmonary disease

21. Observe for thrombophlebitis on clients receiving fungicidal antibiotics.

Client with cystic fibrosis

22. Give oral antibiotics prophylactically.

23. Monitor for hemoptysis.

Client with cystic fibrosis

24. Place in private room.

25. Postop monitor closely for fluid overload.

26. Teach the client about daily immunosuppressive therapy regimen.

27. Teach the importance of follow-up visits.

Using the following illustration, review the physiology of expiration and inspiration with water-seal chest drainage and to help answer questions 35–43.

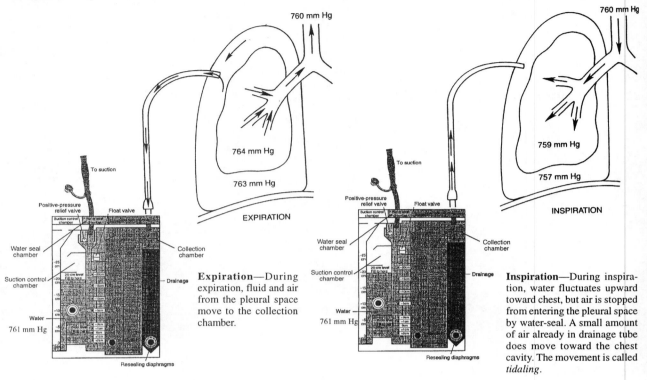

Chambers of Chest Drainage System

Collection chamber—The collection chamber collects drainage and allows monitoring of volume, rate, and type of drainage.

Water-seal chamber—The water seal chamber provides a one-way valve. It allows air and fluid to leave the intrapleural space but prevents backflow into the pleural space.

Suction chamber—The suction chamber uses suction to move drainage from the pleural space at a faster rate than just gravity drainage or when the client's cough and respirations are too weak to force air out of the pleural space.

Match the nursing interventions for management of chest tubes in Column A with the rationale in Column B.

Column A	**Column B**
28. _____ Assess chest drainage.	A. Normal fluid movement
29. _____ Observe water-seal chamber for tidaling.	B. Prevents backflow of fluid and air
30. _____ Observe for bubbling in the water-seal chamber.	C. Lung reexpansion
31. _____ Keep chest drainage system below the client's chest.	D. Possible hemorrhage
32. _____ Check tubing for patency.	E. Increases pleural pressure
33. _____ Strip or milk the tubing cautiously.	F. Kinks and clots
34. _____ Encourage coughing and deep breathing.	G. Indicates air leak
35. _____ Keep petroleum gauze within easy access.	H. Facilitates drainage
36. _____ Observe the suction control chamber for absence of bubbling.	I. Accidental dislodgment of chest tube

63

Management of Clients with Acute Pulmonary Disorders

Acute pulmonary disorders include any disorder that leads to respiratory failure. Examples are pulmonary edema, chest trauma, near-drowning, and carbon monoxide poisoning. There are two types of respiratory failure: hypoxemia and ventilatory. Hypoxemia respiratory failure occurs with disorders such as pulmonary edema where oxygen and carbon dioxide exchange at capillary membrane is altered. Ventilatory respiratory failure includes neuro and neuromuscular impairments. Mechanical ventilation is the standard treatment for acute pulmonary disorders for clients with respiratory failure. At one time, mechanically ventilated clients were cared for in the intensive care unit. However, today it is common to see ventilator-dependent clients in regular nursing units as well as long-term care facilities and at home. Nurses play a major role in the care of clients with respiratory disorders. Therefore, it is essential to have an understanding of normal structure and function of lung parenchyma and pleura and the pathophysiology of each acute disorder. In addition, nurses working in critical care must have a good understanding of ARDS (adult respiratory distress syndrome) because it is a frequent complication of acute lung injury.

OBJECTIVES

63.1   Describe the incidence, etiology, risk factors, clinical manifestations, diagnostic tests, and complications associated with acute pulmonary disorders.

63.2   Discuss the nursing management of acute pulmonary disorders.

63.3   Discuss the nursing management of clients being mechanically ventilated.

THINKING CRITICALLY: ACUTE PULMONARY DISORDERS

Match descriptions in Column A with the correct disorder in Column B.

Column A	**Column B**
1. _____ Mediastinal shift	A. ARDS
2. _____ Dyspnea on exertion	B. Pleural effusion
3. _____ Reduced capillary oncotic pressure	
4. _____ Accumulation of fluid in pleural space	
5. _____ Chest percussion dull or flat	
6. _____ Severe dyspnea and diffuse infiltrates	
7. _____ Sudden onset and progressive	
8. _____ Increased permeability of alveolar membrane	
9. _____ Mechanical ventilation	
10. _____ Poor prognosis	
11. _____ Often follows trauma to lungs	

THINKING CRITICALLY: EVALUATION

List how you will know if the mechanically ventilated client has met the goals for the selected nursing diagnosis.

Altered respiratory function

12.   Goal: Improved respiratory function

Risk for infection

14.   Goal: Remain infection-free

Anxiety

13.   Goal: Exhibit decreased anxiety

Altered nutrition: Less than body requirements

15.   Goal: Exhibit adequate nutritional intake

U N I T 14

Sensory Disorders

ANATOMY AND PHYSIOLOGY REVIEW: THE EYES AND EARS

Vision and hearing are two senses that bring information about our environment to our perception. Vision requires accurate transmission and interpretation of the transmitted signals. The ears are complex sensory organs for both hearing and balance. Any disorder of vision, hearing, or balance can greatly impact the client's ability to perform activities of daily living. A basic understanding of normal structure and function of each system is necessary to adequately assess and plan care for clients with vision and hearing and balance disorders. In addition, nurses use this knowledge to identify risk populations and plan health promotion and illness prevention activities.

OBJECTIVES

14.1 Demonstrate an accurate understanding of the structure, function, and vocabulary related to the eyes and ears.

14.2 Discuss the effects of aging on vision and hearing.

REVIEWING THE STRUCTURE AND FUNCTION OF THE EYES

1.   Label the structures of the eye.

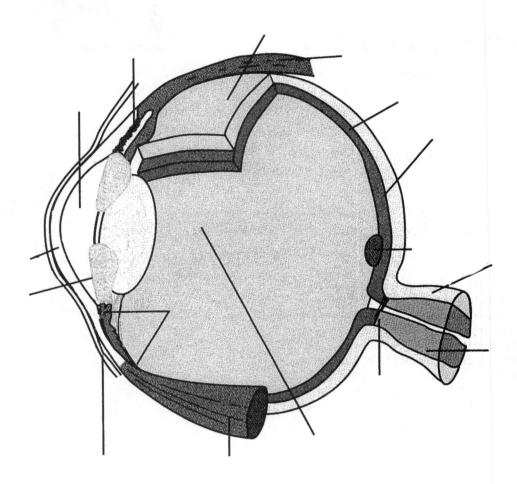

LEARNING THE LANGUAGE: TERMINOLOGY RELATED TO THE EYES

Match the following terms of structure and function of the eye in Column A with the correct definition in Column B.

Column A

2. _____ Aqueous humor
3. _____ Schlemm's canal
4. _____ Ciliary body
5. _____ Conjunctiva
6. _____ Cornea
7. _____ Iris
8. _____ Lacrimal apparatus
9. _____ Lens
10. _____ Meibomian gland
11. _____ Ocular adnexa
12. _____ Optic nerve
13. _____ Retina
14. _____ Sclera
15. _____ Trabecular meshwork
16. _____ Vitreous body

Column B

A. Oil-secreting glands
B. Thin, transparent layer of mucous membranes that lines the eyelids and covers the eyeballs
C. Fluid that circulates from the posterior chamber through the pupil to the anterior chamber
D. Transparent avascular structure that acts as a powerful lens to bend and direct rays of light to the retina
E. Fibrous protective coating for the eye
F. Direct continuity with the iris; is circular and surrounds the lens and secretes aqueous humor
G. Thin, pigmented diaphragm with a central apparatus (the pupil)
H. A structure in the anterior chamber angle where the aqueous humor is filtered before it moves into Schlemm's canal
I. Passageway for aqueous humor as it leaves the trabecular meshwork and is channeled into a capillary network
J. Biconvex, avascular, colorless, almost transparent structure that focuses light on the retina
K. Clear, avascular, jelly-like structure occupying space in the vitreous chamber; accounts for two-thirds of the eye
L. Thin, transparent layer of nerve tissue that forms the innermost lining of the eye; contains sensory receptors for transmission of light
M. Transmits visual impulses from retina to brain
N. Produces tears
O. Accessory structures of the eye (muscles, fat, and bone) that support and protect it

REVIEWING THE STRUCTURE AND FUNCTION OF THE EARS

17. Label the structures of the ear.

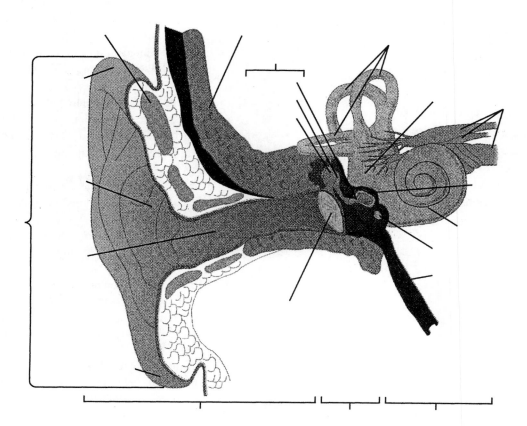

LEARNING THE LANGUAGE: TERMINOLOGY RELATED TO THE EARS

Match the following terms of structure and function of the ears in Column A with the correct area of the ear in Column B.

Column A	Column B
18. _____ Auditory nerve—cranial nerve VIII	A. External ear
19. _____ Bony labyrinth, cochlea, organ of Corti	B. Middle ear
20. _____ Cocha, tympanic membrane	C. Inner ear
21. _____ Eustachian tube equalizes pressure on both sides of the eardrum	
22. _____ Ossicles, eustachian tube, mastoid bone	
23. _____ Produces cerumen (ear wax)	
24. _____ Soundwave conduction, transmit sound to the eardrum	

EFFECTS OF AGING ON VISION AND HEARING

Changes	Effect
25. Eyebrows and lashes turn in	
26. Decrease in tearing	
27. Cataract formation	
28. Decrease in near vision	
29. Decreased tolerance to glare	
30. Decreased ability to adapt to light changes	
31. Ear hair becomes coarser	
32. Changes in the inner ear; loss of auditory neurons and cochlear hair cell degeneration	

64

Assessment of the Eyes and Ears

Sight and hearing are both integral parts in our lives; it would be difficult to overstate the impact that the loss of these senses has on a person. Assessment of these two systems may be simply a general screening or a more specific assessment. Nurses most often do a general screening assessment. The assessment begins with a thorough health history. It is important to know how to correctly assess the eyes and ears. Nurses can play a significant role in educating people about preventable vision and hearing loss. Additionally, understanding and interpreting diagnostic tests helps the nurse care for inpatient and outpatient clients who are undergoing medical and surgical therapy for eye and ear disorders.

OBJECTIVES

64.1 Describe the elements of a complete eye and ear assessment.

64.2 Discuss the pathophysiology, treatment, and nursing care for clients with common disorders of the eye.

64.3 Discuss the pathophysiology and medical and nursing interventions for persons with disorders of the ear.

64.4 Differentiate among the types of hearing loss.

64.5 Discuss pathophysiologies and medical and nursing interventions for clients with balance disorders.

LEARNING THE LANGUAGE : TERMINOLOGY RELATED TO ASSESSMENT OF THE EYES

Match the following terms in Column A with the correct definition in Column B.

Column A

1. _____ Astigmatism
2. _____ Chalazion
3. _____ Cycloplegia
4. _____ Diplopia
5. _____ Hordeolum
6. _____ Hyperopia
7. _____ Miosis
8. _____ Mydriasis
9. _____ Myopia
10. _____ Nystagmus
11. _____ Photophobia
12. _____ Presbyopia
13. _____ Ptosis
14. _____ Strabismus

Column B

A. Pupil dilation
B. Deviation of the eyeball
C. Infection of eyelash follicle or sebaceous gland
D. Granulomatous inflammation of the meibomian gland
E. Pupil constriction
F. Decreased ability to focus at near accommodation; common with aging
G. Intolerance to light
H. Sagging upper eyelids
I. Double vision
J. A rapid, involuntary, oscillating movement of the eyeball that is considered abnormal
K. Nearsightedness; a condition in which the light rays come into focus in front of the retina
L. Farsightedness; a condition in which the light rays come into focus behind the retina
M. A refractive condition in which light rays are not bent equally by the cornea in all directions
N. Causes paralysis of ciliary muscle and iris resulting in papillary dilation and paralysis of accommodation

Match the following eye tests in Column A with the correct description in Column B.

Column A

15. _____ Accommodation
16. _____ Consensual response
17. _____ Corneal light reflex
18. _____ Corneal reflex
19. _____ Direct ophthalmoscopy
20. _____ Ocular motility
21. _____ Slit-lamp examination
22. _____ Snellen's chart
23. _____ Tonometry
24. _____ Visual field

Column B

A. Tests cranial nerve V
B. One pupil constricts when light is shined in opposite eye
C. Pupils respond to changes in distance
D. Tests peripheral vision
E. Examines disc and retinal vasculature
F. Measures intraocular pressure
G. Determines eye alignment
H. Tests visual acuity
I. Tests extraocular muscles, the orbit, and cranial nerves III, IV, and VI
J. A slit beam of light is projected onto the eye, illuminating a cross-section of the anterior chamber

LEARNING THE LANGUAGE: TERMINOLOGY RELATED TO DISORDERS OF THE EARS

Briefly define or describe the following.

25.   Otoscope

29.   Decibel

26.   Romberg test

30.   Tympanometry

27.   Tympanosclerosis

31.   Webber and Rinne Test

28.   Ototoxic drugs

THINKING CRITICALLY: UNDERSTANDING RATIONALES

Provide the rationales for the therapeutic nursing interventions listed below.

	Intervention	**Rationale**
32.	Use the Otologic Health History as a guide for gathering data.	
33.	Be familiar with clues suggesting hearing impairment.	
34.	For an otoscopic examination on an adult, pull the pinna backward and upward.	
35.	Carefully examine the eardrum.	
36.	Test the client for nystagmus.	
37.	Examine the temporomandibular joint when a person presents with otalgia (ear pain).	
38.	Prior to examining tympanic membrane press on the tragus and mastoid bone and ask the client if he/she feels any tenderness or pain.	

CHAPTER

65

Management of Clients with Visual Disorders

Sight plays an integral part in our lives; it would be difficult to overstate the impact that loss of this sense has on a person. Not only do visual disorders affect activities of daily living but they can also affect job performance. Some visual disorders may even result in loss of jobs. The implications are numerous. Nurses need to understand the structure and function of vision, the specific manifestations of visual disorders, as well as the emotional and spiritual impact of the loss of vision. Nurses need to develop a holistic approach to manage clients with actual and potential visual disorders.

OBJECTIVES

65.1   Demonstrate an accurate understanding of the structure, function, and vocabulary related to visual disorders.

65.2   Describe assessment of clients with eye disorders.

65.3   Discuss the pathophysiology, treatment, and nursing care for clients with common disorders of the eye.

LEARNING THE LANGUAGE: TERMINOLOGY RELATED TO GLAUCOMA

Describe the following terms that describe the various types of glaucoma.

1.   Primary or secondary

2.   Acute or chronic

3.   Open (wide) or closed (narrow)

Match the following clinical manifestations in Column A with the correct type of glaucoma in Column B.

Column A

4. _____ Called the "thief in the night"
5. _____ Cupping or indention of the optic nerve disc
6. _____ High-risk group over age 40 and African-Americans
7. _____ Sees rainbow halos around lights; may complain of nausea and vomiting
8. _____ Increased intraocular pressure > 23 mm Hg
9. _____ Most common form of glaucoma
10. _____ No early clinical manifestations
11. _____ Occurs suddenly
12. _____ Severe pain, blurred vision or loss of vision
13. _____ Visual fields defect

Column B

A. Primary open-angle glaucoma
B. Angle-closure glaucoma
C. Both

THINKING CRITICALLY: UNDERSTANDING RATIONALES

State the rationale for the following interventions related to postoperative care.

Intervention	**Rationale**
14. Use of topical miotic medications for glaucoma	
15. Postoperatively, it is very important to prevent constipation.	
16. Caution the client using miotic medications about blurred vision and decreased accommodation.	
17. Postoperatively, for glaucoma, instruct the client not to lie on the operative side.	
18. Report unrelieved pain to the physician after cataract removal.	

■ Eye Medication Orders and Postoperative Care

Write out in which eye(s) the following medications are to be instilled.

19. Methylcellulose, 0.5% OU

20. Phenylephrine hydrochloride (Neo-Synephrine), 2.5% OD

21. Timolol, OS

■ Ophthalmic Medications

Match the drug categories in Column A with the actions in Column B and the specific drugs in Column C.

Column A	Column B	Column C
22. _____ Dye	A. Highlights cornea irregularities	a. Timolol maleate (Timoptic)
23. _____ Beta-blocker	B. Strong contraction of the iris (miosis) and ciliary body	b. Fluorescein sodium
24. _____ Carbonic anhydrase inhibitor	C. Reduces production of aqueous humor	c. Pilocarpine hydrochloride
25. _____ Oral osmotic diuretic		d. Acetazolamide sodium (Diamox)
26. _____ Anticholinergic	D. Emergency treatment of intraocular pressure	e. Glycerin (Osmoglyn)

PUTTING IT ALL TOGETHER

■ Case Studies

Mr. L., 74, has an appointment with the ophthalmologist because of changes in vision. A preliminary diagnosis of cataracts is made.

27. When taking a history from Mr. L., the nurse would expect him to report which of the following?
    A. significant bilateral eye pain
    B. blurred vision and difficulty with night driving
    C. a shadow or curtain across his field of vision
    D. itching and dryness of the eyes

28. Upon ophthalmoscopic examination of Mr. L., the nurse would expect to find
    A. congestion of the retinal vessels.
    B. multiple retinal hemorrhages.
    C. diminished or absent red reflex.
    D. atrophy and cupping of the optic nerve head.

29. Mr. L. is scheduled for an intracapsular cataract extraction (ICCE) in outpatient surgery. Preoperative eye drops include tropicamide (Mydriacyl), a cycloplegic, and cyclopentolate hydrochloride (Cyclogyl), a mydriatic and cycloplegic. The purposes of these medications are to
    A. dilate the pupil and paralyze the ciliary and dilator muscles.
    B. constrict the pupil and paralyze the ciliary and dilator muscles.
    C. increase outflow of aqueous humor and suppress its production.
    D. dilate the pupils and restrict the flow of aqueous humor.

30. Postoperative instructions for Mr. L. would include all of the following *except*
    A. pain management with aspirin.
    B. wear a metal eye protector at night.
    C. how and when to administer eye drops.
    D. limiting activity for the first 24 hours.

Ms. B. is a 63-year-old who comes to the clinic for her annual eye examination. The ophthalmologist measures her intraocular pressure and finds it elevated. Ms. B. is diagnosed with open-angle glaucoma.

31. Ms. B. questions the nurse about glaucoma. Which of the following provides the best explanation of open-angle glaucoma?
    A. Pressure builds in the eye from either over-production of aqueous humor or obstruction of outflow.
    B. Pressure builds in the eye because the lens becomes opaque.
    C. There are multiple hemorrhages in the eye resulting in decreased vision.
    D. There is a sudden build-up of pressure in the eye because of an obstruction of the outflow of aqueous humor.

32. The ophthalmologist prescribes pilocarpine eye drops for Ms. B. In teaching her about the effects of the medication, the nurse will most likely include which of the following?
    A. The medication will dilate her eyes and she will need protective glasses.
    B. The medication will constrict her eyes and cause minimal side effects.
    C. The medication will dilate her eyes and result in decreased accommodation.
    D. The medication will constrict her eyes and may cause blurred vision.

66

Management of Clients with Hearing and Balance Disorders

Some ear disorders may lead to hearing loss or problems with balance, either of which can be a significant problem. In addition, of the 10 million people in the United States over age 65, more than 90% have some hearing loss. These facts lead to the conclusion that nurses in most areas will be working with clients with ear disorders, especially hearing loss. In some cases, such as industrial settings, nurses may be able to have a role in prevention. In other cases, nurses will be caring for clients with whom communication is essential. Bridging this barrier will require the nurse to learn techniques and skills for communicating with people who are hearing impaired, in addition to learning interventions for caring for people with other ear and balance disorders.

Objectives

66.1   Discuss the pathophysiology and medical and nursing interventions for persons with disorders of the ear.

66.2   Differentiate among the types of hearing loss.

66.3   Discuss pathophysiologies and medical and nursing interventions for clients with balance disorders.

LEARNING THE LANGUAGE: TERMINOLOGY RELATED TO DISORDERS OF THE EAR

Match the following terms in Column A with the correct definition in Column B.

Column A

1. _____ Cerumen
2. _____ Conductive hearing loss
3. _____ Mastoiditis
4. _____ Myringotomy
5. _____ Myringoplasty
6. _____ Nystagmus
7. _____ Otitis media
8. _____ Otosclerosis
9. _____ Presbycusis
10. _____ Sensorineural hearing loss
11. _____ Stapedectomy
12. _____ Tinnitus
13. _____ Vertigo

Column B

A. Genetic disorder in which there is repeated resorption and redeposition of abnormal bone

B. Involuntary rhythmic oscillations of the eye

C. Middle ear inflammations

D. Inflammation of the mastoid cavity

E. Incision into eardrum

F. Loss of hearing in which air conduction is worse than bone conduction; involves external and middle ear

G. Secretion from cerumen glands and the fat from sebaceous glands

H. Perception that the person or surroundings are moving

I. Hearing impairment that occurs with aging

J. Ringing in the ears

K. Replacement of stapes with a prosthesis

L. Perceptive or "nerve" hearing loss

M. Closure of tympanic membrane perforation

DIFFERENTIATING BETWEEN CONDUCTIVE AND SENSORINEURAL HEARING LOSSES

Match the etiology and types in Column A with the category of hearing loss in Column B.

Column A

14. _____ Ear obstructions
15. _____ Infections
16. _____ Otosclerosis
17. _____ Tympanosclerosis
18. _____ Tympanic membrane trauma
19. _____ Cigarette smoking
20. _____ Congenital hearing loss
21. _____ Noise induced
22. _____ Benign and malignant tumors
23. _____ Menière's
24. _____ Central auditory dysfunction
25. _____ Presbycusis
26. _____ Ototoxic drugs

Column B

A. Conductive hearing loss

B. Sensorineural hearing loss

THINKING CRITICALLY: UNDERSTANDING RATIONALES

Provide the rationales for the therapeutic nursing interventions listed below.

Intervention	Rationale
27. For an otoscopic examination on an adult, pull the pinna backward and upward.	
28. Carefully examine the eardrum.	
29. Test the client for nystagmus.	
30. Examine the temporomandibular joint when a person presents with otalgia (ear pain).	
31. Treat Menière's disease with diuretics.	
32. Encourage the client on bedrest for vertigo to move slowly.	

Briefly define or describe the following terms.

33. Eighth cranial nerve

34. Tympanosclerosis

35. Ototoxic drugs

36. Decibel

37. Acoustic neuroma

CLIENT EDUCATION: KNOWING WHAT TO TEACH AND WHY

Provide rationales for the following teaching interventions.

38. Turn off hearing aids before removing.

39. After ear surgery, teach the person to blow the nose gently one side at a time, and to cough or sneeze with the mouth open.

40. If attending a rock concert, purchase tickets in the back rows.

THINKING CRITICALLY: KNOWING WHAT TO DO AND WHY

Develop nursing interventions for the following nursing diagnoses.

41. Sensory/perceptual alteration (auditory): diminished hearing related to presbycusis

42. Sensory/perceptual alteration (auditory): total hearing loss related to congenital defect (Data: person signs and reads lips)

43. Risk for injury related to tendency to lose balance

PUTTING IT ALL TOGETHER

■ *Case Study*

Mr. A., a 69-year-old male, was admitted to the medical unit with a diagnosis of bilateral pneumonia. He was started on an IV of 1000 D$_5$W at 100 cc/hour. The physician also ordered gentamycin 80 mg q 8 hours, complete blood count (CBC), electrolytes, and a soft diet.

44. Mr. A. stated at one point in the admission assessment that he didn't hear as well as he used to. Based on this data, the nurse did a complete assessment of his ears. In performing an otoscopic examination of the ears, the nurse would use which of the following techniques?
    A. Hold otoscope in nondominant hand and rest against the client's head. With the other hand, pull the pinna down and back.
    B. Hold otoscope in dominant hand (without resting hand against the client's head) and with the other hand pull the pinna up, back, and out.
    C. Hold otoscope in nondominant hand (without resting hand against client's head) and with the other hand pull the pinna back and down.
    D. Hold otoscope in dominant hand and rest against client's head. With the other hand, pull the pinna up, back, and out.

45. In order to prevent the potential ototoxic effects of the gentamycin that Mr. A. is receiving, the nurse would implement which of the following activities?
    A. Administer the gentamycin over 60 minutes.
    B. Maintain fluid intake at 2000–3000 cc/day.
    C. Limit patient fluid intake.
    D. Administer the gentamycin over 20 minutes.

46. Mr. A. is diagnosed as having presbycusis. Presbycusis is an example of which type of hearing loss?
    A. bone conduction
    B. air conduction
    C. sensorineural
    D. central

47. In order to improve communication with Mr. A., the nurse would do which of the following?
    A. Use one-word answers.
    B. Exaggerate pronunciation of words.
    C. Speak loudly to get his attention.
    D. Face him directly when speaking.

48. Mr. A. recovers from pneumonia and is discharged, but follows up on a recommendation about getting a hearing aid. In teaching Mr. A. about his hearing aid, the clinic nurse would include which of the following instructions?
    A. Wash ear mold weekly.
    B. Open battery compartment at night.
    C. Wear hearing aid at all times.
    D. Check battery if hearing aid "whistles."

Cognitive and Perceptual Disorders

ANATOMY AND PHYSIOLOGY REVIEW: THE NEUROLOGIC SYSTEM

A basic understanding of normal neurologic structure and function is a necessary prerequisite to learning to adequately assess the client with neurologic problems. The central nervous system (CNS) is protected by the skull, vertebrae, meninges, cerebrospinal fluid, and the blood-brain barrier. The neuron, composed of the cell body, one axon, and several dendrites, is the functional unit of the nervous system. Unfortunately, only the axon covered with myelin is able to regenerate after injury. Therefore, it is especially important for the client to have accurate assessments so appropriate interventions can more likely prevent permanent losses of function.

OBJECTIVES

15.1   Describe a neuron, its basic parts, and how it functions.

15.2   Give the general functions of each of the three divisions of the nervous system: central, peripheral, and autonomic.

15.3   List the main parts of the brain with their major functions.

15.4   Name the coverings of the brain and spinal cord, and describe their functions.

15.5   Describe the functions of the cerebrospinal fluid and the blood-brain barrier.

15.6   Describe the reflex arc and how it functions.

15.7   Describe a plexus, and locate and name the major plexuses of the spinal nerves.

15.8   List the names and functions of the cranial nerves.

15.9   Describe the main parts of the autonomic nervous system and how they function.

LEARNING THE LANGUAGE

■ *Terminology Related to Structure and Function of the Nervous System*

Match the following definitions in Column A with the correct term in Column B.

Column A	Column B
1. _____ CNS cells that form scar tissue after injury and contain calcium channels essential to nerve transmission	A. Astrocytes
2. _____ CNS cells that produce myelin	B. Basal ganglia
3. _____ Peripheral nervous system (PNS) cells that produce myelin	C. Corpus callosum
4. _____ Phagocytic scavenger cells	D. Infratentorial
5. _____ Chemicals that send messages from neuron to neuron	E. Lower motor neurons
6. _____ Spaces between neurons	F. Microglia
7. _____ Progression of action potential (resting, depolarization, and repolarization phases) through ion exchanges	G. Myelin
8. _____ Insulating lipid surface that increases speed of nerve impulses	H. Neurotransmitters
9. _____ Bundle of nerve fibers that connects major parts of brain	I. Nerve impulse
10. _____ Has role in controlling major motor activity	J. Oligodendrocytes
11. _____ CNS cells that originate in frontal lobe	K. Schwann cells
12. _____ CNS cells that originate in the spinal cord	L. Supratentorial
13. _____ All brain structures above the brain stem and cerebellum	M. Synapses
14. _____ Brain stem and cerebellum	N. Upper motor neurons

KNOWLEDGE BUILDING: STUDY QUESTIONS RELATED TO STRUCTURE AND FUNCTION OF THE NERVOUS SYSTEM

15. Label the lobes of the brain in the following diagram.

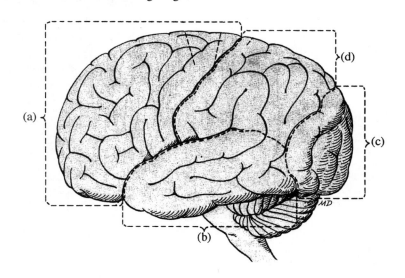

Match the functions in Column A with the lobes of the brain in Column B most associated with them.

Column A

16. _____ Auditory center
17. _____ Emotion and behavior
18. _____ Mental (thinking) activity
19. _____ Vision
20. _____ Motor aspects of speech
21. _____ Inhibiting primitive reflex
22. _____ Motor function
23. _____ Discrimination of sensory impulse (pain, touch, temperature)

Column B

A. Frontal
B. Parietal
C. Temporal
D. Occipital

24. Label the missing parts of the spinal reflex arc.

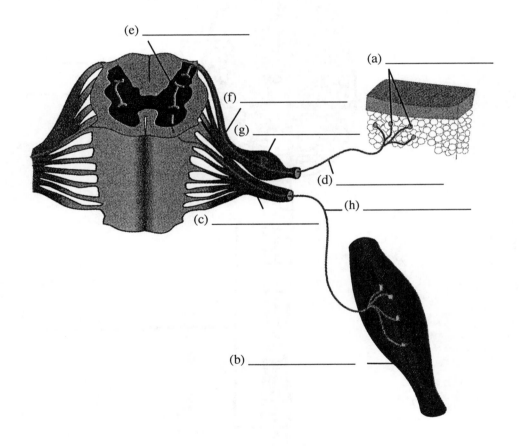

Indicate the appropriate part of the autonomic nervous system responsible for the following responses by marking an (S) for sympathetic or a (P) for parasympathetic.

25. _____ Increased gastrointestinal tract motility

26. _____ Constriction of blood vessels in skin

27. _____ Decreased urinary output

28. _____ Increased blood glucose level

29. _____ Dilation of bronchioles

30. _____ Increased heart rate

31. _____ Increased salivary gland secretion

32. In the diagram below, label the brackets with an (S) for sympathetic or a (P) for parasympathetic to indicate the origins of the two divisions of the autonomic nervous system. Then label the four cranial nerves shown in the diagram.

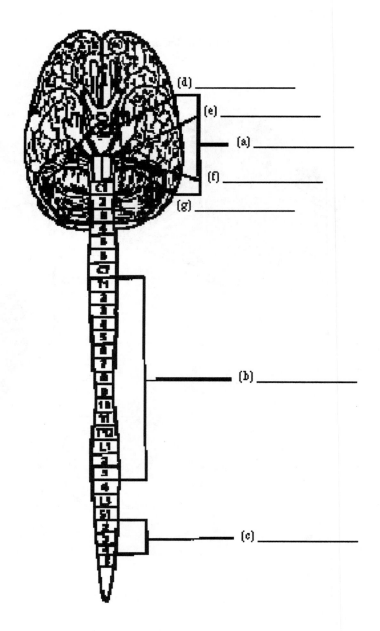

(d) _____

(e) _____

(a) _____

(f) _____

(g) _____

(b) _____

(c) _____

CHAPTER

67

Assessment of the Neurologic System

The focus of the nurse's assessment of the client with neurologic disorders is both anatomic and functional. Because neurologic assessment can be complex, neurologic charts and flow sheets are very useful. It is important to obtain baseline client data when assessing clients with neurologic disorders. In order to assess and report changes in the client's neurologic condition, the nurse must make frequent, careful observations and continually compare these observations with baseline data. Neurologic assessment includes a comprehensive neurologic health history, physical examination, and diagnostic tests.

OBJECTIVES

67.1   Describe the elements of a neurologic health history.

67.2   Identify the purpose and components of a detailed mental status exam.

67.3   Demonstrate the correct test for each cranial nerve.

67.4   List elements to be assessed in the motor examination.

67.5   Give examples of abnormal motor responses.

67.6   List elements to be assessed in the sensory examination.

67.7   Discuss the relationship between the abnormal sensory or motor response and the portion of the nervous system that is damaged.

67.8   Demonstrate the correct tests for major reflexes.

67.9   Differentiate between upper and lower motor neuron damage.

67.10   Interpret the neurologic implications of each section of the neurologic observation chart.

67.11   Give the diagnostic purposes of common neurologic tests.

67.12   Describe common neurologic diagnostic tests in laymen's terminology.

67.13   Identify potential complications of common neurologic diagnostic tests.

67.14   Plan and implement appropriate nursing interventions for clients before, during, and after assessment and treatment procedures.

LEARNING THE LANGUAGE: TERMINOLOGY RELATED TO NEUROLOGIC ASSESSMENT

Match the definitions in Column A with the appropriate term in Column B. Not all items will be used.

Column A

1. _____ Stereotyped movements of the same muscles each time
2. _____ Slow movement
3. _____ Sense of body position
4. _____ Sustained reflex activity
5. _____ Reduced body movements (e.g., swinging arms)
6. _____ Jerky, purposeless movements of hands
7. _____ Paralyzed on one side
8. _____ Stiff and rigid with joint flexion
9. _____ Hypotonic muscles
10. _____ Pushing stimulus away

Column B

A. Akinesia
B. Athetosis
C. Ataxia
D. Battle's sign
E. Bradykinesia
F. Chorea
G. Clonus
H. Dystonic
I. Flaccid
J. Hemiplegia
K. Localization
L. Proprioception
M. Spastic
N. Tic

THINKING CRITICALLY: KNOWING WHAT TO DO AND WHY

■ Neurologic Assessment

11. Can pupillary light response be tested in a client who is blind?

12. Which three cranial nerves control eye movements?

13. Damage to which cranial nerve can result in ptosis (drooping) of the eyelid?

14. Approximately what percentage of the population normally has unequal pupil sizes?

15. What is the condition in question 14 called?

16. Which cranial nerve controls pupil constriction?

17. Which two cranial nerves have you checked when you check for a corneal reflex?

18. How should you check for Babinski's reflex?

19. What is the difference between normal two-point discrimination on the forearms and fingertips?

20. Which lobe of the brain must be functioning normally for discrimination tests to be normal?

21. Do pain and temperature sensations travel on the same pathways?

22. What implication does question 21 have for testing in a neurologic examination?

23. What is the significance of nystagmus?

PUTTING IT ALL TOGETHER

■ Nursing Care Plan for a Client Having a Neurologic Test

24.   Develop a nursing care plan for Ms. B., who is
       having a magnetic resonance imaging (MRI)
       diagnostic test. Ms. B. is a 45-year-old white
       female admitted to the hospital for a neurologic
       work-up. Her signs and symptoms include ataxia,
       numbness and paresthesia of all extremities, hand
       tremors, muscle and joint pain, and blurred vision.
       She is scheduled for an MRI—a procedure that she
       has not had before—and she has some questions.
       As this is a relatively new diagnostic test in this
       hospital, there is no procedure developed for
       preparing the client. Therefore, you need to
       develop a care plan that would be appropriate for
       Ms. B.

CHAPTER

68

Management of Comatose or Confused Clients

When protective functions normally provided by the nervous system are lost, clients may exhibit a range of symptoms from the inability to blink to coma, depending on the degree of impairment to the nervous system. Nursing care is aimed toward substituting for the protective functioning that has been lost. An increase in intracranial pressure can permanently damage the central nervous system and can result in death. It is essential that nursing assessment be aimed toward early detection of increased intracranial pressure rather than later when intervention is futile.

OBJECTIVES

68.1 Differentiate between the two major kinds of physiologic disorders that can produce sustained unconsciousness as to etiology and clinical manifestations.

68.2 Identify levels of consciousness and discuss advantages of using a tool like the Glasgow Coma Scale to determine the level of consciousness (LOC) versus charting descriptions like "unconscious," "obtunded," or "in a deep coma."

68.3 Describe variations in breathing patterns that could indicate neurologic dysfunction.

68.4 Describe six areas of assessment in "neuro checks": level of consciousness, breathing pattern, eye movement, pupillary changes, motor response, and vital-sign changes.

68.5 Relate the importance of the six components of the "neuro checks" to cerebral functioning.

68.6 Discuss immediate assessment and interventions needed for an unconscious client.

68.7 Plan detailed nursing interventions and set priorities in providing nursing care for the unconscious client.

CRITICAL POINTS TO REMEMBER

■ *Physiologic Coma*

Etiology

Structural lesions (tumors, hemorrhage from trauma, or ruptured aneurysm)

Metabolic disorders beginning in another system and affecting the brain through hypoxia, ischemia, or accumulation of waste products

Toxins

Pathophysiology

Impairment/destruction of reticular activating system

Reduction of cerebral oxygen

Accumulation of waste products

Impaired metabolism of neurons

Clinical Manifestations

Structural Lesions:

Supratentorial lesions (above the cerebellum): symptoms vary depending on area of cerebral hemisphere damaged; e.g., damage to area in right parietal lobe results in numbness in corresponding area on left side of body controlled

Intact oculovestibular reflexes

Infratentorial lesions (cerebellum and brain stem): usually produce coma early

Oculovestibular abnormalities

Abnormal respiratory patterns

Pupillary changes

Metabolic Disorders or Toxins

Usually produce confusion first

Bilateral manifestations: e.g., tremor of both hands

Generalized seizures

Normal pupillary responses unless drug overdose

Nursing Care

Apply stiff collar (assume cervical spine injury if trauma present)

Clear airway and maintain

Lateral position

Hyperventilate

Maintain systolic blood pressure between 100 and 160 mm Hg

Use IV diazepam (Valium) to control seizures

Normalize body temperature

Maintain hydration without fluid overload (intake = output, stable body weight)

Maintain nutrition (enteral or parenteral feeding p.r.n.)

Use oscillating bed to prevent complications of bed rest

Assist with diagnosis and treatment of cause of coma (notify physician of change in neurologic status)

Stimulate patient to improve prognosis

Understand that vigorous treatment is not appropriate with poor prognosis

Poor Prognosis

Early and sustained absence of pupillary, corneal, or oculovestibular responses

Coma lasting more than one week with metabolic disorders

Assess families to determine possibility of organ donation (approachability)

LEARNING THE LANGUAGE: TERMINOLOGY RELATED TO COMATOSE PATIENTS

Match the following definitions in Column A with the correct term in Column B. Not all items will be used.

Column A

1. _____ Impaired judgment and decision making
2. _____ Decreased activity and alertness
3. _____ Inability to recognize time, place, and people
4. _____ Sleeps unless stimulated by speech or touch
5. _____ Unresponsive except to vigorous, sometimes painful, stimuli
6. _____ No motor or verbal response
7. _____ Irreversible brain damage resulting in permanent inability to support body functions
8. _____ Movement of eyes in opposite direction to the way that the head is turned—a normal response in an unconscious patient
9. _____ Flexion of the upper extremities and extension of the lower extremities, which occur with increased intracranial pressure at the cortical level
10. _____ Decreased pulse, increased systolic blood pressure, widening pulse pressure, and decreased respirations, which occur with increased intracranial pressure as an attempt to restore normal cerebral blood flow
11. _____ Increasing intracranial pressure toward the brain stem
12. _____ Behavioral disturbances, such as agitation and verbal outbursts, occurring between 3 pm and 7 pm

Column B

A. Brain death
B. Coma
C. Confusion
D. Cushing's changes
E. Decorticate posturing
F. Doll's-eyes reflex
G. Disorientation
H. Glasgow Coma Scale
I. Herniation
J. Lethargy
K. Obtundation
L. Stupor
M. Sundown syndrome

THINKING CRITICALLY: UNDERSTANDING RATIONALES

Provide the rationales for the therapeutic nursing interventions for the unconscious patient. (The complete nursing diagnosis provides the rationale; e.g., Risk for suffocation because the patient cannot swallow due to loss or suppression of gag and cough reflexes is the rationale for inserting an oral airway.)

Intervention	Rationale
13. Oral airway	
14. Suction p.r.n., oral care with patient in lateral position	
15. Oral care every 8 hours	
16. Special oscillating bed, reposition every 2 hours, keep skin clean	
17. Enteral feeding if GI tract functions, otherwise parenteral feeding	
18. I & O, daily weights, assessing condition	
19. Bed rails up with bed in low position, seizure precautions	
20. Bowel retraining, prevent diarrhea/constipation	
21. Family with patient, talk with patient	

69

Management of Clients with Cerebral Disorders

Seizure disorders, intracranial tumors, hemorrhagic cardio-vascular disorders, and neurologic infections are the cerebral disorders discussed in this chapter. Intracranial tumors and neurologic infections can produce seizures. Intracranial tumors, whether benign or malignant, primary or secondary, are among the most destructive lesions of the central nervous system. Epilepsy, a chronic disorder of recurrent seizures, is usually idiopathic. Even though the last two decades have brought significant advances in the understanding, diagnosis, and treatment of epilepsy, there still is an attached social stigma. Intracranial surgery may be a treatment option for clients with seizure disorders and is primary therapy for most clients with intracranial tumors.

OBJECTIVES

69.1 Identify pathophysiology of the following neurologic disorders: seizures, tumors, hemorrhagic cardiovascular disorders, and infections.

69.2 Relate the signs and symptoms of the above listed disorders to the pathophysiology by recalling normal functioning of the neuroanatomy involved.

69.3 Discuss the nursing interventions for the nursing diagnosis Potential for injury due to generalized seizure.

69.4 Discuss the social stigma that continues to be attached to a diagnosis of epilepsy.

69.5 Discuss the action, side effects, and nursing implications for medications given to treat epilepsy.

69.6 Discuss interdisciplinary management of the patient with an intracranial tumor.

69.7 List items to be included in the preoperative preparation for intracranial surgery that are different from those for general surgery.

69.8 Identify the potential intraoperative complications with intracranial surgery.

69.9 Utilize nursing care plans in caring for clients who have had intracranial surgery to prevent complications postoperatively.

69.10 Give rationale for nursing interventions for clients having intracranial surgery.

69.11 Recognize the signs and symptoms occurring with migraine headache.

69.12 Implement appropriate measures for individuals with migraine headache.

LEARNING THE LANGUAGE: TERMINOLOGY RELATED TO SEIZURES, INTRACRANIAL TUMORS, AND NEUROLOGIC INFECTIONS

Match the definitions in Column A with the correct term in Column B.

<table>
<tr><td colspan="2">**Column A**</td><td colspan="2">**Column B**</td></tr>
<tr><td>1. _____</td><td>Rigidity of the neck, a sign of meningeal irritation</td><td>A.</td><td>Absence seizure</td></tr>
<tr><td></td><td></td><td>B.</td><td>Aura</td></tr>
<tr><td>2. _____</td><td>Period during seizure</td><td>C.</td><td>Brudzinski's sign</td></tr>
<tr><td>3. _____</td><td>Sudden abnormal electrical discharge from brain that results in changes in sensation, behavior, movements, perception, or consciousness</td><td>D.</td><td>Clonic phase</td></tr>
<tr><td></td><td></td><td>E.</td><td>Encephalitis</td></tr>
<tr><td></td><td></td><td>F.</td><td>Epileptic cry</td></tr>
<tr><td></td><td></td><td>G.</td><td>Glioblastoma</td></tr>
<tr><td>4. _____</td><td>Inflammation of the brain</td><td>H.</td><td>Glioma</td></tr>
<tr><td>5. _____</td><td>Period of generalized seizure beginning with jerky muscle contractions</td><td>I.</td><td>Ictus</td></tr>
<tr><td></td><td></td><td>J.</td><td>Kernig's sign</td></tr>
<tr><td>6. _____</td><td>Gastric ulcers produced by hyperacidity of gastric secretions and decreased mucus</td><td>K.</td><td>Meningitis</td></tr>
<tr><td>7. _____</td><td>Precise localization of target tissue by computer using three-dimensional coordinates</td><td>L.</td><td>Nuchal rigidity</td></tr>
<tr><td></td><td></td><td>M.</td><td>Seizures</td></tr>
<tr><td>8. _____</td><td>Most lethal form of malignant brain tumor</td><td>N.</td><td>Status epilepticus</td></tr>
<tr><td>9. _____</td><td>Emergency condition in which patient has continuous seizures without regaining consciousness for at least 30 minutes</td><td>O.</td><td>Stereotactic</td></tr>
<tr><td></td><td></td><td>P.</td><td>Stress ulcer</td></tr>
<tr><td>10. _____</td><td>Subjective sensation before seizure; for example, strange smell or noise</td><td></td><td></td></tr>
<tr><td>11. _____</td><td>Brief period of altered consciousness lasting 5–30 seconds</td><td></td><td></td></tr>
<tr><td>12. _____</td><td>Pain and spasm of hamstring muscles when client's lower leg is extended with client supine, thigh flexed at right angle to abdomen, and knee flexed at a 90-degree angle to the thigh</td><td></td><td></td></tr>
<tr><td>13. _____</td><td>Cry that may occur with tonic-clonic seizures early in tonic phase</td><td></td><td></td></tr>
</table>

THINKING CRITICALLY: UNDERSTANDING RATIONALES

■ *Drug Therapy for Seizure Disorders*

Listed below are some important considerations of medication therapy for treating seizure disorders with specific drugs. Write the rationales for these considerations. Use Table 69-1 in Chapter 69 of the textbook and your pharmacology text.

Implication	Rationale
Anticonvulsant: Phenytoin (Dilantin)	
14. Good oral hygiene	
15. Intravenous use with cardiac monitor	
16. Slow rate of IV administration	
17. IV—use with saline solutions only	
18. Routine blood cell counts/drug levels	
Anticonvulsant: Phenobarbital	
19. Drug accommodation/drowsiness with initial therapy	
20. Avoiding sudden withdrawal of the drug	

THINKING CRITICALLY: KNOWING WHAT TO DO AND WHY

■ *Caring for Clients Having Intracranial Surgery*

21.   Why might clients having intracranial surgery be hyperventilated?

22.   Give at least one sign that could indicate cerebrospinal fluid leak postoperatively.

23.   What is the most common cause of hyperthermia postoperatively?

24.   Gastric pH should be kept above _____ to prevent stress ulcer. Which medications are given to increase the pH?

25.   How is the client's head usually positioned following supratentorial surgery? Infratentorial surgery?

■ *Caring for Clients with Epilepsy*

26. Is there a danger of the client becoming hypoxic during status epilepticus? Why or why not?

27. List two medications that are often given for status epilepticus.

28. Why is a social stigma often associated with seizure disorders and how can this be eliminated?

29. List observations to include when assessing seizure activity.

■ *Caring for Clients with Neurologic Infections*

30. What do nuchal rigidity, Brudzinski's sign, and Kernig's sign have in common?

31. Nursing interventions for the client with viral meningitis are related to symptom management. What are the usual symptoms?

■ *Caring for Clients with Intracranial Tumors*

32. What is an acoustic neuroma and what is the prognosis?

33. Why does a client with an intracranial tumor require interdisciplinary medical management?

■ *Caring for Clients with Migraine Headaches*

34. Describe symptoms of the classic (typical) migraine headache.

35. List two medications used to prevent migraine headaches.

70

Management of Clients with Stroke

Because cerebral disorders can be life-threatening and complex, neurologic nursing is one of the most challenging areas. In the United States, stroke (cerebrovascular accident [CVA]) is the third most common cause of death. Nursing care centers on helping the client maintain cerebral perfusion and maximize the level of functional rehabilitation while helping the client and family deal with the emotional reactions.

OBJECTIVES

70.1 Describe pathophysiology of stroke (CVA) and transient ischemic attack (TIA).

70.2 Identify three common causes of stroke.

70.3 Recognize the signs and symptoms occurring with the acute phase of stroke.

70.4 Implement appropriate measures for individuals with the acute phase of stroke.

70.5 Discuss the limitations caused by a stroke and the impact on family caregivers of a person who has had a stroke.

LEARNING THE LANGUAGE: TERMINOLOGY RELATED TO NEUROLOGIC DISORDERS

Match the terms in Column A with the correct definition in Column B.

Column A

1. _____ Agnosia
2. _____ Aneurysm
3. _____ Arteriovenous malformation
4. _____ Apraxia
5. _____ Cerebrovascular accident
6. _____ Homonymous hemianopia
7. _____ Transient ischemic attack

Column B

A. Visual loss in same half of visual field of each eye so client cannot see past midline without turning head toward that side

B. Condition in which client can move affected part, but cannot use it for purposeful actions

C. Neurologic changes caused by brain ischemia (a stroke)

D. Congenital, traumatic, arteriosclerotic, or septic weakening in vessel walls

E. Disturbance in interpreting visual, tactile, or other sensory information so client cannot recognize objects

F. Temporary decreased brain blood supply producing temporary hemiparesis, loss of speech, and/or paresthesias on one side of body

G. Congenital defect consisting of tangles of thin-walled artery and vein without capillaries

THINKING CRITICALLY: KNOWING WHAT TO DO AND WHY

Write short answers to the following questions.

8. Describe the emotional or behavioral reactions that often occur in clients after a CVA.

9. What are the two primary causes of death after a stroke?

10. List four specific interventions that may help in communication with aphasic clients.

11. What is the difference between a TIA and a CVA?

12. Why does hydrocephalus sometimes develop after a subarachnoid hemorrhage?

13. List four specific nursing interventions to help a client who is on aneurysm precautions avoid Valsalva's maneuvers.

CRITICAL POINTS TO REMEMBER

■ Stroke (CVA)

Etiology

Occlusion (thrombus-atherosclerotic plaque or embolus) or hemorrhage (hypertension or aneurysm causing rupture of vessel) resulting in brain ischemia and infarct

Pathophysiology

Decreased blood supply, hypoxia, ischemia, infarction

Clinical Manifestations

Transient ischemic attacks (TIAs)—early warning signs of stroke caused by thrombus

Headache, dizziness, fainting, paresthesias, and nosebleed may precede hemorrhage in hypertensive clients

No warning signs with emboli

Signs must persist longer than 24 hours to be diagnostic of stroke. They vary depending on area of brain damaged. Some signs include hemiparesis and hemiplegia, apraxia, aphasia, dysphagia, visual changes, agnosia, kinesthesia, abstract thought changes, emotional lability, and incontinence.

Emergency Care

Airway maintenance, turn patient on side if unconscious, loosen shirt collar, elevate head, avoid neck flexion, keep quiet

Critical Care

Hypervolemic hemodilution, anticoagulant if hemorrhage is not cause, edema, seizure, and blood pressure (B/P) control

Aneurysm Precautions

Dim lights, limit visitation, decrease noise, private room, elevate head of bed, avoid Valsalva's maneuver, administer analgesics (codeine) and sedatives (phenobarbital)

Acute and Subacute Care

Multidisciplinary services such as physical, occupational, and speech therapy

Nursing Care

Assess p.r.n. and report changes indicative of increased ICP.

Maintain airway and prevent aspiration.

Increase mobility (exercises, wheelchair, braces, physical therapy).

Maintain normal body temperature.

Protect skin.

Prevent corneal abrasion (eye patch and artificial tears p.r.n.).

Prevent contractures, "frozen shoulder," foot drop (range of motion [ROM] exercises, position with joints in extension, arm sling p.r.n., high-top tennis shoes).

Be patient and encourage self-care (teach family its importance).

Prevent injury from falls and burns.

Provide adequate nutrition (use feeding principles for clients with dysphagia).

Use communication techniques for clients with aphasia.

Provide orientation.

Be understanding and kind.

Community and Self-Care

Use individualized unit-dose containers and medication charts to help client learn self-medication.

Provide list of specific community resources.

Use rehabilitation home visits to assess client's ability to be mobile at home and be able to use home appliances.

CHAPTER 71

Management of Clients with Peripheral Nervous System Disorders

This chapter includes painful conditions of the lower back, cranial nerve disorders such as Bell's palsy and trigeminal neuralgia, and peripheral neuropathies. Restoring function and relieving pain are important goals. Understanding the psychological component is also important as it affects the client's ability to cope with the disorder.

OBJECTIVES

71.1 Describe assessment findings with a ruptured lumbar and a cervical intervertebral disc.

71.2 Differentiate among the signs and symptoms resulting from injuries to the following peripheral nerves: radial, median, ulnar, sciatic, common peroneal, axillary, and long thoracic.

71.3 Describe clinical manifestations associated with the cranial nerve disorders trigeminal neuralgia and Bell's palsy.

71.4 Describe nursing care for the client having a laminectomy and spinal fusion.

PATTERNS OF SENSORY LOSS OCCURRING WITH NEUROLOGIC DISORDERS

Match the patterns of sensory loss (A through L; see figure below) that occur with the specified neurologic disorder.

1. _____ Lesion of left side of spinal cord
2. _____ Complete transverse spinal cord lesion
3. _____ Radial nerve lesion
4. _____ Lesion of left side of brain stem
5. _____ Femoral nerve lesion
6. _____ Lateral femoral cutaneous nerve lesion

7. _____ Polyneuropathy
8. _____ Sciatic nerve lesion
9. _____ Left cerebral hemisphere lesion
10. _____ Common peroneal nerve lesion
11. _____ Median nerve lesion
12. _____ Ulnar nerve lesion

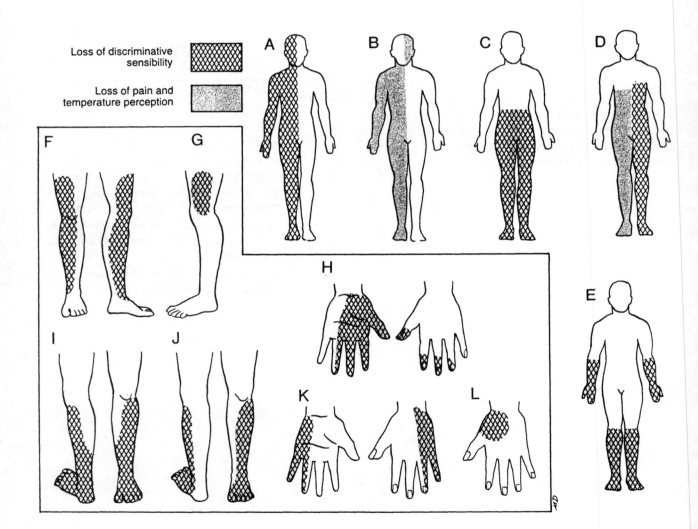

Loss of discriminative sensibility

Loss of pain and temperature perception

Management of Clients with Degenerative Neurologic Disorders

Degenerative neurologic disorders have a profound effect on the client and his/her family. Usually, these disorders are progressive, affecting the client's physical or mental ability. Because there currently is no known cure, the nurse needs to focus care on the management of clinical manifestations and prevention of complications. Supportive care for the client and family is essential.

OBJECTIVES

72.1   Identify pathophysiology of the following neurologic disorders: Alzheimer's disease, multiple sclerosis, Parkinson's disease, myasthenia gravis, amyotrophic lateral sclerosis, Huntington's disease, and Guillain-Barré syndrome.

72.2   Relate the signs and symptoms of the above listed disorders to the pathophysiology by recalling normal functioning of the neuroanatomy involved.

72.3   Discuss the profound physical and psychosocial adjustments required of clients (and their significant others) experiencing permanent or progressive neurologic problems.

72.4   Locate or develop standardized care plans for clients with the following common neurologic disorders: Alzheimer's disease, multiple sclerosis, Parkinson's disease, myasthenia gravis, amyotrophic lateral sclerosis, Huntington's disease, and Guillain-Barré syndrome.

72.5   Discuss the action, side effects, and nursing implications for medications given to treat Parkinsonism and myasthenia gravis.

PUTTING IT ALL TOGETHER: PATHOPHYSIOLOGY OF NEUROLOGIC DISORDERS

Using the chart below, connect the normal function to the disruption to the resulting signs and symptoms and then finally, to the disease. For example, number 1, disruption B, signs/symptoms I, and disease O.

Normal Function	Disruption	Signs/Symptoms	Disease
1. Substantia nigra and basal ganglia provide for purposeful, coordinated movements	A. Degeneration of myelin sheath	F. Atrophy of muscles of hands, forearms, and legs	K. Alzheimer's disease
	B. Decrease in concentration of dopamine		L. Guillain-Barré Syndrome
2. Myelin sheath insulates to promote normal conduction	C. Autoimmune disease that destroys acetylcholine receptor site	G. Sequence of loss of higher cognitive functions, with memory loss first	M. Myasthenia gravis
			N. Multiple sclerosis
3. Motor neuron cells conduct impulses to muscles or organs	D. Neurofibrillary tangles and plaques	H. Muscle weakness, paresthesia, gait difficulties, visual changes	O. Parkinson's disease
4. Nerve impulse travels through axon of motor nerve; acetylcholine is released from sacs in myoneural junction to react with muscle fiber to stimulate contraction	E. Degeneration of motor cells in spinal cord, brain stem, cortex, and some motor tracks	I. Various degrees of tremor and akinesia	
		J. Fluctuating weakness of striated muscle: ocular, facial, lingual, swallowing, and mastication	
5. Normal neurons and cytoplasm in association areas			

THINKING CRITICALLY: UNDERSTANDING RATIONALES

■ Drug Therapy for Neurologic Disorders

Listed below are some important considerations of medication therapy for treating various neurologic disorders with specific drugs. Write the rationales for these considerations.

Consideration	Rationale
Myasthenia Gravis	
Pyridostigmine bromide (Mestinon)/neostigmine bromide (Prostigmin)	
6. Medicate 45–60 minutes a.c.	
7. Individualize dosage/schedule	
8. Observe for increased myasthenia symptoms	

Prednisone
9.   Use antacids liberally

10.   Hospitalize to begin treatment

11.   Give at the same time each day

Parkinson's Disease
Levodopa (Larodopa)
12.   Monitor blood pressure

13.   Add carbidopa (Sinemet)

14.   Avoid vitamin B$_6$

Putting It All Together

■ Outline Summary of a Neurologic Disorder

Use the following example of an outline summary of a neurologic disorder, which includes definition, normal physiology, pathophysiology, usual signs and symptoms, diagnostic tests, and usual nursing care, to make similar summaries of other neurologic disorders.

Myasthenia Gravis

I.   Definition
   A.   Chronic disorder of neuromuscular transmission that results in weak skeletal muscles

II.   Pathophysiology
   A.   Normally, depolarization occurs as motor nerve terminals release acetylcholine that leads to muscle contraction
   B.   Abnormally (in myasthenia gravis), antibodies directed against acetylcholine receptors impair depolarization and, therefore, muscle contraction

III.   Usual signs and symptoms
   A.   Extreme muscular weakness
      1.   Worsens with use
      2.   Relieved with rest
   B.   Weakness of muscles innervated by cranial nerves
      1.   Diplopia (double vision)
      2.   Ptosis (drooping eyelids)
      3.   Masklike expression
      4.   Dysphagia (difficulty swallowing)
      5.   Dysarthria (difficulty speaking)
   C.   Weakness of respiratory muscles
      1.   Decreased vital capacity
      2.   Dyspnea

IV.   Diagnostic tests
   A.   Anticholinesterase tests
      1.   Edrophonium chloride (Tensilon): injection of 2 mg is given IV. If there is no improvement in muscle strength within 1 minute, repeated doses may be given at 2-minute intervals until a total of 10 mg has been given or a response has been demonstrated.
      2.   Neostigmine methylsulfate (Prostigmin): 0.5–1 mg IV may also be used.

B. Nerve stimulation studies
  1. Electrical stimulation of nerves leads to progressive weakness of affected muscles (Jolly's reaction).
C. Serum antibody tests
  1. Radioimmunoassay reveals increased serum antibody titers.
D. Radiologic studies
  1. Thymus scan reveals thymoma or enlarged thymus.
  2. Chest x-ray reveals enlarged thymus.

V. Usual nursing care
A. Diagnosis: Ineffective airway clearance due to dyspnea and impaired ability to cough and swallow. Assess for weakness of cough and ability to handle secretions
  1. Check vital signs including respiratory rate, quality, and pattern.
  2. Assess breath sounds for decreased aeration or obstruction.
  3. Assess for dyspnea on exertion and at rest.
  4. Monitor vital capacity.
  5. Encourage deep breathing and coughing, give chest physiotherapy.
  6. Keep suction equipment at bedside.
  7. Administer oxygen as prescribed.
  8. Teach avoidance of respiratory infections.
B. Diagnosis: Altered nutrition: less than body requirements
  1. Observe for dysphagia and regurgitation of fluid through the nose.
  2. Follow daily calorie count.
  3. Provide small, frequent meals of semisolid food.
  4. Tube feedings or IV infusions may be necessary.
  5. Adjust medications so doses are given about 1 hour before meals.
C. Diagnosis: Impaired physical mobility due to muscular weakness
  1. Assess cranial nerve functioning.
  2. Check muscle strength of all groups with repetitive activity.
  3. Administer anticholinesterases, corticosteroids, and other medications precisely on time.

4. Correlate assessment of muscle strength with time of medication (peak effect is usually 1–2 hours after administration).
5. Plan activities around peak effect levels of medications.
6. Provide rest periods between activities.
7. Minimize emotional stress.
D. Diagnosis: Knowledge deficit regarding disease
  1. Assess level of understanding regarding treatment and prognosis.
  2. Provide realistic information.
    a. How to avoid precipitating factors in crisis (fatigue, stress, infection)
    b. Importance of nutrition (regular, well-balanced diet) and sleep (at least 8 hours every night)
    c. Detailed medication information
    d. Avoidance of all over-the-counter medications
    e. Signs/symptoms of myasthenia crisis and cholinergic crisis (See Box 72-2 in the text.)
    f. Emergency measures (medical alert identification, working telephone in home with emergency number visible at all times, knowledge of how to obtain emergency medical assistance)
    g. Appropriate resources, including Myasthenia Gravis Foundation
    h. Proper use of therapeutic devices
    i. Importance of regular medical check-ups
  3. Promote maximal independence.
E. Diagnosis: Altered family processes
  1. Assess level of anxiety and knowledge level of patient and family.
  2. Provide realistic information. (See interventions listed in "D" above.)
  3. Encourage verbalizations of concerns, fears, and questions.
  4. Reassure patient and family that the best control occurs with their knowledge of the disease and their participation in the appropriate management of the disease so that they may work toward maximal independence.

73

Management of Clients with Neurologic Trauma

Each year approximately 10,000 individuals sustain a spinal cord injury, with the majority occurring to young people. Every 15 seconds, someone in the United States sustains a head injury.

Because brain and spinal cord injuries have such devastating consequences, which are often permanent, it is essential to work toward preventing accidents that can result in these types of injuries. It is also crucial to give appropriate care in the acute phase of an injury to prevent further damage to the brain or spinal cord. It is very important to teach and give the best rehabilitative care available in order to prevent complications and provide the most functional, highest quality of life possible for the victims.

OBJECTIVES

73.1 Describe the neurologic signs of herniation syndromes.

73.2 List the advantages of increased ICP monitoring.

73.3 Discuss in detail the use of the Glasgow Coma Scale.

73.4 Describe immediate assessment and interventions needed for a client with an onset of increased ICP.

73.5 Identify nursing responsibilities in interventions for clients with increased ICP.

73.6 Recognize the signs and symptoms occurring with head injury.

73.7 Compare the initial signs and symptoms of clients with spinal injuries at C3–C4, C5–C6, and L4–L5 levels.

73.8 Describe the signs and symptoms and the physiologic bases of autonomic dysreflexia (hyperreflexia).

73.9 Discuss emergency treatment for a victim of a suspected spinal cord injury.

73.10 List nursing interventions and their rationales for clients who are experiencing autonomic dysreflexia.

73.11 Identify nursing diagnoses and interventions for commonly occurring problems for clients with spinal cord injuries.

OBJECTIVES (CONTINUED)

73.12   Explain, in general terms, medical-surgical interventions to stabilize cervical, thoracic, and lumbar spinal fractures.

73.13   Discuss the profound physical and psychosocial (including sexual) adjustments required of clients, and their significant others, experiencing spinal cord injury.

THINKING CRITICALLY: KNOWING WHAT TO DO AND WHY

Choose the correct answer to the following questions.

1.   Monitoring for increased intracranial pressure (ICP) is ordered. Which of the following pressures indicates an onset of increased ICP and is a symptom of a serious underlying problem?
   A.   60 mm Hg
   B.   100 mm Hg
   C.   160 mm Hg
   D.   260 mm Hg

2.   Herniation syndromes could occur late in the course of increased ICP. Which of the following signs is more likely to result from an early stage of central transtentorial herniation (compression of the cerebral hemisphere that displaces the diencephalon and midbrain through the tentorial notch)?
   A.   dilated pupil
   B.   change in level of consciousness
   C.   generalized seizures
   D.   decorticate posturing

3.   Which of the following signs is more likely to result from a late stage of lateral transtentorial herniation (compression of the temporal lobe that displaces the uncus through the incisura, compressing the third cranial nerve, the midbrain, and the posterior cerebral artery)?
   A.   central neurogenic hyperventilation
   B.   dilation of the ipsilateral pupil
   C.   decerebrate posturing
   D.   generalized seizures

4.   What is the uncus?
   A.   the medially curved anterior part of the hippocampal gyrus
   B.   the central portion of the temporal lobe
   C.   the third cranial nerve
   D.   part of the brain stem

Write short answers to the following questions.

5.   List four advantages of intracranial pressure monitoring.

6.   What is the rationale for using mechanical hyperventilation as a treatment for increased ICP?

7.   What effect does hyperthermia have on increased ICP?

8.   What effect does seizure activity have on increased ICP?

PUTTING IT ALL TOGETHER

■ Case Study: Use of Neurologic Flow Sheet: Patient Situation

Use the following patient situation and Neurologic Flow Sheet on the next page to determine what is occurring with the changes in neuro status and decide which nursing actions are appropriate. Give the rationale for the nursing actions.

Mr. T. is a 26-year-old male brought to the emergency department following a motor vehicle accident. He is alert and oriented x 3 but has no recall of the accident and complains of a headache. The skull x-rays show a hairline fracture in the left temporal region. He is admitted to the neuro unit for observation with a diagnosis of closed head injury. His orders include: NPO, CT in am, and neuro checks with vital signs (B/P, P, R) q 30 min x 4, q hour x 2 then q 2 h.

9.   Suspected problem?

10.   Nursing actions and rationales?

MISSION HOSPITAL
REGIONAL MEDICAL CENTER

ADULT NEURO FLOW SHEET

TIME

GLASGOW COMA SCALE		Eyes Open	
		Best Motor	
		Best Verbal	
		TOTAL	
VOLUNTARY	**MOTOR**	Right	upper extremity
			lower extremity
		Left	upper extremity
			lower extremity
CRANIAL NERVES	**PUPILS**	Right	Size
			Reaction
		Left	Size
			Reaction
	EOMS	Conjugate	
		Dysconjugate	
		Tracking Right	
		Left	
	Blink Reflex		
	Gag Reflex		
	Facial Symmetry		

TIME

KEY

MOTOR
5+ Normal Power
4+ Weakness
3+ Anti-gravity
2+ Not anti-gravity
1+ Trace
0 No movement

Pupil B = Brisk
Size S = Sluggish
       A = Absent

2mm 3mm 4mm 5mm

6mm 7mm 8mm

✔ = Present
O = Absent
S = Symmetrical
A = Asymmetrical

Date

Speech Patterns: _____

_____

Comments: _____

_____

_____

_____

_____

_____

_____

_____

_____

_____

GLASGOW COMA SCALE	Eyes Open	4	Spontaneously
		3	To verbal command
		2	To Pain
		1	No Response
	Best Motor Response	6	Obeys Commands
		5	Localize Pain
		4	Flexion to pain withdraw
		3	Flexion Decorticate
		2	Extension to pain (decerebrate)
		1	No Response to pain
	Best Verbal Response	5	Oriented
		4	Confused
		3	Inappropriate words
		2	Incomprehensible sounds
		1	No Response

Unit _____

R.N. Signature _____ Shift: _____

R.N. Signature _____ Shift: _____

R.N. Signature _____ Shift: _____

ADDRESSOGRAPH

Adult Neuro Flow Sheet

#408 10/89

THINKING CRITICALLY: KNOWING WHAT TO DO AND WHY

■ Spinal Cord Injury

11. What are the main causes of spinal cord injuries?

12. What group represents the largest percentage of people in the cord-injured population?

13. What might be done to help decrease the number of individuals who receive this type of injury?

14. List the care needed by the injured at the site of an accident, including care before movement.

15. What can happen if the injured individual does not receive appropriate management at the time of the accident, or later, before knowledgeable professionals take over care?

16. What are the usual manifestations of a cord injury during the period of spinal shock?

17. If the ascending tracts of the cord are severed, what are the results of the injury?

18. If ascending tracts on only one side of the cord are involved, what are the results of the injury?

19. If the descending tracts of the cord are severed, what are the results of the injury?

20. The phrenic nerve is composed of fibers from the third, fourth, and fifth cervical spinal nerves. If the spinal cord is crushed above this area, what would happen to the client? If the nerve is damaged, what therapy will the client need? Why?

21. When the period of spinal shock is over, what type of paralysis develops in most clients?

25. Who is at greater risk for a urinary tract infection, the client with an indwelling catheter or the client who does intermittent catheterization?

22. What is the objective for the use of Crutchfield tongs? Where are they placed?

26. What is the main cause of decubitus ulcers?

23. If the fracture and cord injury are in the thoracic or lumbar region, would traction be used? How would you turn the client? Why?

27. What can be done to lessen the development of contractures?

28. What state facilities provide care for the rehabilitation of the spinal cord–injured client?

24. Why is a high fluid intake so important for these clients?

■ *Activities Possible with Level of Injury*

Match the following activities that could be accomplished by clients with spinal cord injuries in Column A with the specific level of injury in Column B. There may be more than one answer (activity) for each level of injury. Check your answers by referring to Table 73-3 in the text.

Column A	Column B
29. _____ C5	A. Transfer to and from wheelchair
30. _____ C6	B. No independent use of hands
31. _____ C7	C. Total dressing independence
32. _____ T1	D. Ambulation with short leg braces
33. _____ T12	E. Turn self in bed with arm slings
34. _____ L4	F. Dress upper trunk
	G. Independent self-feeding
	H. Total wheelchair independence
	I. Some ambulation with bilateral long leg braces and crutches

PUTTING IT ALL TOGETHER

■ *Case Study: A Client with Hyperreflexia*

Describe the physiologic basis for hyperreflexia, identify potential causes, and set priorities for emergency treatment.

Mr. J. is a 26-year-old male with quadriplegia at the C6 level. The injury occurred 11 months ago. Mr. J. has been readmitted to the hospital with a kidney infection. The nurse answers Mr. J.'s call light; he is complaining of severe headache, his face is flushed, and he has blurred vision. The nurse takes his vital signs and the results are: B/P 250/150, P 60, R 30.

35. Physiologic basis for hyperreflexia?

36. Potential causes?

37. Emergency treatment in order of priority?

CRITICAL POINTS TO REMEMBER

■ *Brain Injuries*

Etiology

Sudden force to head (blunt or penetrating trauma)

Pathophysiology

Concussion (no visible damage, biochemical damage), contusion (bruise), hematoma (bleeding) which may be epidural or subdural

Clinical Manifestations

Concussion results in loss of consciousness for 5 minutes or less. Contusions and hematomas cause brain damage. Signs of cerebral contusion vary depending on area of brain affected. Brain stem injuries usually render a client immediately unresponsive with respiratory, pupillary, eye movement, and motor abnormalities. Clients may have cerebrospinal fluid (CSF) leak from their nose or ear, blood behind tympanic membrane, periorbital ecchymoses, bruise over mastoid (Battle's sign) with basilar skull fracture. Epidural hematoma usually produces unconsciousness shortly after injury, brief period of recovery, and then rapid deterioration into coma. Subdural hematomas may be acute or chronic with the acute type producing symptoms similar to epidural hematomas.

Emergency Care

Assume cervical spine injury and treat accordingly until lateral cervical spine radiographs are obtained. Cover head wounds, do not attempt to remove penetrating objects, and provide ventilatory support.

Critical Care

Continue ventilatory support, observe for increasing ICP and control (see ICP above). Observe for and treat diabetes insipidus or syndrome of inappropriate secretion of antidiuretic hormone (SIADH), neurogenic pulmonary edema, which is similar to adult respiratory distress syndrome (ARDS).

Recovery Phase

Observe for post-traumatic response and be supportive.

■ *Increased Intracranial Pressure (ICP)*

Etiology

Hemorrhage, tumor, hydrocephalus, cerebral infarction, abscess, toxin

Pathophysiology

Expansion of brain tissue, increase in blood or cerebrospinal fluid within skull that cannot expand

Herniation

Displacement of brain tissue, occurs late in increased ICP, body's last attempt to adapt, always an emergency regardless of type

Clinical Manifestations

Subtle changes that vary with each patient, most important change is any alteration in level of consciousness.

Signs

Restlessness, irritability, confusion, decrease in Glasgow Coma Scale score, changes in speech or vision, abnormal pupillary reactions, motor or sensory changes, changes in cardiac rate or rhythm, nausea or vomiting, headache, increase in systolic blood pressure with a widening pulse pressure, decreasing respirations, abnormal breathing patterns, changes in body temperature

Emergency Care

Airway maintenance, intubation with oxygenation ($pO_2 > 90$ mm Hg) and hyperventilation, osmotic diuretics (mannitol IV), steroids (Decadron IV), elevation of head (30 degrees), sedative p.r.n. (Versed IV), drain cerebrospinal fluid (keep ICP < 20), maintain fluid status (normal serum sodium and osmolality)

■ *Spinal Cord Injuries*

Etiology

Most common cause is trauma.

Flexion injury: for example, head hits steering wheel or windshield and rupture of posterior ligaments results in forward dislocation of the vertebrae; may damage blood vessels leading to ischemia of cord

Hyperextension injury: for example, chin hits object and head is thrown back, rupturing anterior ligament and fracturing posterior elements of vertebral body; may result in complete transsection of the cord

Compression injury: person lands directly on head, sacrum, or feet after falling or jumping a great distance; force of impact fractures vertebrae and fragments compress cord, causing incomplete cord lesions

Pathophysiology

Most injuries occur at C1–2, C4–6, and T11–L2, as these are the most mobile segments of the spine.

Microscopic bleeding occurs at time of injury, edema follows within 1 hour of injury and peaks after 2–3 days and usually subsides after 7 days.

Fragmentation of axonal covering and loss of myelin may occur; tissue necrosis may follow with macrophages engulfing debris, leaving central cavity in injured spinal cord (called post-traumatic syringomyelia) as early as 9 days after injury.

Physiologic generalized stress response; an automatic spinal reflex activity that produces spasticity, may occur as recovery progresses.

Clinical Manifestations

Complete transsection results in immediate paralysis, paresthesia, bowel and bladder function below level of injury, hypotension, and loss of temperature control (client assumes temperature in environment).

Incomplete injury results in partial loss.

Cervical injury results in quadriplegia.

Thoracic or lumbar injury results in paraplegia.

Injury above C4 may be fatal because of innervation of diaphragm.

Autonomic hyperreflexia

After spinal shock resolves, exaggerated sympathetic responses to noxious stimuli below level of injury produce hypertension, diaphoresis, piloerection, dilated pupils; baroreceptors stimulate parasympathetic nervous system in an effort to decrease blood pressure (B/P), resulting in bradycardia, flushing, and headache.

Emergency Care

Assess baseline deficits; immobilize spine using spine board, hard neck collar, and safety straps around torso and legs; maintain patent airway and oxygenation; skeletal traction with skull tongs; cervical spine x-rays; normal saline IV; nasogastric tube to suction; Foley catheter

Critical Care

Transfer to Stryker frame or RotoRest bed, continue with above treatment and add steroids and vasoactive medication as needed; suction p.r.n. to prevent aspiration; enteral or parenteral feedings as indicated to maintain nutrition if oral intake insufficient.

Acute and Subacute Care

Establish functional goals; promote mobility (wheelchair, back brace), and prevent contractures; improve bladder and bowel control (Credé maneuver, catheterization methods, conditioned reflex activity); prevent pressure ulcers (AHCPR guidelines); reduce respiratory dysfunction (incentive spirometry); promote expression of sexuality (education and counseling); reduce pain (non-narcotic analgesics and transcutaneous nerve stimulators); promote self-care; treat autonomic dysreflexia if it occurs (elevate head of bed to sitting position, check B/P; check for stimulus and remove, administer antihypertensive medication if necessary); prevent injury; help client adjust to life changes (be realistic).

U N I T 16

Protective Disorders

ANATOMY AND PHYSIOLOGY REVIEW: THE HEMATOPOIETIC SYSTEM

To care for the client with a hematologic disorder, nurses must have an understanding of the anatomy and physiology of the hematopoietic system. This chapter describes the characteristics of blood, the formation of the cellular elements of blood, blood groups and types, and the processes involved in homeostasis.

Knowledge of the immune system's structure and function is growing exponentially. The immune system is an intricate system—unique to each individual—which protects the individual from hostile invasions by bacteria, viruses, fungi, and parasites. The "killer" T cells, components of the immune system, seek out and destroy malignant cells. With an ineffective immune system, people are at increased risk for the development of overwhelming infection and malignant disease. In contrast, if the immune system is excessively active then autoimmune diseases, hypersensitivity states, or immune-complex diseases are the consequences.

OBJECTIVES

16.1   Discuss normal structure and function of blood and the components of blood.

16.2   Explain the hematopoietic process.

16.3   Discuss blood groups and blood typing.

16.4   Explain the relationship among the ABO, Rh, and HLA systems and blood compatibility.

16.5   Discuss the three phases of homeostasis.

16.6   Discuss the effects of aging on the hematologic system.

16.7   Differentiate between active and passive immunity.

16.8   Compare and contrast humoral and cellular immunity.

16.9   Identify the organs of the immune system.

16.10   Describe the relationship of B lymphocytes and T lymphocytes, Class I and II MHC molecules, and CD4 and CD8 surface markers.

16.11   Distinguish between features of primary and secondary immune responses.

16.12   Discuss, in general terms, the characteristics of immunoglobulins (antibodies).

16.13   Describe the functions of the four types of T lymphocytes.

16.14   Describe the roles of the cytokines.

16.15   Identify the factors that affect the immune response.

LEARNING THE LANGUAGE: TERMINOLOGY RELATED TO BASIC CONCEPTS OF HEMATOLOGY

Complete the following sentences.

1. Blood is a mixture of _____ and plasma. _____ is the liquid portion of blood. The blood is propelled through the body by the _____ pumping action.

2. The blood supplies _____ from the lungs and absorbed _____ from the gastrointestinal tract to cells. The blood removes _____ products from the tissues and takes it to the _____, _____, and skin for excretion.

3. _____ is the normal process that repairs vascular breaks to reduce blood loss and maintain vascular blood flow.

4. In adults, the process of hematopoiesis is performed primarily in the _____ _____ of flat bones.

5. The normal erythrocyte has the shape of a(n) _____.

6. _____ causes the kidneys to release _____.

7. _____, _____, and _____ determine the proportion of each of the five types of white blood cells (WBCs) in a sample of 100 WBCs. A WBC with a differential is the total amount of WBC and the _____ of the five types of WBCs.

Match the blood cells in Column A with the correct precursor cell in Column B (some may have more than one answer).

Column A	Column B
8. _____ Thrombocyte	A. Lymphoblast
9. _____ B Lymphocyte	B. Monoblast
10. _____ T Lymphocyte	C. Megakaryoblast
11. _____ Monocyte	D. Myeloblast
12. _____ Erythrocyte	E. Rubriblast
13. _____ Platelet	
14. _____ Basophil	
15. _____ Eosinophil	
16. _____ Neutrophil	
17. _____ Agranulocyte	
18. _____ Granulocyte	

Match the functions described in Column A with the correct blood component listed in Column B.

Column A	Column B
19. _____ Liquid portion of blood	A. Platelets
20. _____ Perform phagocytosis	B. Erythrocytes
21. _____ Mediate exchange of oxygen and carbon dioxide	C. Neutrophils
22. _____ Promote thrombin formation	D. Albumins
23. _____ Maintain colloidal osmotic pressure	E. Plasma

Match the functions described in Column A with the correct coagulation factor listed in Column B.

Column A	Column B
24. _____ Common pathway	A. Vessel or blood injury
25. _____ Produces thrombin	B. Fibrinogen
26. _____ Initiates the extrinsic pathway	C. Calcium
27. _____ Activates the intrinsic pathway	D. Prothrombin
28. _____ Produces fibrin to stabilize clot	E. Stable factor
	F. Tissue thromboplastin

Match the functions in Column A with the correct lymphocyte in Column B.

Column A	Column B
29. _____ Inhibits T and B cells	A. Killer T Cell
30. _____ Directly destroys antigens	B. Helper T Cell
31. _____ Remembers antigen for future	C. Supressor T Cell
32. _____ Stimulates T and B cells	D. Memory T Cell
33. _____ Antibody-mediated immune response	E. B Lymphocyte
34. _____ Cell-mediated immune response	F. T Lymphocyte
35. _____ Defends against some viruses, kills some tumor cells	G. Null Lymphocyte

THINKING CRITICALLY: THE HEMATOPOIETIC SYSTEM

36. Describe the major characteristics of blood: color, viscosity, pH, volume, and composition.

37. Explain the terms *Rh positive* and *Rh negative*.

38. Discuss the nutritional factors and metabolites needed for hematopoiesis.

39. Discuss the roles of the liver and spleen in hematopoiesis.

40. What is the role of cytokines and interleukins in hematopoietic regulation?

■ *Organs of the Immune System*

41. In the diagram below, label the organs of the
    immune system.

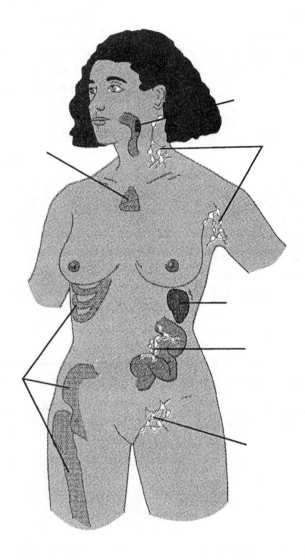

42. Which two organs in the diagram above are
    considered primary organs of the immune system?

43. What is the specific immune function of each of
    these two primary organs?

■ *Cell Cooperation in the Immune Response*

Read the description of the structure and function of the immune system in Unit 16 of the text and study the diagram below to gain an understanding of immune system physiology. Then answer the following questions.

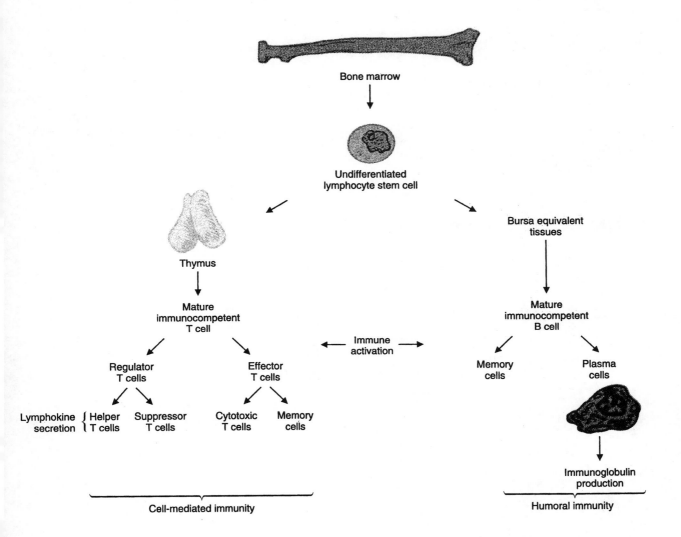

PUTTING IT ALL TOGETHER: STUDY QUESTIONS

44. What is the function of the human leukocytic antigens (HLA), which are present on all body cells?

45. What is the difference between active and passive immunity?

46. What is the main function of macrophages?

47. What is an immature macrophage called?

48. What are the four types of activated T cells?

49. Which type of cell stimulates the release of cytokines, which assist B cells to mature and produce antibodies?

50. Name the five distinct classes of immunoglobulins produced by the B cells and list one effect of each.

74

Assessment of the Hematopoietic System

Hematologic disorders cover a wide range of problems that can affect every body system. Assessment of clients with hematologic disorders includes a thorough health history, physical assessment, and diagnostic tests. Assessment incorporates data from the health history, including past medical history, family medical history, psychosocial history, and lifestyle analysis. The physical exam can entail both a complete head-to-toe examination and examinations of specific systems, depending on the nature of the client's problem. In addition to the health history and physical examination, diagnostic tests are ordered. Diagnosis of blood disorders depends primarily on laboratory analysis. Therefore, the nurse must have a thorough understanding of the common laboratory tests and the nursing responsibilities.

OBJECTIVES

74.1 Identify normal values for adult complete blood count (CBC) and differential count.

74.2 List the four basic pathophysiologic disturbances that characterize hematologic disorders.

74.3 Describe aspects to include in the nursing history and physical assessment of clients with hematologic disorders.

74.4 Describe the diagnostic studies and associated nursing interventions used to confirm or differentiate hematologic disorders.

74.5 Obtain a health history to determine possible allergies, including food, medication, insect, or pollen sensitivities.

74.6 Review the client's health history to identify previous problems and signs/symptoms of immune system dysfunction.

74.7 Perform a physical examination of the client and focus on the area that is target for the allergen or other immune system problem.

74.8 Differentiate among the following tests: CD4 cell counts, lymphocyte and immunoglobulin assays, bone marrow biopsy, and skin testing. Provide a brief description of the tests, and pre- and postprocedure care if applicable.

LEARNING THE LANGUAGE: TERMINOLOGY RELATED TO BASIC CONCEPTS OF HEMATOLOGY

Use a medical dictionary or basic nursing text as a reference to match the definitions in Column A with the correct term in Column B.

Column A		**Column B**	
1. _____ Placed before words to show relationship		A.	Cyte
2. _____ Same, like		B.	Emia
3. _____ Cell		C.	Pneia
4. _____ State or condition		D.	Osis
5. _____ Added to word to alter the meaning		E.	A, an
6. _____ Blood condition		F.	Pan
7. _____ Lack of or deficiency in		G.	Oma
8. _____ The part that indicates essential meaning		H.	Suffixes
9. _____ All		I.	Root word
10. _____ Without, lack of		J.	Prefixes
11. _____ Blood		K.	Poiesis
12. _____ All, entire		L.	Homo, homeo
13. _____ Iron		M.	Hema, hemo
14. _____ Bone marrow		N.	Poly
15. _____ Many, much		O.	Mye
16. _____ Tumor		P.	Heme

Match the values and descriptions in Column A with the correct lab test in Column B.

Column A		**Column B**	
17. _____ Men: 40–45%		A.	Red blood cell count (RBC)
18. _____ 4000–9000/mm^3		B.	Hemoglobin level
19. _____ 150,000–450,000/mm^3		C.	Hematocrit level
20. _____ Women: 4–5 million/mm^3		D.	Red blood cell indices
21. _____ Measures red blood cell (RBC) size and hemoglobin content		E.	White blood cell count (WBC)
22. _____ Measures hemoglobin content of RBCs		F.	Platelet count
23. _____ Measures volume of RBCs in whole blood		G.	Differential count
24. _____ Inflammation, infection, and response to therapy			
25. _____ Number of thrombocytes in whole blood			
26. _____ Percent of the five types of WBCs in a sample of 100 WBCs			

Match the purposes described in Column A with the appropriate diagnostic study in Column B.

Column A	Column B
27. _____ Measures functional fibrinogen available	A. Bleeding time
28. _____ Measure of coagulation process in venous blood	B. Prothrombin time
29. _____ Tests normalcy of intrinsic coagulation process, monitors heparin therapy	C. Thrombin time
	D. Fibrinogen level
30. _____ Measures ability to stop bleeding	E. Clot retraction
31. _____ Indicates function and number of platelets	F. Partial thromboplastin time
	G. Activated clotting time

Match the disorders in Column A with the type of pathophysiologic disturbance in Column B.

Column A	Column B
32. _____ Polycythemia	A. Disorders of the spleen
33. _____ Thrombocytopenia	B. Coagulation mechanism defects
34. _____ Splenomegaly	C. Overproduction of normal or defective cells
35. _____ Hypoprothrombinemia	D. Decrease in the number of cells
36. _____ Myeloma	
37. _____ Leukopenia	
38. _____ Anemia	
39. _____ Myeloproliferative	
40. _____ Hemorrhage	
41. _____ Neutropenia	
42. _____ Disseminated intravascular coagulation	
43. _____ Leukemia	
44. _____ Multiple myeloma	
45. _____ Lymphoproliferative	
46. _____ Hypersplenism	

THINKING CRITICALLY: KNOWING WHAT TO DO AND WHY

Give the rationale for the following actions.

■ Diagnostic Tests

Test	Informed Consent	Pretest Nursing Care	Post-Test Nursing Care
Bone Marrow Aspiration	47.	48. Clean skin with Betadine	49. Sandbag to puncture site for 1 hour
		50. Anesthetize puncture site	51. Observe site for bleeding for 2–3 days

Identify symptoms of hematologic disorders that are associated with each of the following systems.

52. Integumentary

53. Sensory

54. Respiratory

55. Cardiovascular

56. Gastrointestinal

PUTTING IT ALL TOGETHER: ASSESSMENT OF CLIENTS WITH IMMUNE DISORDERS

57. When obtaining a health history from a client with an allergy, what types of information should be sought regarding the chief complaint in order to analyze the symptom?

58. Which lymph nodes are checked more easily with the client in the prone position?

59. List three types of skin tests for specific allergens.

60. How should negative reactions to skin testing for allergens be interpreted?

75

Management of Clients with Hematologic Disorders

This chapter discusses disorders affecting the red blood cells, white blood cells, the lymphoid system, and platelet and clotting factors. Since it may be difficult to remember every disease process, focus your study on the factors common to disorders in each group. Recall normal physiology and base your nursing care on the physiologic changes that are occurring as a result of the disease.

OBJECTIVES

75.1   Describe the two basic pathophysiologic alterations that underlie all red blood cell disorders.

75.2   Describe etiology, pathophysiology, clinical manifestations, diagnostic studies, and complications of selected erythrocyte disorders.

75.3   Describe the medical and surgical management of clients with various hematologic disorders.

75.4   Describe nursing care of clients with various hematologic disorders.

75.5   Provide rationales for nursing care of the client requiring a blood transfusion.

75.6   Evaluate effectiveness of care based on expected outcomes.

LEARNING THE LANGUAGE: TERMINOLOGY RELATED TO HEMATOLOGIC DISORDERS

Match the definitions in Column A with the correct hematologic disorder in Column B.

Column A

Column B

1. _____ Widespread clotting in arterioles, organ hemorrhage

2. _____ Reduction in red blood cells (RBCs) and oxygen-carrying capacity of blood

3. _____ Genetically transmitted bleeding disorder in males

4. _____ Cancer of the plasma cells

5. _____ Extravasation of small amounts of blood into tissue

6. _____ Inherited, chronic, hemolytic anemia

7. _____ Increase in RBCs and hemoglobin concentration

8. _____ Abnormal Hgb that assumes a crescent shape when blood oxygen decreases

9. _____ Vitamin B_{12} deficiency

10. _____ Contagious and self-limiting, known as the "kissing disease"

A. Disseminated intravascular coagulation

B. Pernicious anemia

C. Purpura

D. Thalassemia

E. Anemia

F. Hemophilia

G. Infectious mononucleosis

H. Multiple myeloma

I. Polycythemia vera

J. Sickle cell anemia

THINKING CRITICALLY

Match the assessment data in Column A with the appropriate pathogenesis in Column B.

Column A

Column B

Pernicious Anemia

11. _____ Tingling; numbness of hand

12. _____ Indigestion; weight loss

13. _____ Jaundice

A. Hemolysis of abnormally large erythrocytes

B. Degeneration of peripheral nerves

C. Reduced secretion of hydrochloric acid

D. Decreased leukocyte count

Hemolytic Anemia

14. _____ Hepatomegaly

15. _____ Jaundice

16. _____ Pigment gallstones

A. Accumulation of bilirubin within the blood

B. Reduced secretion of hydrochloric acid

C. Excessive accumulation of bilirubin within gallbladder

D. Increased phagocytosis by macrophages

Polycythemia Vera

17. _____ Painful, swollen joints

18. _____ Ruddy complexion

19. _____ Thrombosis formation

20. _____ Hypertension; headache

A. Increased blood volume

B. Increased viscosity of blood

C. Increased nucleoprotein in blood

D. Congestion of capillaries

Aplastic Anemia

21. _____ Fatigue; lassitude
22. _____ Increased susceptibility
23. _____ Bleeding into skin

A.   Decreased leukocyte count
B.   Decreased secretion of bilirubin to infection
C.   Decreased erythrocyte count
D.   Decreased platelet count

Sickle Cell Anemia

24. _____ Osteoporosis; osteosclerosis
25. _____ Pain in extremities; leg ulcers
26. _____ Elevated bilirubin

A.   Occluded microcirculation
B.   Hemolysis of sickle cells
C.   Proliferation of bone marrow

Blood Transfusion Reaction

27. _____ Chills, high fever, vomiting, diarrhea, marked hypotension, and shock
28. _____ Dry cough develops
29. _____ Oliguria occurs
30. _____ Urticaria, flushing, itching, no fever
31. _____ Chills and fever within an hour of starting transfusion
32. _____ Dyspnea, pulmonary congestion, tachycardia
33. _____ Most commonly caused by ABO incompatibility
34. _____ Usually develops in clients with renal or cardiac impairment

A.   Hemolytic reaction
B.   Allergic reaction
C.   Circulatory overload
D.   Febrile nonhemolytic reaction
E.   Septicemia

THINKING CRITICALLY: KNOWING WHAT TO DO AND WHY

Provide the rationales for the following nursing interventions related to disorders of platelets and clotting factors.

Intervention	Rationale
35. Teach client to refrain from flossing during acute phase.	
36. Use lightweight blankets.	
37. Teach client to avoid Valsalva's maneuver.	
38. Teach client to monitor skin condition.	

Provide the rationales for the following nursing interventions related to multiple myeloma.

Intervention	Rationale
39. Force fluids: 3000–4000 mL per day.	
40. Administer pamidronate disodium (Aredia).	
41. Closely monitor intake, output, and blood studies.	

Indicate the compatible donor blood for each of the following blood types.

Blood Type	Compatible Donor Blood
42. A	
43. B	
44. AB	
45. O	

Provide the rationales for the following nursing interventions related to blood transfusions.

Intervention	Rationale
46. Check physician's order.	
47. Obtain transfusion history.	
48. Confirm compatibility.	
49. Verify client's identity.	
50. Use large-bore needle for IV.	
51. Use normal saline for flush solution.	
52. Take vital signs before, during, and after transfusion.	
53. Begin infusion slowly (1 mL/kg/hr).	
54. Begin transfusion soon after receiving from blood bank.	
55. Store blood in refrigerator designated only for such purposes.	
56. Infuse within a 4-hour time limit.	

Provide the rationales for the following nursing interventions related to the anemias.

Intervention	Rationale
57. Adjust environmental temperature to meet the client's needs.	
58. Teach basics of proper nutrition.	
59. Provide for periods of rest.	
60. Assess cardiovascular status.	

Putting It All Together

■ Case Study: Iron Deficiency Anemia

Ms. N., a 30-year-old Caucasian female, has been diagnosed with endometriosis. She makes an appointment to see her physician because she is experiencing shortness of breath and fatigue. She tells her physician that her menstrual flow has become very heavy and that it lasts for 7–8 days. The physician assesses a heart rate of 132, blood pressure of 102/86, and respirations of 32. Initial laboratory results are: hemoglobin 8 g/mL, hematocrit 30%, total red blood cell count 52,000, serum iron level 35 µg/100 mL.

61. Which one of Ms. N.'s clinical signs reflects her body's attempt to compensate for the anemia?
  A. fatigue
  B. tachycardia
  C. shortness of breath
  D. tachypnea

62. Which of the following is the most likely cause of Ms. N.'s anemia?
  A. dietary iron deficiency
  B. malabsorption syndrome
  C. blood loss
  D. intestinal parasite

63. Which of the following food combinations would increase the client's iron intake?
  A. milk, cheese, chicken
  B. potatoes, pork, egg whites
  C. apples, oranges, raisins
  D. kidney beans, lean meat, carrots

64. The client is started on an oral iron preparation. She should be taught to
  A. take the medication after meals.
  B. decrease the fiber in her diet.
  C. decrease her fluid intake.
  D. crush the iron tablet and mix it with food.

CHAPTER 76

Management of Clients with Immune Disorders

Since the immune system is an interrelated system that affects the whole body, the care of clients with altered immune systems requires a comprehensive approach. The client often has a wide variety of problems that may require complex interventions. It is especially important that the risks of infection and injury be reduced for the client with an altered immune system. All clients need understanding and support, but these needs are even greater for the client with HIV infection.

OBJECTIVES

76.1   Describe the four types of hypersensitivity reactions.

76.2   Describe self-care for the client with allergies.

HYPERSENSITIVITY REACTIONS

Match the reactions in Column A with the type of hypersensitivity in Column B.

Column A

1. _____ Contact dermatitis
2. _____ ABO incompatibility
3. _____ Anaphylaxis
4. _____ Drug-induced hemolytic anemia
5. _____ Acute glomerulonephritis
6. _____ Transplant rejection
7. _____ Atopic diseases such as hay fever
8. _____ Tuberculosis
9. _____ Serum sickness

Column B

A.   Cell-mediated—delayed
B.   Immediate
C.   Immune complex
D.   Cytolytic/cytotoxic

Read through Table 76-3 in the text. List one of the most common agents from each category causing anaphylaxis.

10.   Drugs

14.   Blood products

11.   Foods

15.   Allergen extracts

12.   Insect venoms

16.   Diagnostic agents

13.   Biologicals

List four specific interventions to prevent anaphylactic hypersensitivity.

17.

19.

18.

20.

Management of Clients with Autoimmune Disorders

Connective tissue disorders often occur during young adulthood, impairing mobility and functional capacity. Many of the connective tissue disorders are difficult to diagnose as they are characterized by remissions and exacerbations. These disorders have many overlapping signs and symptoms because connective tissue throughout the body may be affected. Nursing interventions are aimed primarily at pain control and maintenance of joint mobility. It is most important to be sensitive to the psychosocial impact of the disorders while at the same time teaching the client to manage self-care.

OBJECTIVES

77.1 Discuss the immune dysfunction as it relates to autoimmune disease.

77.2 Discuss the immune dysfunction related to the etiology of rheumatoid arthritis.

77.3 Describe the pathologic changes in the joint that occur with rheumatoid arthritis.

77.4 Describe physical and laboratory findings (diagnostic criteria) with rheumatoid arthritis.

77.5 Identify the main intervention goals for clients with arthritis.

77.6 Discuss management for clients with arthritis.

77.7 Administer medications prescribed to decrease inflammation and reduce pain with knowledge of the action, toxicity, and nursing considerations of each medication.

77.8 Discuss types and characteristics of unproven remedies for arthritis.

77.9 Describe types of surgical procedures used in the treatment of arthritis.

77.10 Discuss the etiology and pathophysiology of systemic lupus erythematosus.

77.11 Describe physical assessment findings with systemic lupus erythematosus.

77.12 Describe laboratory findings with systemic lupus erythematosus.

77.13 Discuss interventions for clients with systemic lupus erythematosus.

LEARNING THE LANGUAGE: TERMINOLOGY RELATED TO CONNECTIVE TISSUE DISORDERS

Match the definitions in Column A with the correct term in Column B.

Column A		**Column B**	
1. _____	Connective tissue inflammation	A.	Ankylosis
2. _____	Inflammation of synovial membrane	B.	"Butterfly rash"
3. _____	Fibrous scar in joint	C.	Collagen
4. _____	Inflammation of voluntary muscles	D.	CREST
5. _____	Connective tissue scleroprotein	E.	Fibrosis
6. _____	Arthritis hand deformity	F.	Hemiarthroplasty
7. _____	Calcium skin deposits	G.	Myositis
8. _____	Replacement of femoral head and acetabulum	H.	NSAIDs
9. _____	Femoral head or acetabulum is replaced	I.	Pannus
10. _____	Firm union	J.	Scleroderma
11. _____	Characteristic skin lesion with lupus	K.	Subcutaneous nodules
12. _____	Anti-inflammatory drugs	L.	Calcinosis
13. _____	Systemic sclerosis	M.	Synovitis
14. _____	Characteristic lesion of rheumatoid arthritis (RA)	N.	Total hip replacement
15. _____	Hardening of skin and internal organs	O.	"Ulnar drift"

CRITICAL THINKING: UNDERSTANDING RATIONALES

■ Medications for Arthritis

Listed below are some important implications of medication therapy for treating arthritis with specific drugs. Write the rationale for these considerations.

Implication	**Rationale**
Aspirin	
16. Use cautiously with anticoagulation therapy.	
17. Give aspirin with food or milk, or use buffered or enteric-coated aspirin.	
18. Counsel persons to be alert for signs of tinnitus or dizziness.	
Ibuprofen (Motrin)	
19. Use cautiously in persons with impaired renal function.	
20. Advise client to inform dentist or surgeon that the drug is being taken.	
21. Tell client to report any onset of GI disturbances or jaundice.	
22. Inform client to avoid alcohol and aspirin unless otherwise advised by physician.	

PUTTING IT ALL TOGETHER

■ *Case Study*

Ms. T., 56, who has had rheumatoid arthritis for 15 years, is admitted for a total hip arthroplasty on the right side. She had the same surgery on her left hip 3 years ago with good results. She is looking forward to having this surgery so that she will be relieved of pain and can be more independent. The following questions concern her postoperative care.

23. Which of the following signs or symptoms might be indicative of dislocation of the prosthesis?
    A. rapid, sharp hip pain
    B. excessive Hemovac drainage
    C. temperature of 101° F
    D. external rotation of right leg

24. Which of the following positions is allowed 2 days after surgery?
    A. flexion of right hip by bending forward slightly at waist
    B. adduction of right lower extremity with toes turned inward
    C. external rotation of right lower extremity
    D. abduction of right hip

25. How often should Ms. T. do quadriceps-setting exercises?
    A. ten times, twice a day in physical therapy
    B. five times, every four hours
    C. ten times, every hour during the day
    D. for a few minutes while sitting up in the chair

26. What is the primary purpose of quadriceps and gluteal exercises?
    A. strengthen the quadriceps muscles for ambulation
    B. prevent dislocation of prosthesis and thromboemboli
    C. decrease postoperative pain and muscle spasms
    D. involve client in her care immediately after surgery

27. Which of the following medications is likely to increase the amount of drainage collected from the Hemovac?
    A. cefazolin sodium (Kefzol)
    B. meperidine hydrochloride (Demerol)
    C. dextran
    D. aspirin

28. Which of the following would be inappropriate to include in Ms. T.'s discharge instructions?
    A. "Do not sit continuously for longer than one hour."
    B. "Sleep only on your back or left side."
    C. "Wear support stockings."
    D. "Use a raised toilet seat."

Management of Clients with Leukemia and Lymphoma

This chapter discusses cancers of the hematopoietic system; leukemia, a cancer of the bone marrow; and lymphoma, a cancer of the lymph system. The terms *acute* and *chronic* have a different meaning when used with these diseases and refer to the maturity of the cells. Leukemia is uncontrolled proliferation of the leukocytes (myelocytes or lymphocytes). With acute leukemia, at least half of the marrow cells are immature. With chronic leukemia, most of the cells are normal except during a blast crisis. Most lymphomas are tumors of lymphoid tissue outside the bone marrow and involve the lymph nodes and spleen. Two major types of lymphoma are Hodgkin's lymphoma and non-Hodgkin's lymphoma. Bone marrow involvement occurs more often in non-Hodgkin's lymphoma than in Hodgkin's lymphoma. During therapy for leukemia or lymphoma, symptom management is an important goal of nursing care.

OBJECTIVES

78.1 Differentiate between leukemia and lymphoma and the major types of each.

78.2 Discuss the etiology and risk factors for leukemia and lymphoma.

78.3 Differentiate between acute and chronic leukemia.

78.4 Differentiate between Hodgkin's and non-Hodgkin's lymphoma.

78.5 Describe clinical manifestations, including diagnostic testing, for leukemia and lymphoma.

78.6 Discuss treatment for leukemia and lymphoma.

78.7 Discuss symptom management for clients undergoing treatment for leukemia or lymphoma.

LEARNING THE LANGUAGE: TERMINOLOGY RELATED TO LEUKEMIA AND LYMPHOMA

Match the definitions in Column A with the correct term in Column B.

Column A

1. _____ Uncontrolled proliferation of lymphocytes
2. _____ Chronic progressive cancer characterized by painless, enlarged lymph nodes
3. _____ Proliferation of abnormal, immature leukocytes
4. _____ Immature and undifferentiated leukocytes
5. _____ Potentially fatal metabolic complications associated with rapid destruction of large number of WBCs
6. _____ Removal of specific blood element and returning remaining cells and plasma to the patient
7. _____ Used to estimate the client's risk for infection
8. _____ Used to stage Hodgkin's lymphoma
9. _____ Night sweats, fever, and weight loss occurring with lymphoma
10. _____ Bone marrow from the intended recipient

Column B

A. Absolute neutrophil count
B. Allogenic bone marrow
C. Apheresis
D. Autologous bone marrow
E. B symptoms
F. Blast cells
G. Cotswold Staging Classification
H. French-American-British (FAB) Classification
I. Hodgkin's disease
J. Leukemia
K. Lymphadenopathy
L. Lymphoma
M. Reed Sternberg cells
N. Tumor lysis syndrome

THINKING CRITICALLY

Match the assessment data in Column A with the appropriate pathogenesis in Column B.

Column A

Leukemia

11. _____ Lymphadenopathy
12. _____ Hyperuricemia
13. _____ Headache
14. _____ Splenomegaly

Column B

A. Abnormal white blood cells (WBCs) infiltrating CNS
B. High number of white blood cells accumulating in organs
C. Destruction of large numbers of leukocytes
D. Excessive number of WBCs accumulating in lymph nodes
E. Increased metabolic rate

Hodgkin's Disease

15. _____ Jaundice
16. _____ Cough; stridor
17. _____ Cyanosis of face
18. _____ Anemia; fatigue

A. Shortened erythrocyte lifespan
B. Neoplastic involvement of internal nodes
C. Mediastinal lymph node enlargement
D. Obstruction of bile ducts
E. Pressure on veins

THINKING CRITICALLY: KNOWING WHAT TO DO AND WHY

Provide the rationales for the following nursing interventions related to leukemia.

Intervention	Rationale
19. Institute proper hand-washing techniques.	
20. Provide client with a low-bacteria diet.	
21. Use cotton swabs for oral hygiene.	
22. Avoid overinflation of the blood pressure cuff.	

PUTTING IT ALL TOGETHER

■ Case Study: Chronic Myelogenous Leukemia

Ms. S., 68, has been diagnosed with chronic myelogenous leukemia. Her disease was initially diagnosed when routine laboratory tests showed leukocytosis and thrombocytosis. For approximately 5 years, she was treated symptomatically with steroids. She is being seen now because her condition has deteriorated. She has splenomegaly and hepatomegaly; her food intake has decreased and she has begun to have repeated infections. In addition, she has become quite depressed. The physician orders additional diagnostic studies and schedules the client for radiation therapy.

23. Which one of Ms. S.'s clinical signs is probably the cause of her decreased food intake?
   A. repeated infections
   B. depression
   C. hepatomegaly and splenomegaly
   D. thrombocytosis

24. The physician orders the radiation therapy to
   A. decrease the size of the spleen and liver.
   B. reduce the leukocytosis.
   C. increase platelet production.
   D. achieve long-term remission in the condition.

25. Nursing care of this client should include
   A. proper hand-washing techniques.
   B. administration of medication by intramuscular route.
   C. three high-caloric meals a day.
   D. a planned exercise program.

Multisystem
Disorders

CHAPTER

79

Management of Clients with Acquired Immunodeficiency Syndrome

HIV (human immunodeficiency virus) kills more people than any other infectious disease. Worldwide it is the fourth leading cause of death and it is the second leading cause of death among 25- to 44-year-olds. Although there have been great advances in diagnosing and treating HIV, it is still poorly understood by the general public and many health care providers. The cost of caring for a client with HIV is approximately $12,000 annually, thus access to care is a major problem. Nurses must have a good understanding of the disease process HIV illness trajectory as well as knowledge of resources to effectively manage the care of clients infected with HIV and with AIDS (acquired immunodeficiency syndrome).

OBJECTIVES

79.1 Describe the following characteristics of HIV infection: definition, incidence, etiology, risk factors.

79.2 Discuss the pathophysiology and resulting clinical manifestation of HIV infection.

79.3 Discuss the HIV illness trajectory.

79.4 Identify various pharmacologic agents used in treating clients with HIV infection.

79.5 Describe the various opportunistic infections according to causative agent, symptomatology, and treatment.

79.6 List HIV-associated malignancies.

79.7 Describe central and peripheral HIV neurologic disease.

79.8 Discuss nursing care for the client with HIV infection.

79.9 Describe universal precautions.

LEARNING THE LANGUAGE: TERMINOLOGY RELATED TO HIV AND AIDS

Match the terms in Column A with the correct definition in Column B.

Column A

1. _____ CD4+ cell counts
2. _____ HIV classification system for adolescents and adults
3. _____ HIV illness trajectory
4. _____ NNRTIs (Non-nucleoside reverse transcriptase inhibitors): Nevirapine (Viramune)
5. _____ NRTIs (Nucleoside reverse transcriptase inhibitors): Retrovir, AZT
6. _____ PGL
7. _____ PIs (Protease inhibitors): Indinavir (Crixivan)
8. _____ Viral load

Column B

A. Block HIV replication by protecting noninfected cells

B. Measures viral activity in a person infected with HIV

C. Persistent generalized lymphadenopathy

D. Prognostic indicator to identify whether a patient infected with HIV is at risk for developing opportunistic infections

E. Render HIV particles noninfectious

F. The CDC's classification system that is divided into laboratory and clinical categories

G. The course of the disease progression from caring for the person with HIV disease to AIDS

H. Works similar to nucleoside analogs; blocks RNA and DNA disrupting the enzymes site

THINKING CRITICALLY

Use Box 79-1, Human Immunodeficiency Virus (HIV) Classification System for Adolescents and Adults, to classify the following:

9. _____ Asymptomatic infection with CD4+ > 500 mm³

10. _____ Candidiasis, oropharyngeal (thrush) CD4+ > 500 mm³

11. _____ Fever or diarrhea lasting more than one month CD4+ < 200 mm³

12. _____ History of acute infection

13. _____ Kaposi's sarcoma CD4+ > 500 mm³

14. _____ Wasting syndrome due to HIV

A. Category A
B. Category B
C. Category C

For each of the following nursing diagnoses, list specific nursing interventions. Include those interventions necessary in collaboration with medications.

Risk for infection related to immunocompromised state.

15. Prevent by:

17. If problem occurs, treat with:

16. Monitor for:

Altered nutrition: less than body requirements related to diarrhea from infections, malabsorption from GI involvement of Kaposi's sarcoma, anorexia from fear and anxiety, difficulty in eating because of oral candidiasis, fever and malaise, and accompanying weight loss either from the disease itself or an opportunistic infection

18. Prevent by:

19. Monitor for:

20. If problem occurs, treat with:

Social isolation related to stigma attached to AIDS diagnosis and inadequate support systems

21. Prevent by:

22. Monitor for:

23. If problem occurs, treat with:

Fear and anxiety related to unknown but potential problems and poor prognosis

24. Prevent by:

25. Monitor for:

26. If problem occurs, treat with:

Knowledge deficit regarding discharge plans including preventing the spread of the disease

27. Prevent by:

28. Monitor for:

29. If problem occurs, treat with:

Management of Clients Requiring Transplantation

Organ transplantation is an option for clients with end-stage organ failure. The number and type of organ donors and organ transplantation has consistently risen over the last decade. Improved immunosuppressive therapy advances in organ preservation, and newer surgical techniques have all contributed to the success and survival of transplant recipients. Ongoing research related to total transplantation process has contributed important data to identify risk factors that affect survival.

It is important for the nurse to have a good understanding of the organ donation, recovery, and transplantation process. Potential organ donors have suffered an injury leading to brain death. In situations where death is expected or when death occurs, nurses are often the ones to identify potential donors and approach the family members concerning organ donation. Nurses coordinate the organ donation and recovery process by collaboration with the family, healthcare team, and the OPO (organ procurement organization). Thus, the nurse must be articulate, caring, and sensitive to the needs of the client and family or significant others. Being aware of the religious, ethical, and legal considerations concerning organ donation and methods and mechanisms of organ donation and recovery/procurement can help the nurse deal more effectively with clients and family members.

The other part of the organ donation and recovery process is the transplant recipient. Nurses prepare clients for the transplant, provide postoperative care and ongoing education and follow-up.

OBJECTIVES

80.1 Discuss the basic concepts of histocompatibility and the immunologic aspects of transplant rejection.

80.2 Describe the signs and symptoms of graft rejection and graft-versus-host disease.

80.3 Identify the basic criteria for transplantation.

80.4 Discuss nursing care for the client having a transplant.

80.5 Identify major medications used in immunosuppression.

80.6 Discuss ethical, religious, and cultural considerations associated with transplantation.

THINKING CRITICALLY: LEGAL ASPECTS AND ORGAN TRANSPLANT DONORS

Match the terms in Column A with the definition in Column B.

Column A

1. _____ The Omnibus Budget Reconciliation Act (OBRA) of 1986
2. _____ The National Transplant Act of 1984
3. _____ Organ Donation Request Act of 1987
4. _____ The Uniform Anatomical Gift Act of 1968 (and revised in 1987)
5. _____ Organ Procurement and Transplant Network (OPTN)
6. _____ Organ Procurement Organization (OPO)
7. _____ Uniform Determination of Death Act

Column B

A. Family members who can legally make the decision can give consent for organ donation.

B. Established a national client registry to coordinate organ allocation and distribution

C. Defines *brain death*. An individual is considered dead if sustaining either 1) irreversible cessation of circulatory and respiratory function, or 2) irreversible cessation of all function of entire brain including brain stem.

D. Requires that hospitals have written policies and procedures for identification and referral of potential donors

E. Required national registries and declared it illegal to buy and sell organs

F. A nonprofit organ-recovery service in the United States that coordinates organ recovery and transplant procurement

G. Mandated consideration of the donor's religious beliefs and provided guidelines for attaining the next of kin for donor consent

8. Use Box 80-1 to list three general contraindications to organ transplant.

Are these clients candidates for organ donors?

9. 24-year-old healthy male who was thrown from a horse and sustained a massive head injury.

10. 34-year-old female who is in a chronic vegetative state following a head injury sustained in a motor vehicle accident.

11. 22-year-old admitted to emergency department following an all-terrain vehicle accident. He has signed the organ donation section of his driver's license. He is a Jehovah's Witness.

12. A 21-year-old male sustained a massive head injury from "car surfing." He is on a ventilator and has brain stem activity.

Thinking Critically: Client Family Education After Transplantation

Give the rationale for teaching the following:

Teaching Point	Rationale
13. When to call the transplant coordinator	
14. Immunosuppression therapy	
15. Signs and symptoms of rejection	
16. Infection	
17. Routine screening and immunizations	
18. Activities	
19. Wearing medical identification bracelet and card	
20. Yearly evaluations of transplant	

THINKING CRITICALLY: KNOWING AND UNDERSTANDING RATIONALES

What is the rationale for the following nursing interventions?

Type of Transplant	Nursing Interventions	Rationale
21. Renal transplant	Ongoing assessment of renal function: BUN, serum creatinine, intake and output, weights and serum electrolytes	
22. Pancreas and pancreas-kidney transplant	Urine amylase, blood glucose, BUN and serum creatinine; Monitor for graft thrombosis (GT)	
23. Heart transplant	Auscultation of heart and lung sounds; Assessment of pedal pulses and neck vein distention (NVD)	
24. Liver transplant	Monitoring fever, elevation of liver enzymes, Protime-INR change in color, amount and consistency of bile drainage through T-tube	
25. Lung transplant	Meticulous use of chest percussion, postural drainage, and incentive spirometer.	

Use Table 80-1 to determine the following religious and cultural groups' beliefs concerning organ donation and transplantation. Mark D for organ donation permitted, T for organ transplant permitted, NA for no official position or information not available, or NE for not encouraged. (More than one category may be used.)

Cultural Group

26. _____ African-American
27. _____ American Indian
28. _____ Black Muslim
29. _____ Chinese-American
30. _____ Hispanic
31. _____ Japanese-American
32. _____ Southeast-Asian–American
33. _____ West Indian

Religious Group

34. _____ Adventist
35. _____ Baptist
36. _____ Mormon
37. _____ Jehovah's Witness
38. _____ Presbyterian
39. _____ United Methodist
40. _____ Roman Catholic
41. _____ Pentecostal

81

Management of Clients with Shock and Multisystem Disorders

Regardless of the cause of shock, the result is inadequate tissue perfusion and death of cells as shock progresses. It is essential that the nurse recognize the signs and symptoms of shock in the early compensatory stage so that interventions can be initiated to prevent cell death. Of course, it is always best to prevent shock and this is accomplished by identifying clients at risk for developing shock and intervening before symptoms progress. If untreated, shock results in multisystem disorders as cell and organ death occurs.

OBJECTIVES

81.1   Discuss basic etiologies of shock.

81.2   Identify similarities and differences among various types of shock.

81.3   Describe generally recognized stages of shock and possible consequences of each.

81.4   Explain the systemic effects of shock.

81.5   Recognize the early assessment findings indicating shock.

81.6   List potential nursing diagnoses for the client in shock.

81.7   Implement appropriate interventions for people in shock.

81.8   Discuss how each body system is affected by shock.

PUTTING IT ALL TOGETHER: STUDY QUESTIONS RELATED TO SHOCK

1.   Regardless of the cause of shock, what is the end result?

2.   How can blood pressure (B/P) be normal for a person in the compensated stage of shock? Why is monitoring changes in pulse pressure crucial?

3. How is the respiratory system affected as shock progresses and complications result?

9. What is the modified Trendelenburg position?

10. Why is the measurement of central venous pressure (CVP) useful in early hypovolemic shock? Why are the measurements of pulmonary artery pressure and capillary wedge pressure used for assessment of persons in shock in many instances?

4. Why is disseminated intravascular coagulation (DIC) associated with progressive shock?

5. Treatment for shock should normally begin with which two of the following three changes in vital signs? (1) systolic blood pressure of 80 mm Hg, (2) pulse pressure of 40 mm Hg, and (3) pulse rate of 120 or more.

11. What is the major difference between crystalloid and colloid IV fluids?

12. How should a person in shock, who is also hypothermic, be warmed? Why?

6. What is the first step in assessing a person in shock?

13. Why is nasogastric suction used during treatment for shock?

7. What is the purpose of an anti-shock garment? What are contraindications for its use? Should it be removed to obtain physical assessment data and x-rays?

14. Why is urine output measured every 15 minutes?

8. What is the purpose of the intra-aortic balloon pump?

15. Why are vasoconstrictor medications used in shock to raise blood pressure to about 80 mm Hg systolic and no higher?

16. Should a person in shock and in pain receive analgesics or narcotics? Why or why not?

17. What is the concentration and dose of epinephrine given subcutaneously to treat anaphylactic shock?

18. What is the pathophysiologic basis for the following characteristic manifestations of septic shock: (a) warm, flushed skin; (b) decreased urine output; and (c) edema?

19. Give specific examples of nursing interventions that will provide emotional support to the client in shock.

20. How can the nurse support the significant others of the client in shock?

VASOACTIVE MEDICATIONS USED IN SHOCK MANAGEMENT

Match the drug effects in Column A with the appropriate name(s) of the medication(s) in Column B. (Medication names in Column B may be used more than once.)

Column A	Column B
21. _____ Systemic constriction of veins and arterioles	A. Adrenalin chloride (epinephrine)
22. _____ Increases myocardial contractility	B. Low-dose dopamine (Intropin)
23. _____ Extravasation may cause tissue necrosis	C. High-dose dopamine (Intropin)
24. _____ Elevates systemic blood pressure	D. Phenylephrine HCl (Neo-Synephrine)
25. _____ Increased heart rate	E. Nitroglycerin (Tridil)
26. _____ Systemic vasodilation	F. Norepinephrine (Levophed)
27. _____ Dilates renal blood vessels	G. Sodium nitroprusside (Nipride)
	H. Amrinone lactate (Inocor)
	I. Dobutamine (Dobutrex)
	J. Isoproterenol HCl (Isuprel)

■ *Case Study*

Ms. T., 45, is injured in an automobile accident and is being transported to the emergency department. The dispatcher on the ambulance relays that Ms. T. appears to have sustained a fracture of her right femur and no other apparent injuries. She is conscious, apprehensive, her right thigh is markedly swollen, has a pulse of 110, B/P of 118/70, and her skin is moist. Her right lower extremity has been splinted. She has no preexisting medical conditions, is currently taking no medications, and says she is allergic to penicillin. She is now being transported; her expected arrival is in 20 minutes.

28. Which assessment item from the dispatcher gives the best indication that Ms. T. might be at high risk for developing shock?
    A. She is apprehensive.
    B. Her thigh is markedly swollen.
    C. Her pulse is 110, her B/P is 118/70.
    D. Her skin is moist.

29. Which of the following types of shock is Ms. T. most likely to have?
    A. hypovolemic
    B. cardiogenic
    C. distributive
    D. anaphylactic

30. Which of the following changes will Ms. T. exhibit in the early compensatory stage of shock?
    A. decrease in urinary output to less than 30 cc/hour
    B. significant decrease in lying B/P: 10–15 mm Hg decrease
    C. increased heart rate: increase of 15–20 beats/minute or greater
    D. mental confusion

31. If assessment findings indicate an early compensatory stage of shock, which of the following interventions is the most important for treating Ms. T.?
    A. prevent chilling, but don't overheat
    B. restore blood volume
    C. allay apprehension
    D. relieve pain

32. What is the main goal for Ms. T.'s care plan?
    A. preserve kidney function
    B. prevent aspiration
    C. improve tissue perfusion
    D. maintain adequate vascular tone

CRITICAL POINTS TO REMEMBER: SHOCK

Types and Etiologies: Hypovolemic (hemorrhage, burns, dehydration), cardiogenic (myocardial infarction [MI], pulmonary embolus), distributive (anaphylactic—acute allergic reaction, neurogenic—acute phase of spinal cord injury, septic—severe infection with sepsis)

Pathophysiology: Early compensatory stage (with decreased perfusion, sympathetic nervous system is stimulated and blood flow is redistributed to brain and heart), decompensation stage (decreased cardiac output with continued vasoconstriction, decreased tissue perfusion, anaerobic metabolism and lactic acidosis, dilation of microcirculation), progressive stage (cellular ischemia and necrosis, organ failure)

Clinical Manifestations: Early compensatory stage (normal blood pressure then narrowing of pulse pressure, tachycardia, restlessness, agitation, confusion, decreased urine output to less than 20 cc/hour, tachypnea), decompensation to progressive stage (severely low blood pressure, weak and thready pulse, dysrhythmias, lethargy, stupor, coma, decreasing urine specific gravity, anuria). Skin and mucous membranes may be flushed, warm, and moist in early septic shock; cool, pale, and moist in progressive shock; and flushed with macular or papular lesions in anaphylactic shock. (See Figure 81-7 in the text for a graphic illustration.)

Management: Maintain perfusion with titrating vasoconstrictors and vasodilators (see Table 81-2 in the text.). Improve oxygenation with oxygen and mechanical ventilation with positive-end expiratory pressure (PEEP) if needed. Assist circulation with modified Trendelenburg's position. Replace fluid volume with colloids, blood, and crystalloids as needed; and prevent renal failure by maintaining urine output greater than 40 cc/hour. Prevent GI bleeding by using gastric suction, antacids, and histamine blockers. (See Tables 81-3, 81-4, and 81-5 in the text for more details.)

It is critical to recognize shock in the early compensatory stage and to treat it early in order to prevent the decompensation and progressive stages from occurring. If left untreated, the progressive stage of shock, called irreversible shock, leads to multiple organ failure.

82

Management of Clients in the Emergency Department

The Emergency Nurses Association defines *emergency nursing care* as the assessment, diagnosis, and treatment of perceived, actual, or potential, sudden or urgent, physical or psychosocial problems that are primarily episodic or acute.

Nursing care in the emergency department has both challenging and routine aspects. When the client's care is truly an emergency, the nurse and team are required to make accurate, rapid assessments and implement appropriate interventions. Knowing protocols and standards for emergency situations will assist the nurse in making assessments and carrying out interventions thoroughly and rapidly. Obviously, caring for a client in an emergency situation is stressful and requires attention to the ABCs of client care. However, the psychosocial and spiritual needs of the client and his or her family are also important and need special consideration from the nurse. When the nursing care required is of a more "routine" nature, there are multiple opportunities for client teaching and even primary prevention teaching activities.

In addition to being able to quickly assess, prioritize, and intervene in emergency situations, emergency nurses need to be aware of ethical and legal situations. These situations include consent to treatment, right to privacy and confidentiality, mandatory reporting, and proper handling of physical evidence; for example, bullets and specimens. Emergency nurses are confronted with acute physiologic and psychological situations, thus astute assessment, communication, and technical skills are important. Written documentation must be concise, but thorough, and legible.

OBJECTIVES

82.1 Discuss situations that hospitals, nurses, and physicians are required to report to appropriate agencies.

82.2 Explain the proper handling of evidence such as bullets and specimens.

82.3 Discuss laws governing client admission and transfer.

82.4 Discuss initial nursing assessment, triage categories, documentation, secondary nursing assessments, and discharge teaching in the emergency department.

82.5 Discuss death and dying in emergency settings.

89.6 Discuss primary assessment and priority nursing interventions in emergency situations.

89.7 Discuss secondary nursing assessments in emergency situations.

82.8 Identify signs and symptoms associated with selected medical-surgical emergencies.

82.9 Describe appropriate medical management and priority discharge teaching of clients with medical-surgical emergencies.

LEARNING THE LANGUAGE: TERMINOLOGY RELATED TO BASIC CONCEPTS OF EMERGENCY CARE

Match the descriptions in Column A with the correct term in Column B.

Column A		**Column B**
1. _____ The process of determining priorities		A. Emergency
2. _____ Interventions focused on emergent care		B. Emergent
3. _____ Life-threatening: the client may die without immediate interventions		C. Urgent
4. _____ Requires intervention within a few hours		D. Nonurgent
5. _____ A complete focused assessment		E. Telephone triage
6. _____ Occurs when the emergency department is called for help with a crisis		F. Triage
7. _____ Interventions may be delayed beyond a few hours		G. Priority nursing interventions
8. _____ Any sudden illness or injury that is perceived to be a crisis that threatens the physical or psychological well-being of a person or group		H. Secondary nursing interventions

Label the following examples with the correct triage category—E (emergent), U (urgent), or N (nonurgent).

9. _____ Airway obstruction		15. _____ Vomiting		
10. _____ Cardiac arrest		16. _____ Persistent nausea		
11. _____ Chest pain		17. _____ Multiple bruises and abrasions		
12. _____ Sprained ankle		18. _____ Fracture without circulatory comprise		
13. _____ Sudden loss of vision		19. _____ Open chest wound		
14. _____ Severe pain		20. _____ Diarrhea		

Label the following situations Y (for those that are required by law to be reported to the appropriate agency) or N (for those that are not required to be reported).

21. _____ Rape		26. _____ Overdoses	
22. _____ Suspected child abuse		27. _____ Poisonings	
23. _____ Suspected elder abuse		28. _____ Sexually transmitted diseases	
24. _____ Suspected spousal abuse		29. _____ Food poisonings	
25. _____ Animal bites		30. _____ Attempted suicides	

KNOWLEDGE BUILDING

31. Describe how emergency care can be given when the client is unconscious or unable to give consent.

32. Describe assessment of the airway and appropriate interventions in an emergency situation.

33. List four types of deaths that must be reported by
    the emergency department to the medical examiner.

LEARNING THE LANGUAGE: TERMINOLOGY RELATED TO CLIENTS WITH MEDICAL-SURGICAL EMERGENCIES

Match the descriptions in Column A with the correct term in Column B.

Column A	**Column B**
34. _____ Causes a break in the integrity of the skin	A. Peritoneal lavage
35. _____ A core body temperature of 34.4° C or 94° F	B. Acute abdomen
36. _____ Ecchymosis (bruising) in the mastoid area	C. Penetrating injuries
37. _____ Nonpenetrating injuries caused by accelera- tion-deceleration forces	D. Blunt injuries
38. _____ Results from dehydration	E. Champion Trauma Score
39. _____ Periorbital bruising	F. Ocular avulsion
40. _____ Sudden onset of abdominal pain	G. Contusion
41. _____ Removal of the eye from its socket	H. Battle's sign
42. _____ An injury that does not break the skin but causes discoloration of the skin	I. Kehr's sign
	J. Sexual assault
43. _____ Performed to determine the presence of blood in the abdomen	K. Heat exhaustion
44. _____ The stress of heat exposure increases the demand on the heart; sweating doesn't occur	L. Classic heat stroke
	M. Exertional heat stroke
45. _____ Injury to one or more body systems	N. Hypothermia
46. _____ A violent shaking or jarring caused by an explosion or a blow to the head	O. Raccoon eyes
	P. Mechanism of injury
47. _____ Shoulder pain unrelated to trauma; sugges- tive of diaphragm irritation	Q. Immersion syndrome
	R. Multiple trauma
48. _____ Used to categorize and determine severity of injury	S. Concussion
49. _____ Term applied to victims of rape	
50. _____ Term used to describe how an injury oc- curred	
51. _____ Term used to describe near-drowning	
52. _____ Common in laborers, farm workers, and athletes who are exposed to heat; sweating occurs	

Match the descriptions in Column A with the correct type of chest injury in Column B.

Column A	Column B
53. _____ Air enters the pleural space and becomes trapped	A. Hemopneumothorax
54. _____ Contents of the mediastinum are pushed toward the unaffected side	B. Tension pneumothorax
55. _____ Air in the pleural space	C. Mediastinal shift
56. _____ Blood in the pleural space	D. Open pneumothorax
57. _____ Fractures of two or more ribs on the same side	E. Paradoxical motion
58. _____ Chest moves opposite of normal respiratory pattern	F. Flail chest
59. _____ Occurs with a sucking chest wound	G. Hemothorax
60. _____ Blood and air in the pleural space	H. Pneumothorax

THINKING CRITICALLY: UNDERSTANDING RATIONALES

List the rationales for the following nursing interventions for clients with altered level of consciousness.

Intervention	Rationale
61. Draw blood for complete blood count, calcium, electrolytes, drug screen, and alcohol level.	
62. Naloxone (Narcan) 2 mg IV	
63. IV dextrose	
64. Position head in neutral alignment.	
65. Hyperventilate with 100% oxygen prior to suctioning	
66. Refrain from discussing the client's condition at the bedside.	
67. Administer glucose paste per orders.	
68. Thiamin 100 mg IV	
69. Position the unconscious victim in a side-lying position.	
70. Administer artificial tears and tape eyelids shut on an unconscious client.	

List the rationales for the following nursing interventions.

	Intervention	Rationale
71.	Insert two large-bore IVs in trauma victim.	
72.	Remove all the clothes of a trauma victim.	
73.	Do not massage affected part in clients with frostbite.	
74.	Avoid flexion of the neck in head-trauma victims.	
75.	Administer broad-spectrum antibiotics and tetanus prophylaxis to clients with human bite wounds.	
76.	Draw, type, and cross-match blood on multiple-trauma victims.	

List the rationales for the following discharge teaching.

	Teaching Point	Rationale
77.	For head-trauma victim: Wake the client every two hours (for the next eight hours) to check level of consciousness (LOC) and orientation.	
78.	For sexual assault victim: Schedule follow-up care in 4–6 weeks for test results, a pregnancy test, and psychosocial support.	
79.	Care of sutured lacerations: Keep the wound and dressing clean. You may take a shower. Do not expose the wound to moisture for prolonged periods of time.	

Determine the Glasgow Coma Scale for the following situation.

80. Mr. E. is a 24-year-old college student who was brought to the emergency department following a head injury and possible abdominal injury he received during an intramural basketball game. Witnesses reported that he ran into the official's table chasing a loose ball. He hit his head on the table and fell to the floor and another player landed on top of him. He did not lose consciousness immediately but appeared "rattled." However, he insisted on finishing the game. He continued to play ball until he collapsed on the floor about 10 minutes after the injury.

    Upon admission he opened his eyes when his name was called but answered questions inappropriately. He obeys commands. He guards his left abdomen. Vital signs are B/P 110/80, R 24 with normal expansion, P 98, temperature 98.4° F, and capillary refill is normal (> 3 seconds).

Provide a short answer for the following question.

81. Differentiate between penetrating and nonpenetrating chest injuries.

What are the predicted injuries for the following situations?

82. Automobile accident: driver unrestrained

83. Automobile accident: passenger (front seat with restraints)

84. Motorcycle accident: motorcyclist impacting with a nonmovable object

85. Fall or jump greater than 10 feet: victim lands on feet

86. Fall or jump greater than 10 feet: victim lands on buttocks or in sitting position

87. Altercation or beating: victim hit with a blunt object

KNOWLEDGE BUILDING: NURSING CARE OF CLIENTS WITH MEDICAL-SURGICAL EMERGENCIES

88. What is the drug of choice used when narcotic overdose is suspected?

89. Describe the purpose and process for gastric lavage.

90. Describe the primary assessment and priority interventions for chest injuries.

91. What are the effects of a mediastinal shift?

92. When a client is admitted to the emergency department with chest pain, what assessment questions are asked?

93. If a client comes to the emergency department with complaints of abdominal pain, what are important history questions to ask?

94. Why do emergency department nurses refer to rape as alleged sexual assault?

95. If a person comes to the emergency department with a "dirty" soft tissue wound, who has had his or her series of three tetanus immunizations and a booster six years ago, what, if any, tetanus prophylaxis would he or she likely receive?

96. What is the usual treatment for heatstroke?

97. What is the usual treatment for frostbite?

■ *Case Study*

Mr. K. is a 30-year-old male brought to the emergency department following a motor vehicle accident. He was the driver of the car involved in a low-speed head-on collision. He was not wearing his seat belt. Mr. K. is on a back board and has an 18-gauge intravenous needle in place with 1000 cc lactated Ringer's running at 150 cc/hour. Mr. K. was not responding verbally to the paramedics at time of transport.

98. Initial assessment by the nurse would include which of the following as highest priority?

    A. airway, breathing, circulation

    B. Glasgow Coma Scale

    C. Champion Trauma Score

    D. neurological assessment

99. Based on the type of accident that Mr. K. was in, the nurse would assess for what signs of blunt chest injury?

    A. wheezes over upper thorax

    B. diminished sensation over the chest wall

    C. bruising over the chest wall

    D. hyperresonant lung sound

100. Mr. K. should also be examined for what other types of injuries?

    A. patellar and vertebral compression

    B. cardiac contusions and facial fractures

    C. Waddell's triad and patellar fractures

    D. wrist fractures and lacerated solid organs

101. The nurse has to notify Mr. K.'s wife about his accident and condition. General points to consider when the nurse calls include which of the following?

    A. Share immediately the seriousness of his condition.

    B. Do not give out your name.

    C. Ask about the handling of Mr. K.'s valuables.

    D. Present the facts chronologically.

102. Mr. K. is sent to radiology for skull series and computed tomography scan. The nurse accompanies him to provide continuous assessment. Of the following symptoms exhibited by Mr. K., which would be the most serious?

    A. complaining that the ride was too bumpy

    B. sleeping intermittently in radiology

    C. shallow breathing at a 40-per-minute rate

    D. complaining of pain during transfer from the stretcher

Answer Key

1. Signs: objective data.

2. Symptoms: subjective data reported by the client.

3. Syndrome: a group of signs and symptoms resulting from a single cause.

4. Germ theory: Specific microorganisms cause infectious disease.

5. Multicausal theory: Many factors specific to each individual can cause illness.

6. Adaptation: A change or response to stress.

7. Psychosocial theory: Physiologic, psychologic, and social factors cause disease and illness.

8. Cognitive appraisal: How one interprets problems.

9. Daily hassles: Minor life events that everyone experiences. They are irritating, frustrating, and distressing demands of everyday life.

10. Daily uplifts: Buffers to daily hassles. There are three types: *breathers:* things that interrupt the intensity or frequency of hassles such as reading a novel or seeing a movie; *sustainers:* daily psychological nourishment needed to continue coping with life such as spending time with loved ones or friends; and *restorers:* things that replenish that which has been depleted or lost. Examples of restorers are prayer, meditation, and talking out problems with friends.

11. Biopsychosociospiritual: The person's body, mind, and environment all function together to determine whether illness develops.

12. B

13. E

14. D

15. A

16. C

17. B

18. C

19. B

20. E

21. C

22. C

23. B

24. G

25. A

26. H

27. E

28. F

29. G

30. A

31. General Adaptation Syndrome (GAS): Selye's term for responses to illness that involve generalized changes in several body systems mediated by the sympathetic nervous system and adrenal cortices. They include loss of appetite, weight loss, feeling and looking ill, and various muscle aches and pains. The Local Adaptation Syndrome (LAS) takes place in a single organ or specific section of the body such as inflammation or a blood clot. The three stages include:

    1. Alarm reaction: first contact with the stressor called the "fight or flight" stage.

Catecholamines (epinephrine and norepinephrine) are excreted, heart rate increases, strength of heart contractions increases. Cortisol is released to increase glucose energy. The body cannot stay in stage 1 without experiencing pathologic changes.

2. Stage of resistance: when the body starts to react and to return to a homeostatic state. Parasympathetic nervous system returns hormones to normal levels. The stressor is removed or the body learns to adapt to the stressor.

3. Stage of exhaustion: The stressor continues and the body cannot continue to produce hormones as in stage 1 or when damage has occurred to other organs.

32. The increase in serum glucose in a GAS response of cortisol is released in response to the stressors caused by the pneumonia.

33. Type A: Constant mobilization of inner resources to combat real or imagined stresses. Type A behaviors are aggressive, hostile, and deadline-driven. Diseases associated with type A personalities are high cholesterol and heart disease. Type B personalities put all of life's stresses in perspective. They are not deadline-driven. They are calm, optimistic, and self-confident.

34. *Biocultural factors* refers to multiple and frequently interrelated factors that are responsible for differing susceptibilities to conditions. Examples are natural and acquired immunity, intermarriage, geographic and climate conditions, ethnicity, race, and hereditary predisposition, and religious practices.

35. Describe in your own words.

Health Promotion

36. Health: A state of complete physical, mental, and social well-being and not merely the absence of disease or infirmity.

37. Health promotion: The process of fostering awareness, influencing attitudes, and identifying alternatives to achieve optimum physical and mental health.

38. Wellness: Quality or condition of well-being that incorporates positive mental, physical, and spiritual states.

39. Self-responsibility: Developing an awareness and ability to take action to achieve or maintain individual freedom, health, and well-being.

40. Primary prevention: Health promotion activities that prevent the actual occurrence of a specific illness or disease.

41. Secondary prevention: Activities that promote early detection (screening) and treatment of disease and limitation of disability.

42. Tertiary prevention: Activities directed toward rehabilitation after a disease or condition has already developed.

43. Risk factors: Anything that affects health. Classified according to six categories: genetic, age, biologic characteristics, personal health habits, lifestyle, and environment.

44. C
45. A
46. A
47. B
48. B
49. C
50. A
51. C
52. E
53. A
54. F
55. E
56. B
57. E
58. A
59. D
60. D

61. Nurses are charged with the responsibility of altering client attitudes toward health rather than altering the system itself. However, the very nature of nursing dictates that nurses be involved in all aspects of the system that they have the ability to affect. The ANA social policy statement delineates involvement in social reform.

62. Dunn's high-level wellness is "an integrated method of functioning that is oriented toward maximizing the potential of the individual. Wellness is an ongoing process directed toward a higher potential."

Travis' model emphasizes that wellness requires attention; it does not happen automatically. Using this model, people can move from the point of illness or disease to neutrality into high-level wellness. Both models emphasize health promotion and illness prevention rather than just treating diseases.

63. The *Healthy People 2000* report lists objectives and specific activities for achieving the objectives. It prompted agencies to focus on prevention and promotion through strategies of institutional change, legislation, and public policy, not merely in the realm of personal behavior changes. An

example of how this could be implemented is by offering incentives in the workplace and lower insurance rates for nonsmokers.

64. Nursing is the diagnosis and treatment of human responses to actual and potential health problems. The human responses to potential health problems are the main focus of health promotion.

65. *Recognizing and believing*: Understanding and accepting that we are more than individual members of groups; we are members of a global family. What one does can affect another.

    Conserving: Turning off lights conserves energy.

    Water: Repairing a leaking faucet conserves water. Eliminating residential lawn watering which accounts for 30-80% of water usage in the United States.

    Consuming: Individuals can develop creative ways to make recycling more effective. They can support agencies and groups that focus on conserving natural resources.

    Eating: Using less pesticides and insecticides, which indirectly affect the food chain.

    Moving: Developing more efficient ways to use fuel would reduce the amount of air pollution.

    Stepping forward: Nurses must act individually and collectively on global problems that affect health.

Chronic Conditions

66. In general there are three stages: (1) prediagnostic, (2) diagnostic, and (3) chronic. Some conditions have a fourth stage—terminal.

67. One physiologic change (depending on the chronic condition) could be decreased ability to ambulate (for instance, after a stroke). An adaptive challenge would be learning to use a cane or walker (acquiring a skill in using techniques or devices). Nursing interventions could focus around teaching or reinforcing teaching about the use of a cane; additional interventions could focus on safety issues in the home.

    One psychological change (again, a person who has had a stroke) could involve loss of independence when the person can no longer drive (restructuring one's life around the chronic condition). A corresponding adaptive challenge would involve adjusting to changes in roles in terms of depending on others to drive and/or learning to use public transportation that is handicap-accessible (adapting to changes in physical abilities). Nursing interventions could involve open discussions with the client and family about these changes to provide an opportunity for discussion and planning in regard to them. Additionally, information could be provided about

public transportation and other services available in the community that assist with transportation.

Social adaptive changes could involve changes in employment (loss of or the need for a different position). The adaptive challenges center around retraining for a new job or adjusting to loss of position (developing new skills and networks). Nursing interventions could involve providing information about rehabilitation facilities. These facilities would provide information about job retraining. Additionally, nursing interventions could involve supporting the client and family as they adjust to these changes.

68. Assessment includes a detailed health history with a thorough analysis of manifestations (what makes them better, what makes them worse, when did they start, what relieves them, do they interfere with activities), complete history and physical assessment, psychological assessment, and social assessment. Assessment tools for physical and cognitive functioning might provide valuable data.

69. Further assessments involve determining Mr. J.'s understanding of the purpose of the medications, important side effects, when and how to take the medications, safety precautions, and medical follow-up.

70. A physician consult would be important to obtain before developing a specific exercise plan. Other considerations to examine are the difficulty of the exercise program, amount of time required, and amount of exertion required.

Putting It All Together

Student A has correctly appraised the stressors and demands of nursing school. She has developed or strengthened coping mechanisms. Student B's cognitive appraisal of the stressor is distorted. She seems to have more daily hassles that increase her stress and hinder her ability to cope. She has fewer daily uplifts.

71 Answers will vary.

72. Student B.

73. Will vary with the individual. Some examples: too many things to do, managing many different roles at one time, finding a parking space, and financial concerns.

74. First gather more data to identify the real problem. Socialization into nursing school requires many adjustments compared to traditional college courses. Both students have a "B" average in the course but student B is exhibiting stress-related behaviors. Student B's prior coping mechanisms are not working. Some coping mechanisms:

    • Provide time for problem solving and venting of feelings.

- Encourage the development of relationships with peers.
- Join study groups.
- Improve time management and organization skills by:
  — Developing a time-management grid. Block out *fixed activities* such as travel time, class time, sleep time, and required family and household duties. Next block out the *flexible time*. Evaluate the management grid and make adjustments. Remember to make time for daily uplifts.
  — Study in 20- to 30-minute time blocks rather than 2- to 3-hour blocks.
  — Read the course syllabus and schedule, keep a calendar.
  — Ask questions when something is not clear.

75 & 76. Individual answers.

Case Study

77. C Arteriosclerotic heart disease is linked to hyperlipidemia and hypercholesteremia. These are considered *biologic* characteristics.

78. B According to the textbook, the demise of the extended family and the loss of family support systems are a component of health lifestyle behaviors.

79. A These factors are age-related health risks because they were caused by self-medication errors that occur frequently in the elderly client.

80. B All the nursing diagnoses listed are realistic for Mr. G. However, Fluid volume excess is the only one evident now; the client is *at risk* for developing the others.

81. D Only identification of an adequate support system will help with health promotion for Mr. G. The nurse needs to find someone who lives close enough that they can help to monitor the client's drug therapy. In addition, contact with the outside by way of this other individual may help to improve Mr. G.'s mental processes.

82. B Improved technology is resulting in survival from acute illnesses that may become chronic. (Also, the increase in older adults is increasing the numbers of chronic conditions.)

83. C Revising life goals is a behavior seen in the integration phase.

84. B Mr. M. has paralysis of his lower body resulting in disuse, which places him at risk for pressure sores.

85. A Hospice care is focused on the care of people in the last six months of life.

86. D Dealing with genetic concerns would be a social challenge rather than a physiologic challenge.

CHAPTER 2: HEALTH PROMOTION IN YOUNG AND MIDDLE-AGED ADULTS

1. Motor vehicle accidents
2. • Confine the incidence of HIV infection to no more than 100/100,000
   • Reduces unplanned pregnancies to no more than 30% of all pregnancies
3. False, the percentage of obese people is consistently rising.
4. Obesity is a body mass index of 30 or higher.
5. Type 2 diabetes, heart disease, degenerative joint disease, hypertension, sleep apnea, and gallbladder disease
6. Good question. I wish I knew the answer! There are no guidelines for the words *sparingly* or *moderately*. Thus, everyone interprets these differently. The pyramid (textbook Figure 2-1) is used along with the dietary guidelines for Americans (textbook Table 2-2).
7. No answer provided.
8. No answer provided.
9. CAGE is a tool used to screen all clients for drinking problems.
   AUDIT is a ten-item tool that is highly sensitive and specific to problem drinking. A score of 8 or greater indicates a more in-depth assessment of the drinking problem.
10. Low-birth-weight babies, cancer, peptic ulcer disease, and osteoporosis
11. "I can understand your frustration but please realize that your health and well-being are our main concern. Our staff is required to ask these questions at each visit." Then review the client's health history and gently explain which problems are directly related to smoking and the health risks generally related to smoking.
12. • Tetanus-diphtheria booster every 10 years
    • Proven immunity to rubella or rubella vaccine
    • Hepatitis B for people at high risk (see Table 2-8)
13. E
14. B
15. D
16. C

17. A
18. C
19. B
20. E
21. D
22. A
23. People often worry more about imagined problems than actual problems. Helping clients to identify real versus imagined problems is the first step of problem solving.
24. The focus is to change the perception of the problem. If it is not a problem, try cognitive reappraisal techniques.
25. Some problems such as death, a catastrophic illness, or something legally mandated are beyond control. For these problems resolution is not possible so effective coping is directed toward acceptance.
26. Hypertension
27. Obesity
28. Coronary heart disease risk
29. Cervical cancer
30. Colorectal cancer
31. Breast cancer
32. Nonimmune status
33. Problem drinking
34. Prostate cancer

CHAPTER 3: HEALTH PROMOTION IN OLDER ADULTS

1. E
2. A
3. J
4. I
5. K
6. M
7. L
8. O
9. F
10. H
11. G
12. C
13. B
14. D
15. N
16. T
17. F   Ethnic people over 65 are increasing proportionately.
18. F   Life expectancy for men is 72.7 years.
19. T

20. T
21. F   Eighty percent of people over 65 have at least one chronic illness.
22. T
23. F   Hearing and vision are the most common senses to diminish.
24. F   Studies have shown that 10-15% of older adults in the community have serious problems related to alcohol.
25. F   Only 5% of people over 65 are living in nursing homes.
26. T
27. Personal care, intermediate, skilled
28. Stomach emptying, changes in gastric pH, and gastrointestinal motility may affect absorption. Altered cardiac output and sluggish circulation may delay transport of drugs to target sites and slow elimination of the drug or its by-products from the body. Decreases in total body water alter cellular distribution of drugs, which can result in higher than usual blood levels. Fat content increases and results in storage of lipid-soluble drugs, thus extending and possibly elevating drug levels. Liver clearance is diminished and this slowed metabolism results in the drug remaining in the body longer. Changes in the kidneys affect both the length of time the drug is in the body and its half-life, with possible toxic effects. Changes in the sensitivity of the CNS may result in exaggerated or idiosyncratic reactions to hypertensive drugs.
29. Box 3-2 in the text contains guidelines for teaching older adults. Be cautious not to assume that these guidelines would be necessary without a thorough initial assessment of your client.
30. Particular attention needs to be paid to assessing for adverse reactions to medication due to the potential for delayed excretion, slowed metabolism, and increased storage.
31. Your assessments of the client would include visual acuity, hearing, attention span and energy level, literacy, and background knowledge about diabetes. Assessment of job history or hobbies might be helpful in order to draw analogies.
32. Important sensory assessments would include hearing, vision, touch, pain, and balance.
33. B   Aging actually results in decreased amounts of HCl.
34. C   Joining groups provides for companionship and support.
35. A   Dementia is characterized by gradual onset.
36. D   Congregate housing is individual housing within a multiunit dwelling. It is appropriate for a person who is independent with most ADLs but

needs some assistance with meals, transportation, and social and recreational activities.

37.   D   Approximately half of the physical deterioration in older adults is caused by disuse, not from aging or disease.

CHAPTER 4: OVERVIEW OF HEALTH CARE DELIVERY

1.   D
2.   E
3.   F
4.   B
5.   G
6.   A
7.   H
8.   I
9.   C
10.   *Period of Expansion*: The major focus was to develop health care programs that made health care more accessible to the people.

Period of Regulation and Cost Containment: The major focus of this period was to develop ways to control the rising cost of health care and coordinate health care services. Prior to this period, the focus was reactive rather than proactive.

Period of Reform: The focus is on trying to fix the problems created in the first two periods by developing creative ways to decrease health care costs and meet the health care needs of all people.

11.   Social Security Act of 1935 established as social policy the right of the aged to financial security. It later became the vehicle for meeting the health care needs of the aged and poor.

12.   The Hill-Burton Act was passed to eliminate shortages of hospitals, especially in rural and economically depressed areas.

13.   National Health Planning Resources Act of 1974. The purpose of this Act was to control health care costs by combining health planning and regulation. States were required to develop a statewide health plan for the use of resources. The Act also requires states to review health care providers' requests to initiate or expand health services. This review process is known as Certificate of Need (CON). If the provider could not demonstrate sufficient need for the services, the request was denied.

14.   Tax Equity and Fiscal Responsibility Act (TEFRA) of 1983 directed the Secretary of Health and Human Services to develop a prospective payment system (PPS) for the Medicare program. Blue Cross and other insurers began to restructure their payment systems to protect themselves.

15.   Prospective payment systems (PPSs) and diagnosis-related groups (DRGs) in 1983 replaced the cost-based retrospective (after the care was provided) payment system for Medicare clients with a prospective payment system. Under this system, hospitals were paid a designated amount for each DRG regardless of the actual cost of health care.

16.   Quality, cost, and access to care

17.   Nurses represent the largest single group of health care providers. The American Nurses' Association (ANA) collaborated with other professional nursing organizations to develop *Nursing's Agenda for Health Care Reform.*

CHAPTER 5: AMBULATORY HEALTH CARE

1.   C
2.   G
3.   H
4.   B
5.   D
6.   A
7.   E
8.   F
9.   H
10.   I
11.   B
12.   E
13.   D
14.   F
15.   C
16.   A
17.   G
18.   J
19.   K
20.   Financial: The government and private payers will not pay hospitals for services that can be done in an ambulatory care setting.

21.   They do not provide sleeping accommodations and they are not for clients incapable of self-care after the procedure.

22.   Answers will vary.

23.   Recovery from anesthetic agents, orientation to time and place, ability to move all extremities, ability to void, no allergic reactions, ability to ambulate.

24.   In the medical model nurses assume a subordinate role to the physician. The nurses have less autonomy. In the nursing model, nurses assume a leadership role and provide primary care. They generally have a broader scope of practice.

25. The criterion includes Baccalaureate degree in nursing and meets the hours of experience in ambulatory care nursing. To maintain certification nurses must practice a certain number of hours in an ambulatory care setting and show evidence of a specified number of continuing education hours.

CHAPTER 6: ACUTE HEALTH CARE

1. K
2. G
3. H
4. J
5. D
6. B
7. I
8. M
9. F
10. A
11. L
12. N
13. C
14. E
15. The Great Depression, the advent of prepayment insurance (the Blue Cross Plan); and as a result insurance, sounder hospital financial standing.
16. Monitoring or nursing care.
17. Government-owned, voluntary (nonprofit, tax-exempt organizations), and for-profit (proprietary).
18. Designed to fill the gap between acute care hospitals and long-term care facilities. Clients who are out of the fragile stage of their illnesses but still need monitoring and rehabilitation.
19. Direct care provider, educator, and/or manager.
20. Four common categories: (1) the client's ability to perform activities of daily living, (2) general health, (3) emotional support, and (4) treatment modalities. More specific categories are eating, grooming, comfort, excretion, general health, treatments, medications, and teaching and emotional support. The client is rated on a four-point scale on his or her ability or care needs in these areas.
21. Efficacy, appropriateness, availability, timeliness, effectiveness, continuity, safety, efficiency, respect, and caring.
22. A   Disadvantages of team nursing are that it is expensive because there is a fragmentation of personnel, a lack of delegation skills by nurses may reduce efficiency, and some duplication may occur between members of different teams.
23. B   The most important consideration in delegation is the task itself and whether this task must be legally performed by an RN.
24. D   One of the primary purposes of a patient classification system is to identify the numbers and kinds of health care providers needed for a particular shift. The system can also be used to determine cost of nursing care and to track case-mix changes or changes during a certain time of year.
25. A   Medication errors are one of the top five risk areas in the hospital. The others are complications from diagnostic or treatment procedures, falls, patient or family dissatisfaction, and refusal of treatment or refusal to sign consent for treatment.

CHAPTER 7: HOME HEALTH CARE

1. Nursing care provided to clients admitted to the hospital.
2. Nursing care provided to clients in any setting other than the hospital or long-term care setting.
3. Nursing care provided in the client's place of residence.
4. A framework for providing care, documentation, evaluation, and information management used in community-based settings.
5. Software that improves communication between instructors and students in community-based settings. It allows direct verbal and visual communication between the instructor and students by means of a portable computer, TV, and modem. The Nightingale Tracker was released in 1998, and is used by schools and colleges that use the Omaha System.
6. One major trend impacting home health care is the aging population. The number of Medicare reimbursements for home health care services doubled between 1991 and 1994.
7. Clients have both rights and responsibilities. They must be knowledgeable about their own health care and actively involved in decisions regarding their care. When the nurse enters the home, it is the client, not the nurse, who is in charge. The nurse is there to assist the client.
8. The home health care nurse does not have extra help available to assist or retrieve extra supplies. They must anticipate and plan for every possible situation. For example, proper lighting, extra supplies, different-sized Foley catheters, and so forth.
9. Medicare
10. Neither
11. Medicare
12. Neither
13. Medicaid

CHAPTER 8: LONG-TERM CARE

1. •   The Social Security act of 1935 afforded older adults the means to purchase care privately. An informal long-term care system emerged.

    •   The 1946 Hill-Burton Hospital Survey and Construction Act provided funds for the construction of hospitals and nursing homes provided they meet certain criteria.

    •   1965 Medicare and Medicaid ensured a minimum level of care for the aged and poor.

    •   The Omnibus Budget Reconciliation Act of 1987 produced reform in nursing home care. Facilities that do not meet standards described in the regulations can have their Medicare and Medicaid reimbursements terminated.

2. A registered nurse must be on duty for at least 8 consecutive hours, 7 days per week; a full-time director of nursing must be on staff if the facility has more than 60 beds; and the facility must provide 24-hour nursing services. The proportion of other nursing staff is not stated. They must be sufficient to meet total nursing care needs.

3. The requirements for the MDS. The RN must coordinate the completion of the minimum assessment within 14 days of admission. Following this, the client is reassessed annually or when health status has changed.

4. The MDS is a minimum assessment database that does not assess the resident's self-concept, spirituality, sense of power, knowledge of health conditions, self-care practices, patterns of solitude, sexuality, immunity, stress management, use of alternative therapies, attitudes regarding health status and death.

5. See Box 8-1 in the textbook.

6. They have to adapt to new surroundings, they no longer have access to their own refrigerator, and their personal space is reduced from a house or apartment to one room.

7. Routines are centered on the facility instead of the resident. Meals are served at specific times, baths and showers are regimented. Hours of sleep are scheduled.

8. Residents have to adjust to many new people and faces.

9. There is a sense of loss of independence when people become residents. Many decisions concerning ADLs are made for the residents thus compounding the problem.

10. See Box 8-4 in the textbook.

CHAPTER 9: HEALTH HISTORY

1. D
2. F
3. C
4. A
5. F
6. G
7. B
8. B
9. C
10. A
11. D
12. E
13.-31.   Refer to Table 9-2, textbook pp. 148–154.

32. Subjective data are collected by interviewing the client. It is what the client *tells* the nurse. Objective data are collected by the nurse during the physical assessment. Objective data also include laboratory and diagnostic test results.

33. Psychological patterns are nonphysical components of a client, such as thoughts, feelings, motivation, mental status, and personal strengths and weaknesses.

    Social experiences are the parts of a client's life that are affected by or dependent on others.

34. All client information should remain confidential and be shared only with health care providers involved in managing the client's health. However, when a client reveals illegal practices or practices that may be harmful to self or others, the nurse must report the information to the appropriate people.

35. Using broad statements such as: "Tell me how you would describe your health," or a rating scale: "How would you rate your health on a scale of 1 to 5, with 1 being the worst and 5 being the best?"

36. The purpose of the health risk appraisal is to 1) identify risk factors that affect the client's potential for developing a particular health problem; 2) identify clients who may benefit from timely interventions; and 3) assess the client's willingness to modify or reduce his or her health risks.

37. *Affect* consists of the observable, outward demeanor that depicts a client's current emotional state. It is generally an ongoing assessment that is integrated into all interactions with the client. *Mood* is the client's subjective descriptions of personal emotion that is pervasive and sustained. Affect and mood should be congruent. Any inconsistencies should be validated.

38. If the client has a known altered thought process, a formal mental status examination would be

required. Memory is informally assessed during the interview by asking questions such as what the client had for breakfast that morning and the previous morning.

39. **A**   Biographic information includes data such as age, sex, name, place of birth, race, and religious preference.

40. **C**   Hyperlipidemia, hypercholesterolemia, hyperglycemia, and hypersensitivity reactions are examples of biologic risk factors.

41. **D**   High-risk sexual activity is considered a lifestyle risk factor.

42. **A**   Stressful situations are environmental risk factors. They may occur in the home or workplace.

43. **B**   All of the items are components of the health history interview. However, in this situation the priority is to obtain more information about the chief complaint.

44. **A**   Asking the client to repeat a series of numbers assesses the client's ability to focus or concentrate on a task or activity over time.

45. **B**   Recommendation for women over age 50 is a yearly mammogram.

CHAPTER 10: PHYSICAL EXAMINATION

1. C
2. D
3. B
4. A
5. G
6. A
7. D
8. A & E
9. A
10. A & D
11. D
12. A
13. H
14. A
15. Inspection can provide assessment data about affect, size, shape, color, symmetry, position, and deformities.
16. The diaphragm is used for high-pitched sounds such as lung sounds and blood pressure. The bell is used for low-pitched sounds such as bruits and murmurs.
17. Inspection: The systematic, deliberate visual examination of the entire client or a region of the body. Example: examining facial skin while collecting a history.

18. Light palpation: Depressing the underlying tissue 1 to 2 cm (1/2-3/4 inches). Example: lymph nodes.

19. Deep palpation: Depressing the underlying tissue 4 to 5 cm (1 1/2-2 inches). Examples: breast and internal organs such as the liver and spleen.

20. Percussion: A technique to assess the density of a part by the sound produced by striking the skin. Example: lung fields.

21. Auscultation: Listening to internal body sounds. Examples: heart and lung sounds.

22. Conduct the Webber and Rinne tests.

23. Auscultate voice sounds by using either bronchophony, egophony, or whispered pectoriloquy. Correlate with percussion.

24. Verify landmarks and listen again. If the heart sounds are still muffled have the client lean forward or lie on the left side to place the heart closer to the chest wall. If muffled sounds are still heard, document and report to the nurse in charge or the physician.

25. Validate findings: Listen for *at least* one minute in each quadrant. Gather and review additional data such as contour of the abdomen, percussion and palpation, history, last BM, passing gas, and medications or procedures that affect elimination. If the absence of bowel sounds is verified, document the findings and report the results to the nurse in charge or the physician.

26. Palpate distal pulses.

27. Check technique and retry the reinforcement technique by having the client perform isometric exercises on the muscle group.

28. Conduct a thorough auscultation with the bell and diaphragm.

29. Recheck the reading in both arms. Obtain readings with the client lying, sitting, and standing.

30. Conduct a thorough examination of the mouth. Document and report findings.

31. Document and report to the nurse in charge or the physician.

32. Complete a symptom analysis and conduct a thorough physical examination of lung sounds.

33. Complete a symptom analysis and conduct a thorough physical examination of the throat and neck.

34. Gather more data on other risk factors for breast cancer: last mammogram and self-breast exam.

35. Findings from one side of the body are compared to the opposite side. The nurse compares these findings with a known standard.

36. The nurse compares findings with known standards to determine if the findings are normal for the age, sex, and racial background or if they are abnormal.

37. *Contralateral* means opposite.
38. Lung sounds are clear in all lobes: vesicular sounds in the periphery, no crackles or wheezes.
39. Femoral, popliteal, posterior tibial, and dorsalis pedis pulses 2+ bilaterally.
40. Acetone breath noted.
41. Vital signs: B/P 120/80 (R arm) 124/84 (L arm); T 98.6° oral, P 100, R 18.
42. Bowel sounds active in all quadrants.
43. Shoulder-length, dark brown, thick hair.
44. Visual acuity per Snellen chart with glasses OD 20/30, OS 20/20.
45. Whisper heard bilaterally at 3 feet.
46. B
47. A
48. C
49. D
50. A
51. D
52. B

CHAPTER 11: DIAGNOSTIC ASSESSMENT

1. N
2. E
3. D
4. J
5. M
6. C
7. K
8. B
9. A
10. F
11. G
12. L
13. H
14. I
15. E
16. D
17. C
18. B
19. A
20. F
21. They may damage tissue as they move in the strong magnetic field.
22. To ensure excretion of the dye
23. Food and fluid would obstruct visualization.
24. To enhance elimination of the barium
25. Explain that some clients feel claustrophobic during the test. Emphasize that the client can communicate with the technician during the exam. Clients who have claustrophobia may not tolerate the exam. Clients with mild claustrophobia may be sedated.
26. The dye has a diuretic effect. Encourage fluids to flush the dye and prevent injury to the kidneys.
27. Agitated clients may require sedation so they can tolerate the test. The test may last up to 4 hours.
28. No specific postprocedure instructions
29. Instructing the client on what to expect reduces anxiety.
30. No specific postprocedure care for this test.
31. Contrast dye contains iodine.
32. The extremity is kept immobile to stabilize the clot formed at the puncture site.
33. To provide a baseline for postprocedure assessments
34. A topical anesthetic is sprayed in the back of the throat that affects swallowing and the gag reflex.
35. A biopsy is performed to determine the presence of malignant cells.
36. Biopsies are invasive procedures.
37. To decrease the possibility of contaminating the specimen.
38. Antibiotics given before the blood cultures could alter the test.
39. All urine must be collected during the specified period. If a specimen is omitted during the collection period, the test must be started again.
40. The test is for a specific period.

UNIT 4: FOUNDATIONS OF MEDICAL SURGICAL NURSING

1. C
2. A
3. B
4. C
5. C
6. Basic unit of structure and function in biologic systems.
7. Two important activities are (1) the capacity to select which molecules are to be transported into the cell and (2) the ability to transport substances into and out of the cell.
8. Contains DNA and transcription products produced here provide the means for controlling all metabolic and physiologic activities of the cell.
9. Provides large quantities of energy (ATP).
10. Production of lipids for organelles and transmembrane proteins.

11. Prepares proteins and lipids for storage, excretion, or incorporation into the membrane.

12. Contain the digestive proteins that break down lipids, proteins, certain carbohydrates, and nucleic acids into smaller molecules so that they can be oxidized by the mitochondria.

13. Microfilaments provide a framework for the cytoskeleton. Microtubules function to attach to spindles and centrioles to assist in movement and separation of chromosomes during mitosis and incorporation into eukaryotic cilia and flagella.

14. See Figure 14–1 in textbook.

15. D

16. E

17. B

18. I

19. C

20. A

21. J

22. F

23. G

24. H

25. T

26. F   The cells are nonreplicating and any loss is permanent.

27. T

28. T

29. T

30. T

31. T

32. 1) Changes in gene structure and function; 2) degeneration of normal tissue or infiltration by foreign substances; and 3) disorganization of cell growth, including malignant growth, atrophy, and hypertrophy.

33. *Atrophy* is the decrease in the size of an organ tissue because of a decrease in cell size or number, and *hypertrophy* is an increase in the size of an organ or tissue cells because of an increase in the cell size. Precancerous changes are characterized by cell changes of dysplasia (deranged cellular growth occurring with permanent injury or irritation), hyperplasia (an increase in the number of cells in response to hormone secretion), and metaplasia (transformation of one mature cell type to another). Neoplastic growth is characterized by disturbances in cell differentiation and growth.

34. B   Spinal nerve cells do not reproduce, and therefore the injury is permanent.

35. C   Bone-marrow–forming cells are replaced at a high constant rate.

36. D   Endotoxins from gram-negative bacteria are released when the bacterium dies and act directly on macrophages and T lymphocytes stimulating the release of interleukin-1 (IL-1) and tumor necrosis factor (TNF).

CHAPTER 12: CLIENTS WITH FLUID IMBALANCES: PROMOTING POSITIVE OUTCOMES

1. Two-thirds of body water; water inside the cells

2. One-third of body water; water outside the cells

3. Extracellular fluid outside the vascular space and surrounding the cells

4. Fluid in intravascular spaces

5. Total number of dissolved particles (solute) per liter of solvent

6. Pressure created by blood volume inside the vessels

7. Pressure created by protein inside vessels, creating a "pulling force" as water is pulled toward higher oncotic pressure

8. Hydrostatic pressure minus oncotic pressure

9. Two-thirds (66%) is intracellular, interstitial 28%, intravascular approximately 15%

10. An adult needs about 2600 ml of fluid per day (1200 ml as water in beverages, 1100 ml as water in solid foods, and 300 ml as water produced during metabolic processes).

11. They shrink because "water goes where salt is."

12. Confusion, convulsions, coma, irreversible brain damage

13. To prevent hyponatremia. If the client is weighed at the same time of day on the same scale wearing the same clothing, then a change in weight reflects a change in fluid status. One liter of fluid = 1 kg (2.2 lbs) of body weight.

14. Postural systolic blood pressure decrease of more than 25 mm Hg and diastolic decrease of more than 20 mm Hg with pulse pressure of 30 or more

15. A hypertonic fluid causes a sudden acute increase in intravascular volume resulting in pulmonary edema and pleural effusion if the patient is not able to handle the increased intravascular volume. Normal saline must be given very slowly—while constantly observing the patient—if it is used at all.

16. It depends on the cause of deficit; for example, blood loss requires packed red blood cells, or if less than 1 liter is needed, lactated Ringer's solution may be given.

17. Low; ADH signals the kidneys to retain water and since the intravascular volume is increased, aldosterone levels are not increased. Aldosterone would have signaled the kidneys to retain sodium.

CHAPTER 13: CLIENTS WITH ELECTROLYTE IMBALANCES: PROMOTING POSITIVE OUTCOMES

1. Substances in body fluid that dissociate into ions
2. Electrically charged particles formed by electrolytes that dissociate
3. Ion with a positive charge
4. Ion with a negative charge
5. Electrolyte measurement
6. A Because water goes where salt is, water shifts into the intracellular compartment and brain cells swell. (With hyponatremia, extracellular sodium levels are below normal.) The brain can adjust to gradual or moderate changes in serum sodium levels, but not too rapid or severe changes. Because Mr. W. is elderly and large amounts of irrigating fluid had been used during his surgery, he was at increased risk for severe hyponatremia.
7. C Mr. W. may also be weak due to cerebral edema and as intracranial pressure rises, he will have increased neuroexcitability with muscle twitching or tremors deteriorating to delirium, convulsions, and coma.
8. B NS has 0.9% NaCl, 1/2 NS has 0.45% NaCl, $D_5$1/2 NS has 5% dextrose and 0.45% NaCl in water.
9. C Normal saline (0.9% NaCl) is an isotonic fluid which can be given more rapidly than hypotonic or hypertonic fluid, but it is also a replacement rather than a maintenance fluid. It should not be given in large quantities unless sodium and chloride need to be replaced.
10. D As an IV fluid with a high concentration of sodium (such as 3%) is given, it must be given very slowly because it is very hypertonic and will pull fluid into the intravascular compartment with resulting hypervolemia. This could lead to acute pulmonary edema. Mr. W. needs to be monitored for hypernatremia also, but the usual first complication is hypervolemia unless he is dehydrated.

CHAPTER 14: ACID-BASE BALANCE

1. B
2. C Rationale: CO_2 is retained as one holds one's breath. This results in respiratory acidosis for a short period of time. The increased CO_2 will stimulate the respiratory center in the medulla to increase depth and rate of respirations.
3. D
4. A
5. A
6. B Rationale: When hydrochloric acid (HCl) is removed from the stomach, there is an excess of bicarbonate, which results in metabolic alkalosis.
7. C
8. D Rationale: The respiratory center in the medulla is stimulated by the salicylates, which results in respiratory alkalosis as the CO_2 is blown off.
9. D
10. B
11. A Rationale: With diabetic ketoacidosis, ketones are produced as the body uses fats and proteins for energy. Since ketones are acids, a metabolic acidosis results.
12.-15. See the Critical Monitoring section in Chapter 14 of the text. For example, hypocalcemia occurs in alkalosis because calcium does not ionize well in an alkaline environment. The hypocalcemia causes hyperexcitability and increased neuromuscular activity as seen in hyperactive reflexes, tingling around the mouth and in the fingers, positive Trousseau's sign, etc.
16. Normal blood gas values
17. Metabolic acidosis
18. Compensated metabolic acidosis
19. Respiratory alkalosis
20. Mixed respiratory acidosis and metabolic alkalosis with hypoxemia

CHAPTER 15: CLIENTS HAVING SURGERY: PROMOTING POSITIVE OUTCOMES

1. H
2. F
3. J
4. I
5. K
6. D
7. E
8. C
9. L
10. G
11. A
12. B
13. D
14. C
15. A
16. B
17. E
18. D
19. C

20. F

21. E

22. H

23. B

24. G

25. A

26. Assessing nutritional status is important as a compromised nutritional state will increase the risk for intraoperative and postoperative complications. One example is delayed wound healing.

27. Data on smoking is important as the smoker has decreased hemoglobin levels, and therefore there is less oxygen for tissue repair. There is also increased susceptibility to thrombus formation due to hypercoagulability and smokers are more likely to have lung disease.

28. Weight data can indicate obesity which increases the risk of hypertension, congestive heart failure, and metabolic problems such as diabetes mellitus; adipose tissue makes the surgery more difficult and increases the risk of postoperative infections, incisional hernias, wound dehiscence, and evisceration. Obese clients also exhibit problems associated with immobility.

29. The very young and older adults have the lowest tolerance to the stressful effects of surgery.

Case Study

30. Notify the anesthesiologist or nurse anesthetist.

31. Respiratory acidosis.

32. Slow, shallow respirations and retention of CO_2 due to effects of anesthesia

33. Reverse the effects of anesthesia

34. Coma, deepening respiratory acidosis

35.

  __6__   Urine output and color

  __7__   Bile output from T-tube

  __3__   Pulse rate and rhythm, blood pressure, and temperature

  __5__   Dressing intactness and drainage

  __4__   Level of consciousness

  __2__   Respiration rate, depth, and skin color

  __1__   Position of person for alignment, safety, and comfort

36. Patent airway is always the first priority; assessment of breathing is the second priority.

37.

  __1 x__   Check Foley patency.

  __5 x__   Notify the physician.

  _____   Wait 4 hours to see what the urine output is before calling the physician.

  __4 x__   Check mucous membranes and skin turgor.

  __3 x__   Check IV rate, patency, and total intake.

  _____   Give Ms. W. an injection of pain medication.

  __2 x__   Take vital signs.

38. A   There would be protein, vitamin C, and carbohydrates included in this diet.

39. D   Alcohol can change a person's reaction to anesthesia; he/she may require more or less anesthesia and clearance may be impaired if there is liver disease.

40. C   Legally the nurse does not give full disclosures about the surgery or give the alternatives to the surgery; that is the responsibility of the surgeon.

41. B   Demerol is given for sedation and pain relief and Robinul is given to dry up secretions.

42. B   Excessive postoperative blood loss would be assessed by pulse, blood pressure, and respiratory rate.

CHAPTER 16: CLIENTS WITH WOUNDS: PROMOTING POSITIVE OUTCOMES

1. U

2. E

3. S

4. T

5. I

6. V

7. J

8. L

9. F

10. H

11. D

12. K

13. R

14. N

15. G

16. Q

17. P

18. B

19. C

20. A

21. M

22. W

23. O

24. T

25. T

26. T

27. T

28. F   Neutrophils increase in acute inflammation, while lymphocytes and tissue macrophages are the major phagocytes in chronic inflammation.
29. T
30. T
31. T
32. T
33. B
34. A
35. D
36. C
37. Poor nutrition, chronic disease, diabetes mellitus, obesity, anorexia, impaired blood flow, steroid therapy, older age, impaired immunity, smoking
38.

I.   Vascular Response Phase
  A.   Blood vessels
    1.   Constrict to decrease blood flow
    2.   Constrict to decrease exposure to bacteria
  B.   Clotting process begins
    1.   Platelets aggregate to form clot
    2.   Plasma protein systems begin to form fibrin network
    3.   Platelets contract to fibrin network and adhere to form plug
    4.   Platelets release chemicals (e.g., ADP)
      a.   Promote clotting
      b.   Attract other platelets
  C.   Capillaries dilate
    1.   Allows ingress of plasma that dilutes toxins, brings nutrients, and carries phagocytes to the area
    2.   Blood flow slows and extra blood and oxygen brought to area
II. Inflammation Phase
  A.   General
    1.   May last 4-6 days
    2.   Sets up conditions to promote tissue repair
    3.   Response is immediate
  B.   Role of WBCs
    1.   Neutrophils
      a.   First to arrive and most numerous
      b.   Arrive at injury within 4-6 hours
      c.   Role is to phagocytose agents
      d.   Attracted by chemotaxis
      e.   Compose 60% of WBCs

    2.   Monocytes
      a.   Next phagocyte to arrive on scene
      b.   Stimulated by neutrophils and lymphokines
      c.   Arrive about 4 days following injury
      d.   Enter cells and become macrophages
    3.   Macrophages
      a.   Phagocytose large numbers of bacteria
      b.   Have greater role in chronic inflammation
      c.   Secretes angiogenesis factor (AGF)
        (1)   Stimulates formation of new blood vessels at the ends of vessels
        (2)   Stimulates fibroblasts to spew forth collagen
      d.   Secretes cytokines (platelet-derived growth factor, transforming growth factor, interleukin-1, and basic fibroblast factor)
    4.   Lymphocytes
      a.   Formed in lymphoid tissue
      b.   Lymphokines are sensitized lymphocytes
      c.   Controlled by adrenocortical hormones
    5.   Eosinophils
      a.   Secrete antihistamines
      b.   Help control inflammatory response
    6.   Basophils
      a.   Secrete histamines
  C.   Mediators of inflammation phase
    1.   Mast cells
      a.   Filled with histamine and neutrophil chemotactic factors
        (1)   Cause capillary dilation
      b.   Synthesize leukotrienes and prostaglandins
        (1)   Cause same response as histamine, but it lasts longer
        (2)   Prostaglandins cause pain
        (3)   Increase vascular permeability

(4)   Enhance action of neutrophils

2.   Free radicals

a.   Single oxygen atom derived from molecular oxygen and having an unpaired electron

b.   If it attaches to lipids, it enters the cell and organelles and causes damage

c.   If it attaches to hydrogen, hydrogen peroxide is produced, which is toxic to cells

d.   If it attaches to vitamin C, it is stabilized

e.   Mediators of both acute and chronic inflammation

3.   The complement system

a.   Composed of a group of plasma proteins

b.   Promotes inflammation

c.   Promotes movement of leuko-cytes into the area (process of chemotaxis)

d.   Coats microbes to make them vulnerable to phagocytosis

4.   Kinins

a.   Plasma protein

b.   Increase vascular permeability and allow leukocytes to enter tissue

c.   Later in inflammatory process act with prostaglandins to cause pain and smooth muscle contraction

d.   Primary kinin is bradykinin

III.   Proliferative (or Resolution) Phase

A.   Mediators of the proliferative phase

1.   Cytokines

a.   Regulate mobility, differentia-tion, and growth of leukocytes

b.   Best known cytokines are interleukins and interferons

c.   Interleukins account for clinical manifestations of both acute and chronic inflammation, such as fever, anorexia, cachexia, and movements of leukocytes to site of injury

d.   Interferons promote B cell maturation and moderate suppressor T-cell function

2.   Growth factors

a.   Catalysts of wound healing

b.   Released by platelets and macrophages

c.   Prime cells to enter growth phase

d.   Move a cell from growth phase to DNA production phase

e.   Major growth factors

(1)   Platelet-derived growth factor (PDGF)

(a)   Regulates synthesis of fibronectin and fibroblasts in the matrix of the wound-healing bed

(2)   Epidermal growth factor (EGF)

(a)   Stimulates fibroblasts and endothelial cells

(3)   Fibroblast growth factor

(a)   Stimulates collagen synthesis and angiogenesis

(4)   Transforming growth factor alpha (TGF-a)

(a)   Stimulates epithelial cells and macroph-ages

(b)   Controls cell growth and synthesis of matrix component

(5)   Transforming growth factor beta (TGF-b)

(a)   Increases synthesis of matrix perfor-mance

(6)   Colony-stimulating factors

(a)   Secreted by bone marrow, monocytes, fibroblasts, and keratinocytes

(b)   Major function appears to be enhancing the function of WBCs

B.   Overlapping processes of proliferative phase

1.   Collagenation

a.   Fibroblasts synthesize and secrete collagen, elastin, and proteoglycans

b.   Reconstructs connective tissue

c.   Adds strength to wound

2.   Angiogenesis
    a.   Development of new blood vessels
    b.   Begins within hours of injury
    c.   Endothelial cells emerge at ends of new blood vessels
3.   Granulation
    a.   Matrix of collagen, capillaries, and cells begins to fill the wound space forming a scar
    b.   Tissue grows from the wound edges and base of wound
    c.   Tissue is filled with new capillary buds, with a red, bumpy, or granular appearance
    d.   Surrounded by fibroblasts and macrophages
    e.   As granulation tissue forms, the epithelialization begins
4.   Wound contraction
    a.   Mechanism by which edges of wound are drawn together
    b.   Due to the action of myofibroblasts
        (1)   Form a bridge across wound and contract to pull wound closed
5.   Contracture
    a.   Process of contraction in large wounds that can produce deformities
6.   Epithelialization
    a.   Migration of epithelial cells from surrounding skin
    b.   Epithelial migration is limited to about 3 cm
    c.   Can be hastened if wound is kept moist
    d.   Scar in this stage is bright red, thick, and blanches with pressure
7.   The "walling-off" effect
    a.   Occurs in damaged area to prevent the spread of injurious agents to other body tissues

IV.   Maturation Phase
    A.   Remodeling of scar
        1.   Occurs for a year or more after the wound is closed
        2.   Capillaries disappear
        3.   Scar tissue regains about two-thirds of its original strength

4.   Process of collagen synthesis and lysis
5.   As scar matures, it becomes thin and white

39.   As gauze dries, debris, necrotic tissue, exudate, and drainage adhere to it therefore wound healing is optimized in a moist environment
40.   Retains moisture, semipermeable, water resistant, and facilitates autolytic debridement
41.   Provides autolytic debridement of ulcers, retains moisture, semipermeable, water resistant, reduces pain
42.   Have cooling effect, retains moisture, permits autolytic debridement
43.   Retains moisture, absorbent, promotes autolytic debridement
44.   Retains moisture, absorbent, left intact for several days
45.   Keep wound free from pressure and pulling, keep clean but do not wash with water, cover wound with appropriate size sterile dressing, return for suture removal in 7-10 days. Call physician for indications of wound infection: fever over 101° F; redness all around wound, not just along wound edges; purulent drainage; pain; wound edges opening; and malaise
46.   Sterile normal saline is used because it is isomolar and it keeps the wound bed moist.
47.   An all-gauze dressing is needed for wet-to-dry treatment.
48.   A wet-to-dry dressing is used to provide mechanical debridement of the wound. As the dressing dries, debris, necrotic tissue, exudate, and drainage will adhere to it.
49.   Assessment data need to include wound size, color, presence of granulation or epithelial tissue, presence of any sinus tracts, edema, odor, drainage (color and odor, consistency, and approximate amount), pain, and condition of skin around the wound.
50.   Important nutrients include protein; calories; fats; vitamins A, B complex, C, and E; zinc; and iron.
51.   C   Decadron has an anti-inflammatory action that decreases wound strength, inhibits contraction, and impedes epithelialization. Poor nutritional status can result in decreased synthesis of collagen and leukocytes, lack of protein for repair, decreased immune response, and slowed coagulation.
52.   D   The expected finding with a wound infection would be an increase in neutrophils.
53.   A   The purpose of wet-to-dry dressings is to remove the necrotic eschar from the wound.
54.   A   In inflammation, the redness is confined to the wound edges; in infection, the redness is extended around the entire wound.

55.   B   Circumference of the wound is the priority assessment for compartmental syndrome as it will track edema from the inflammatory repines that could restrict vessels and entrap nerves.

CHAPTER 17: PERSPECTIVES ON INFECTIOUS DISORDERS

1.   (1) Infectious agent that is capable of causing disease by growing and multiplying within the host, evading host defenses, penetrating and spreading through host tissues, and producing toxins; (2) source or reservoir of the infectious agent that may be endogenous (originating from the host, such as microbes that colonize the skin) or exogenous (external to the host, such as stagnant water); (3) host susceptibility due to damaged or destroyed defense mechanisms; (4) modes of transmission to host that include contact, airborne, common vehicles (contaminated food), and vectors (insects or animals); (5) portal of entry to host and portal of exit from host.

2.   Sterile technique for catheter insertion and aseptic technique for emptying the urinary drainage bag.

3.   Use aseptic technique and change the dressing at regularly scheduled intervals.

4.   *Escherichia coli* is normal flora in the colon but can cause urinary tract infections if transferred to the urinary tract. Teach females to cleanse perineum from front to back.

5.   Pathologic organisms primarily spread from person to person via the hands. Wash your hands before and after donning gloves. Wet hands, use soap, vigorously rub hands for 15 seconds, rinse, and then dry with a disposable paper towel.

6.   Check the protocol and policy at your institution.

7.   Colonization must occur before infection. *Methicillin-resistant* means the presence of pathogens resistant to all penicillins (including methicillin) and cephalosporins.

8.   Complete series of three doses within six months.

9.   Documented immunity or two doses of vaccine.

10.   Once a year because the virus is different each year.

11.   Easy access to supplies; minimizes contaminating objects in the bag.

12.   To avoid contaminating the nursing bag and exposing other clients.

13.   These are highly transmittable. Taking into the home only the supplies needed for the visit minimizes the possibility of cross-contamination.

14.   One cup full-strength bleach added to regular wash kills infectious organisms.

15.   Same principle of bagging and double-bagging used in acute-care settings. Prevents cross-contamination.

CHAPTER 18: PERSPECTIVES IN ONCOLOGY

1.   Synonymous with the term *malignant neoplasm*—used for describing a large group of diseases characterized by uncontrolled growth and spread of abnormal cells

2.   A harmful tumor capable of spreading and invading other tissues far removed from the site of origin

3.   An abnormal new growth or formation of tissue that serves no useful purpose and may harm the host organism. It can be either benign or malignant.

4.   Harmless growth that does not spread or invade other tissue

5.   Number of new cases occurring in a given population at risk during a specified time

6.   Process of genetically identical cells assuming various structures and functions so that one muscle cell looks like another muscle cell but not like a kidney or liver cell

7.   Normal cells grown on a culture medium spread freely until they contact another cell. Then they adhere to one another and align themselves in parallel.

8.   The ability of neoplastic cells to spread from the original site of the tumor to distant organs

9.   Substances that, when introduced into the cell, cause changes in the structure and function of the cell that lead to cancer

10.   Test used to detect cancer of the cervix, digestive, respiratory, and renal tracts

11.   Tumor staging defines the extent of the tumor. It involves characteristics of the primary tumor, involvement of lymph nodes, and evidence of metastasis.

12.   Tumor grading evaluates the extent to which tumor cells differ from their normal precursors. High grades (III or IV) indicate that the cells are poorly differentiated and the most aberrant compared to normal cells.

13.   Oncogens are small segments of genetic DNA that can transform normal cells into malignant cells—independently or incorporated into a virus.

14.
A.   B
B.   M
C.   B
D.   M
E.   B

F. B

G. M

H. M

I. B

J. B

K. M

L. B

M. B

N. M

O. B

P. M

Q. B

R. B

S. M

T. M

U. M

15. E

16. C

17. C

18. F

19. C

20. F

21. C

22. B

23. C

24. C

25. C

26. A

27. Normal cells are a mixture of stem cells (precursors) and well-differentiated cells.

28. Normal cells exhibit contact inhibition.

29. Normal cells cannot grow in presence of necrosis.

30. Normal cells do not invade adjacent tissue.

31. Normal cells have a specific, designated purpose.

32. Normal cells proliferate in response to specific stimuli.

33. Normal cells have a constant or predictable growth rate.

34. Normal cells have a cell birth rate that equals or is less than the cell death rate.

CHAPTER 19: CLIENTS WITH CANCER: PROMOTING POSITIVE OUTCOMES

1. F

2. J

3. D

4. A

5. G

6. C

7. I

8. L

9. K

10. E

11. B

12. H

13. B

14. C

15. A

16. E

17. C

18. D

19. F

20. G

21. A

22. B

23. Explain to Ms. J. that the hair loss is temporary. Based on the type of cancer she has, discuss the possibility of scalp hypothermia. Discuss the use of scarves, wigs, or turbans. Discuss the disadvantages of frequent, vigorous hair washing and brushing during the time the hair is falling out.

     Rationale: Meet basic information needs of the client; prepare her for the side effects and the ways to manage this sometimes devastating side effect; frequent shampooing and brushing will increase the rate of hair loss.

24. Recall treatments from your fundamentals course; that is, use mild soaps; bathe with Aveeno in the water; report problem to physician for order to obtain an antihistamine such as Benadryl; use moisturizing lotion or emollient cream; drink 3000 cc fluid unless contraindicated; and trim nails.

     Rationale: Many soaps will dry the skin; fluids will help moisturize; antihistamines will provide some relief from the pruritus.

25. Depending on the severity of the neutropenia, Mr. B. needs to avoid raw or uncooked foods; avoid crowds; avoid contact with animal excrement; report an elevated temperature, cough, sore throat, chills, sweating, or frequent or painful urination; maintain personal hygiene, especially good handwashing; get adequate rest and exercise; and avoid indiscriminate use of antipyretics.

     Rationale: These measures are focused on reducing exposure to infection, recognizing the signs of infection, preventing infection, and avoiding the use of antipyretics which might mask the signs of infection. Extra precautions should be taken as the prednisone may mask signs of infection.

26. Begin an oral hygiene program before therapy starts and continue during the therapy; arrange for a dental examination before therapy begins; teach thorough and gentle cleansing of the teeth and gums, moisturizing if mucus is scanty or absent; teach avoidance of alcohol and smoking; assess the oral cavity daily and teach the client to do this; modify diet to avoid extremely hot or cold foods, spicy foods, or citrus fruit and juices.

    Rationale: The oral hygiene program will help ameliorate the effects of the chemotherapy; the dental exam will prepare the oral cavity for the chemotherapy; other interventions are focused on decreasing trauma to oral cavity tissues that can be easily damaged.

27. The nurse should call the radiation therapy institute or have Mr. C. call, because often the recommendation is that no lotion is used.

    Rationale: The metals in some lotions may affect the radiation.

28. Tiredness is common among clients receiving radiation therapy. Ironically, one of the recommendations is moderate exercise, as well as periods of rest, and carefully planning activities by identifying priorities.

    Rationale: Pacing of activities will conserve energy for the most important activities. Moderate exercise will help prevent further fatigue from disuse.

29. With chemotherapy known for causing nausea and vomiting, clients are often premedicated 6-12 hours prior to the administration and then every 4-6 hours afterwards for at least 12-24 hours. Nonpharmacologic interventions may include adjusting oral and fluid intake, relaxation, exercise, hypnosis, biofeedback, guided imagery, and systemic desensitization.

    Rationale: Prevention and control are more effective than treatment after the nausea and vomiting have started. The nonpharmacologic interventions address the anticipatory/emotional aspects of the nausea and vomiting.

30. Active listening and maintaining a noncritical relationship with the client allows for the expression of negative feelings; referrals for counseling may be appropriate. Information needs are high and are usually best facilitated by consistent, accurate information in as much detail as the client requests.

    Rationale: Active listening and openness will encourage a trusting relationship and allow for expression of negative feelings without fear of criticism; in time of high anxiety, teaching that focuses on the basics and is repetitive often is

absorbed best; listening to the client will help the nurse recognize the depth of information that the client is seeking.

31. Assessment factors would include checking for bleeding gums, bruising, petechiae, hypermenorrhea, tarry stools, occult blood, blood in the urine, "coffee-ground" emesis, headaches, blurred visions or visual changes, hemoptysis, or nosebleeds.

    Rationale: Ms. J. is at risk for bleeding. As the platelet count falls, CNS hemorrhage or massive GI bleeding may occur.

32. B   For a 33-year-old female, the American Cancer Society's guidelines for Pap smear tests are annually for three years; then, if negative, the frequency will be recommended by the physician.

33. B   Class IV Pap smear report indicates that the cells examined may be cancerous.

34. C   The biopsy will involve the physician removing a piece of tissue for examination.

35. B   Multiple sex partners, chronic cervicitis, and history of HPV are all risk factors for cervical cancer.

36. F   Annual chest x-ray is no longer recommended.

37. F   Mammography is recommended annually for women over 50.

38. T

39. F   Sexually active women should have a Pap test regardless of age. Pap tests should be performed yearly until there are three negative examinations in a row; at this point, they can be performed yearly or as the physician advises.

40. F   Stool guaiac should be performed annually for people over age 50.

41. T

42. F   BSE should be performed monthly.

43. T

44. A   During the diagnostic and treatment phases of the cancer continuum, one of the main nursing interventions involves giving the client and family information about tests and treatments. Because of the anxiety levels at this point, simple explanations are usually better understood and retained.

45. B   This response indicates that the family and possibly the client need further explanations about external beam radiation; that is, that once the source (the machine) is removed, there is no radiation present with the client.

46. D   Chemotherapy agents and their metabolites are found in the body fluids of clients undergoing chemotherapy; therefore, it is recommended to take

precautions when handling blood or body fluids for 48 hours after chemotherapy.

47. B   Until symptoms develop, the principal action of the nurse is to assess for signs and symptoms.

48. D   Bone pain is the primary side effect in people taking G-CMF.

Chapter 20: Clients with Psychosocial and Mental Health Concerns: Promoting Positive Outcomes

1. Anxiety, stress, coping mechanisms, and self-esteem

2. About 10 minutes

3. The high level of cortisol triggers the hypothalamus and pituitary to cease production of corticotropin-releasing hormone (CRH) and adrenocorticotrophic hormone (ACTH) to end the stress response.

4. Answer questions honestly and maintain a calm, unhurried approach

5. With a flat affect, the client has no expression of feelings, regardless of the variation in topics. With an inappropriate affect, the client has nonverbal signs of feelings that do not match the verbal response.

6. Incongruent communication (when the words and nonverbal behavior do not match) often is the first clue that a client has a psychiatric disorder.

7. The nonverbal behavior

8. Definition of illness, medications and treatment options, and relapse prevention

9. A, D, E

10. B

11. C, G

12. G

13. D, E

14. F

15. B, C, D

16. Because typical antipsychotics target all dopamine receptors, including those affecting movement, muscle side effects known as extrapyramidal symptoms are common.

17. Anticholinergic agents such as benztropine or trihexyphenidyl

18. Neuroleptic malignant syndrome (NMS) is a rare but serious condition that may appear suddenly in a client taking antipsychotics. Symptoms include extreme muscle rigidity, high fever, sweating, and fluctuations in consciousness. The client requires emergency hospitalization with supportive treatment to prevent seizures, coma, or even death.

19. Hopelessness, substance abuse, male gender, living alone, previous attempted suicide

20. Once comfort measures have been provided to your client's wife, a thorough assessment of the family situation would be essential. Some areas to explore include family structure, support systems, financial concerns, and level of family functioning.

21. A nursing diagnosis of Altered family processes should be used for a normally healthy family currently challenged by stress. Data related to verbal outbursts, interference with treatments, absence of family interactions, inappropriate communications, and verbalizations of fear, anxiety, or anger would support this diagnosis.

22. One approach would be to use the therapeutic family communication four-stage process.

    (1) *Engagement*: encourage your client and wife to express their concerns. Remember that your role is neutral and that you need to avoid confrontation and power struggles.

    (2) *Assessment*: as the nurse you would further explore the concerns with your client and his wife to identify specific problems.

    (3) *Intervention*: working with your client and his wife in this stage involves teaching and role-modeling communication techniques and problem-solving strategies.

    (4) *Termination*: the nurse–client relationship is ending in this stage. Your client and his wife need to be encouraged to continue their new communication patterns.

23. A key to applying the nursing process would be to complete a cultural assessment which will provide the data to guide your nursing process interventions. You will likely need the assistance of a family member who speaks English or the services of a hospital interpreter.

24. Nursing interventions could include creating a climate that minimizes guilt and anxiety, education/information, anticipatory guidance, listening, referral for complex situations, and encouraging discussion of fears and concerns.

25. D   An open, nonjudgmental response will give the client the opportunity to explore and express his concerns.

26. B   To assess a client for spiritual distress, broad questions, initially not specifically directed at religion, will provide data for this diagnosis.

27. B   Spirituality may have aspects of religion, but it is a broader concept.

28. B   Altered family process is used with a family who is normally healthy, but is having difficulty coping with an acute or chronic illness.

29. D   A genogram would be a primary assessment tool for a family assessment, not a cultural assessment.

30. A   Assisting clients with sexuality and sexual issues begins with clarification of the nurse's personal values related to sexuality and personal comfort.

CHAPTER 21: CLIENTS WITH SLEEP AND REST DISORDERS AND FATIGUE: PROMOTING POSITIVE OUTCOMES

1. C
2. G
3. A
4. B
5. D
6. E
7. F
8. When collecting a sleep history, determine the following: usual bedtime, usual rising time, rituals used to enhance sleep quality, frequency and duration of naps, daily caffeine intake, and number of awakenings during the night.
9. Visible signs of fatigue and lack of sleep, such as induration of the eyes, lack of coordination, drowsiness, lack of concentration, and irritability
10. Serotonin, norepinephrine, acetylcholine
11. Stage 1 NREM sleep is very light. Respirations begin to slow and muscles relax.

    Stage 2 NREM sleep is still light sleep. More than 50% of sleep occurs in this stage.

    During sleep stages 3 and 4, respirations become slow and even, and pulse rate and blood pressure fall. Oxygen consumption and urine formation is decreased.

    REM sleep stages have the following characteristics: rapid eye movement, erratic respirations, changes in the heart rate, and very low muscle tone. Dreams in REM sleep are vivid, story-like, emotional, and bizarre.

    In adults, each sleep cycle (stages 1 through 4) lasts about 90 minutes.
12. Dyssomnias are sleep disorders in which there is difficulty initiating or maintaining sleep. The parasomnias are disorders that occur during sleep but usually do not produce insomnia or excessive sleep.
13. The elderly take longer to fall asleep, have increased nocturnal wakefulness, and experience more sleepiness during the day. There is a considerable decrease in stage 4 sleep and stage 1 sleep is increased.

14. Inadequate orientation to hospital routines, noise level, unfamiliar environment, excessive lighting
15. Medical conditions that require immobility and/or isolation, and inadequate orientation to hospital routines
16. Lasix is a loop diuretic that inhibits sodium and chloride from being reabsorbed by the kidneys. The result is increased urination. If taken prior to bedtime, frequent urination could interfere with normal sleep patterns.

Goals and Outcome Criteria	Nursing Interventions
17. The client will have improved sleep patterns within 3 nights as evidenced by: 1. Sleeping 6-8 hours per night 2. Verbalizing less fatigue 3. Verbalizing less irritability	1. Complete a thorough sleep history on admission. 2. Adhere to the client's bedtime rituals as much as possible. 3. Schedule nursing interventions to allow 90-120 minutes of uninterrupted sleep. 4. Modify the environment: dim lights, close doors. 5. Offer back massage and relaxation techniques to promote sleep. 6. Assess the client's sleep patterns each morning.

CHAPTER 22: PERSPECTIVES ON END-OF-LIFE CARE

1. When there is a poor prognosis at diagnosis and the client is either not eligible for treatment or elects no treatment and when the prognosis is less than 6 months
2. Morphine
3. Nonsteroidal anti-inflammatory drugs (NSAIDs), steroids, tricyclic antidepressants, anticonvulsants
4. Heat, massage; relaxation technique
5. Fear of addiction to narcotics, fear of what the pain represents and the unknown, concern and worry regarding the side effects of the medications used to control the pain
6. An around-the-clock schedule maintains a therapeutic level of analgesia to relieve baseline pain; i.e., oral morphine requires dosing every 4 hours.

Even with around-the-clock schedules rescue dosing is needed because breakthrough pain will occur. If a client needs more than two rescue doses during a 12-hour period, then the around-the-clock dose needs increasing.

7. The exact mechanism is not known but morphine may blunt the perceptual response to dyspnea or to reduce the respiratory drive.

8. Oxygen should only be used to relieve dyspnea when the oxygen saturation is less than 90% with room air.

9. Mottling and cyanosis, decrease in urine output, tachycardia and irregular heart beat, significant widening in pulse pressure with a decrease in systolic blood pressure, tachypnea and dyspnea progressing to Cheyne-Stokes breathing, incontinence, cannot subjectively respond to verbal stimuli

10. Provide all comfort measures for the client such as pain medications, mouth care, preventive skin care, and proper positioning; tell the family about the signs of impending death, encourage the family to say good-bye and to give permission to the dying person to let go; and help the family plan for the death event such as having the appropriate people present and making funeral arrangements.

11. Avoidance (shock, denial, disbelief), confrontation (extreme emotions), and re-establishment (gradual decline in emotions)

12. Before death occurs, encourage family to say good-bye, allow family to relive the death events by telling their stories, attend the funeral if possible, provide information about the grief response and refer for counseling if needed.

CHAPTER 23: CLIENTS WITH PAIN: PROMOTING POSITIVE OUTCOMES

1. C
2. F
3. I
4. A
5. D
6. J
7. B
8. G
9. E
10. H
11. I
12. A
13. G
14. E
15. H
16. C
17. B
18. D
19. F

20. The word *complains* tends to minimize the client's experience. The word *reports* is more objective and less judgmental.

21. Pain may actually be the cause of the confusion and does not negate the perception of pain in the older client.

22. The back rub through cutaneous stimulation can relieve pain. Cutaneous stimulation is related to the gate-control theory by activating large- and small-diameter fibers that close the gate to painful stimuli.

23. Your rating should match the client's following the definition of pain: Pain is what the client says it is. Additionally, a person's behavior is not always correlated with the level of pain.

24. Where is the pain? Have the patient point to the area.

   Is the pain inside or on the surface?

   Is the pain always in these areas?

   If the pain is in more that one spot, are the pains equal or does one trigger the other?

   Is the pain on both sides of your body? If so, is it the same on each side?

25. Ask the client to rate pain on a scale of 0-10 with 10 being the worst you can imagine. How would you rate the pain at its worst? How would you rate the pain at its best? How would you rate the pain with activity? Rest? Note nonverbal manifestations of pain.

26. Drug allergies

   Body weight

   Individual pain experience

   Other individual characteristics such as age, general state of health, mental status, probable duration of pain.

   Cardiac, respiratory, renal, and nervous system status

   Previous response to analgesics

27. Response to pain medication. Ask her to re-rate her pain on the 0-10 scale, check vital signs, and assess for side effects of Demerol.

28. See Table 23-7 in Chapter 23 of the textbook for a list of IM medications that would be equianalgesic to Demerol 75 mg.

29. Nonpharmacologic interventions could include a back rub (with client consent), progressive relaxation, imagery, and rhythmic breathing.

30. D   Pain threshold is defined as the lowest perceivable intensity of stimuli that is transmitted as pain.

31. A   The SG is proposed as the anatomic location of the "gate" that could either facilitate or inhibit the transmission of pain signals.

32. C   Chronic pain may be associated with withdrawal and depression. It does not always have a definable cause or produce sympathetic nervous system symptoms such as increased pulse and blood pressure and has the characteristics of slow pain.

33. A   "Real" pain, particularly chronic pain, may not have an identifiable cause.

34. B   Guided imagery helps relieve pain by distraction and muscle relaxation.

CHAPTER 24: CLIENTS WITH SUBSTANCE ABUSE DISORDERS: PROMOTING POSITIVE OUTCOMES

1.   B
2.   B
3.   A
4.   A
5.   A
6.   A
7.   A
8.   B
9.   B
10. B
11. C
12. F
13. E
14. A
15. B
16. H
17. C
18. D
19. G
20. E
21. C
22. D
23. A
24. F
25. B
26. D
27. E
28. F
29. G
30. C

31. B
32. A
33. G
34. H
35. I
36. J
37. K
38. A
39. B
40. C
41. D
42. E
43. F

44. Addiction is a complex process that includes physical, psychological, and social factors. Clients are typically defensive and deny that they are addicted. The first step to recovery is to understand the addiction process.

45. Substance abuse affects every body system. It can either increase or inhibit normal processes.

46. Nutritional deficits may be related to decrease in food intake or the effects of the drug on various body systems.

47. Clients with substance abuse problems lack the responsibility for their personal behavior. Constantly blaming and manipulating others are typical behaviors that affect all family members.

48. Substance abuse affects all areas of a person's life. Understanding addiction and how it affects daily living may help the client understand the problems caused by addiction and motivate him or her to adhere to a treatment program.

49. Family members are strongly affected by drug addiction and are important to the recovery process.

50. Informed decisions and problem solving will increase the chance of success in the recovery process.

51. Substance abuse treatment is a lifelong process. The client and family will need strong support systems that are easily accessible.

52. Substance abuse is a complex combination of physical, psychological, and social variables. Typically, the person has low self-esteem and problems communicating with other people and maintaining healthy relationships.

53. Addiction and recovery affect the roles and responsibilities of all family members. These changes may be positive and easily accepted by the family members or they may have negative effects on the family and be sabotaged by family members.

54. Knowing that the client's confidentiality and right to privacy are protected by law may increase compliance to a treatment program.

55. Levels over .10% are considered proof of intoxication in most states.

56. A person can consume alcohol and be intoxicated without exhibiting noticeable behaviors.

57. Low self-esteem, high frustration level, inability to cope, depression, lack of healthy relationships, and involvement in high-risk behaviors.

58. DTs are a result of severe withdrawal from alcohol; they can occur up to 3 days after ingesting the last drink. Early symptoms occur within 6-8 hours.

59. Stimulant abusers are usually very alert, appear euphoric, exhilarated, hyperactive, overenthusiastic, and extremely talkative. The period of overactivity is followed by depression, lethargy, and fatigue.

60. Long-term health effects are increased risk of respiratory, cardiac, and reproductive problems. Marijuana residues in the lungs are considered more carcinogenic than tobacco residues.

61. Direct effects on the heart include decreased mechanical performance; increased heart rate and cardiac output followed by decreased rate and output increases; the slowing heart rate produces an accumulation of lactic acid in the peripheral vascular system that results in vasodilation and tachycardia. A long-term development is cardiomyopathy that results in congestive heart failure. Vascular hypertension and strokes also have a great incidence. Indirect effects include the heavy workload put on the heart during withdrawal, sinus tachycardia, and hypertension. Prolonged, severe withdrawal can lead to extreme fatigue and sudden death.

62. Alcohol interferes with the delivery of folate to the marrow potentially resulting in ineffective cell production, thrombocytopenia, megaloblastic hematopoiesis, leukopenia, and anemia.

63. Disulfiram (Antabuse) is classified as an anti-alcohol agent. It acts as a deterrent to alcohol by inhibiting the enzyme acetaldehyde dehydrogenase that breaks down alcohol in the body. If the client ingests alcohol while on Antabuse the following symptoms may occur: blurred vision, chest pain, confusion, dizziness or fainting, palpitations, flushing, diaphoresis, nausea, vomiting, headaches, and dyspnea. These symptoms last as long as alcohol is in the body.

64. Rohypnol is a benzodiazepine that is not legal in the United States. It is used in conjunction with other drugs, especially alcohol and heroin, to enhance their effects. Substance abuse practitioners predict it will become the drug of choice for high-school– and college-age youth because of the cost and accessibility. Implications include an increase in emergency room admissions because of the side effects. It is ten times more potent than diazepam (Valium). Rohypnol causes memory loss and blackouts for up to 24 hours. Use of this drug has been linked to rapes and gang rapes.

65. The issue of the chemically impaired coworker is especially important for health care workers because of the possible harm to clients. There are no easy solutions. The two major concerns are client safety and the health and safety of the chemically impaired nurse. If a coworker is chemically impaired there is an ethical and legal obligation to inform the nurse manager.

66. B   When Mr. H. had his last drink is the most important information to obtain. With his drinking history, he is at risk for withdrawal and it will be important to know when to anticipate problems.

67. B   Chlordiazepoxide (Librium) is given to decrease the withdrawal symptoms and prevent DTs from occurring.

68. A   Impaired liver metabolism can result in anesthetic agents not being metabolized efficiently, which may result in accumulation in the blood and prolonged sedation. During surgery the client may be more prone to cardiac and respiratory depression, depleted catecholamines, and hemorrhage. Withdrawal from the substance may also occur but be delayed postoperatively, and pain medication dosages may be affected.

69. D   Poor general nutrition (i.e., nutritional deficits) alters metabolic activity of the nervous system. Polyneuropathies and Wernicke-Korsakoff syndrome are directly related to thiamin deficiencies.

70. C   An exact diagnosis of Mr. H.'s problem is inappropriate; however, referral to a community agency for follow-up is appropriate, as his alcohol use falls outside the definition of social use.

UNIT 5: MOBILITY DISORDERS

1. Abduction of shoulder
2. Extension of fingers
3. External rotation of hip
4. Abduction of hip
5. Adduction of shoulder
6. Flexion of fingers
7. Internal rotation of hip
8. Adduction of hip
9. Pronation of forearm

10. Supination of forearm
11. Extension of shoulder
12. Extension of elbow
13. Extension of wrist
14. Extension of hip
15. Extension of knee
16. Extension of ankle
17. Flexion of wrist
18. Flexion of elbow
19. Flexion of shoulder
20. Flexion of knee
21. Flexion of ankle
22. Flexion of hip
23. Ulnar deviation of hand
24. Radial deviation of hand
25. Eversion of foot
26. Inversion of foot

CHAPTER 25: ASSESSMENT OF THE MUSCULOSKELETAL SYSTEM

1. Throbbing
2. Poorly localized
3. Yes
4. Increase
5. Places stress on musculoskeletal system
6. Kyphosis, "humpback"; scoliosis, obvious lateral deformity; lordosis, "swayback"
7. Active range of motion
8. 0 to 5, 0 = paralysis, 1 = muscle contraction with no movement, 2 = full ROM with support, 3 = full ROM with no resistance, 4 = full ROM with moderate resistance, 5 = full ROM with normal resistance
9. Grating sound or feeling occurring with joint injury or degeneration
10. X-ray views of tissue at various planes—as though slices had been made of the tissue
11. About one hour
12. About 30 minutes
13. Endoscopic exam of various joints without the need for a large incision
14. In clients whose joint flexion is less than 50%, and in clients who have a skin or wound infection at the site where the arthroscopy would be performed
15. Walking is okay when sensation returns, but avoid excessive exercise for a few days
16. Using dual-energy x-ray absorptiometry to measure bone density
17. "Tennis elbow" or lateral epicondylitis

18. Decreased
19. C
20. D
21. B
22. E
23. A
24. D
25. B
26. C
27. A
28. E

CHAPTER 26: MANAGEMENT OF CLIENTS WITH MUSCULOSKELETAL DISORDERS

1. Primary osteoporosis occurs among the elderly and has no predisposing secondary condition, such as hyperparathyroidism or long-term steroid therapy.
2. Handrails in the bathroom, removal of scatter rugs, increased lighting
3. Regular weight-bearing exercise, such as walking, preferably 2 miles per day
4. A machine will pass over your wrist to measure your bone density. You will be exposed to minimal radiation for a short period of time. Bone loss of as little as 1-3% can be detected. There is no preparation required for the test.
5. Milk, cheese, broccoli, fish (See Box 26-1 in the textbook.)
6. 1000 to 1500 mg/day before meals
7. Cardiopulmonary complications
8. Acute osteomyelitis responds to a 4- to 6-week course of IV antibiotics whereas chronic osteomyelitis does not and instead requires surgical intervention.
9. Fever usually over 101° F (38° C); localized pain or tenderness, heat, and swelling around the affected bone
10. Sequestrectomy—surgical removal of dead bone. Saucerization—removal of scar or infected tissue, sequestra, and/or necrotic bone leaving a saucer-like depression
11. Breast, prostate, kidney, thyroid, and lung
12. Well-defined borders, slow growth, rare metastasis
13. Osteogenic osteosarcoma
14. Ewing's sarcoma, chondrosarcoma, fibrosarcoma
15. To reduce the tumor size and treat small metastases
16. Tingling or shocklike pain elicited by light percussion over the median nerve at the wrist
17. Ganglion that consists of a round, cystlike lesion overlying or adjacent to the wrist joint or tendon

18. Bone resection of first metatarsal, removing bony overgrowth and bursae
19. Use of pads to cushion the foot from the shoe, removal of corns, and passive stretching exercises
20. Severe burning sensation usually occurring in the web space between the third and fourth toes. The symptoms usually occur with the pressure of walking.

CHAPTER 27: MANAGEMENT OF CLIENTS WITH MUSCULOSKELETAL TRAUMA OR OVERUSE

1. J
2. N
3. U
4. S
5. T
6. R
7. V
8. M
9. G
10. A
11. K
12. O
13. F
14. E
15. D
16. A
17. B
18. H
19. G
20. P
21. L
22. I
23. Elevation facilitates drainage thus decreasing swelling and improving circulation. The improved circulation further facilitates drainage. Elevate the extremity above heart level.
24. A closed fracture could be a comminuted fracture—anything but simple.
25. To avoid acute hip flexion, adduction, and external rotation of the hip, which could happen otherwise; for example, if the client were to sit with legs crossed
26. To prevent thrombophlebitis
27. Infection following a fracture may be from contamination of an open fracture or may be introduced during surgery. Osteomyelitis is a serious bone infection.
28. To promote healing and correct any postinjury or postoperative anemia

29. To compare with the client's normal status in the noninjured extremity

UNIT 6: NUTRITIONAL DISORDERS

1. The LES is not a distinctive sphincter but a zone of increased pressure that provides a physiologic barrier to protect the esophageal mucus from the effects of gastric reflux. It is located at the distal end of the esophagus.
2. Villi are finger-like projections in the small intestine that stir intestinal contents; digested food is absorbed from the villi.
3. Upper part of the stomach
4. Located at the distal end of the stomach, the pyloric sphincter permits flow of chyme from the stomach into the duodenum.
5. Liquefied food in the stomach
6. Produced by the parietal cells of the stomach; necessary for vitamin B_{12} to be absorbed
7. A valve between the end of the ileum and the large intestine that controls flow into the large intestine and prevents reflux into the small intestine
8. GALT: Immune system of the GI tract. Produce up to 80% of the body's immunoglobulin.
9. A
10. A, C
11. D, E
12. A
13. A, D
14. C
15. D
16. E
17. A
18. C
19. F   It means difficulty swallowing.
20. F   It contains the enzyme ptyalin (amylase).
21. T   HCL secretion causes the stomach to be acidic.
22. F   The sympathetic nerves inhibit gastric secretion and motility.
23. F   The small intestine is 22 feet long; the ileum is 12 feet long.
24. T
25. F   The functions of the large intestine include absorption of water, sodium, and chloride; reduction of the volume of chyme; manufacture of vitamins B and K; and formation and expulsion of feces.
26. T   Decreased bile secretion impairs absorption of fat-soluble vitamins.

27. 3
28. 4
29. 6
30. 7
31. 1
32. 5
33. 2
34. 9
35. 8
36. Emetics cause vomiting by stimulating receptors in the stomach and duodenum or by activating the chemoreceptive trigger zone (CTZ) in the brain.

CHAPTER 28: ASSESSMENT OF NUTRITION AND THE DIGESTIVE SYSTEM

1. B
2. A
3. C
4. B
5. G
6. F
7. C
8. H
9. E
10. D
11. A
12. Assessing the chief complaint requires conducting a symptom analysis. Components of this include questions about onset, duration, quality and characteristics, severity (rate the pain), location, precipitating factors (what makes it worse), relieving factors (what makes it better), and any associated manifestations.
13. The order for examination of the abdomen is slightly altered from other systems; it involves inspection, auscultation, percussion, and palpations. During inspection assess the skin, shape of abdomen, and umbilicus. Assess for pulsations or peristaltic movement, and for *diastasis recti abdominis.* When auscultating, listen with the diaphragm of the stethoscope in all four quadrants and with the bell listen for vascular sounds. Percuss the four quadrants of the abdomen for comparison of sounds. Palpate in a circular motion, first using a light pressure and then a deeper pressure, noting for rigidity and guarding.
14. When assessing for bowel sounds, listen in all four quadrants of the abdomen with the diaphragm of the stethoscope. Listen for the frequency and character of the sounds (normal rate is 5–15 per minute; hypoactive would be 1 or fewer per minute) to determine an absence of bowel sounds. Listen for at least one minute in each quadrant.
15. A nutritional screening is an important tool to identify clients who are at high risk for nutritional problems.
16. The abdomen is examined with auscultation following inspection because percussing or palpating before auscultating might alter the bowel sounds.
17. Assessing family history related to GI disorders is important, as there are hereditary GI disorders.
18. Aspirin and nonsteroidal anti-inflammatories can cause gastric bleeding and/or gastritis.
19. Iron can cause changes in the stool color and consistency, and can cause constipation.
20. Caffeine can cause gastritis or irritable bowel; alcohol can cause gastritis and eventually hepatic damage; and nicotine can irritate the GI mucosa and is linked to cancer of the mouth and esophagus.
21. A change of bowel habits can be one of the earliest signs of colon cancer.
22. The total lymphocyte count (TLC) is an indicator of immune function and provides a gross measure of nutritional status. A TLC below $1800/mm^3$ suggests malnutrition.
23. It is important to get detailed information to assess for large doses, possible toxic effects, and drug interactions.
24. Assess his knowledge of Coumadin therapy: Reason for taking, INR/therapeutic range, and contraindications.
25. There is a wide range in nutritional content. Some have a very high carbohydrate count. Also, determine the reason for taking and if there are any contraindications such as diabetes or kidney disease.
26. Decreased absorption of calcium, magnesium, and zinc
27. Increased renal loss of potassium, calcium, magnesium
28. Inhibited fat digestion and absorption
29. Ensure that no medicines containing alcohol are given.
30. Obtain a cultural history to determine food restrictions. Communicate findings with nursing staff. Order a dietary consult.
31. Ensure that no medicines containing alcohol are given.
32. Cheese and fish or other meat substitutes are eaten during Lent.

33. Good communication skills are needed to educate and help devise a plan for clients with diabetes, hypoglycemia, or ulcers. May require between-meal snacks.

34. R of 10 equals medium frame; 100 + (5 x 5 inches) = 125 pounds

35. 106 + (6 x 8 inches) = 154 + (10% large frame) = 169.4 pounds

36. BMI 31.8 = Obesity

37. BMI 26 = Normal range

38. 42 grams of protein per day

39. 43.5 grams of protein per day

40. Upper GI Series

    Test Purpose: visualization of the esophagus, stomach, duodenum, and jejunum to detect strictures, ulcers, tumors, polyps, hiatal hernia, and motility problems. The client drinks radiopaque contrast medium.

    Informed Consent—No

    Pretest Nursing Care—NPO 6–8 hours before the test

    Post-Test Nursing Care—A laxative is usually prescribed to expel the barium and prevent fecal impaction. Instruct that stools may be white for 24–72 hours; increase liquids; report any pain, bloating, absence of stool, or bleeding to physician.

41. Flat plate of the abdomen

    Test Purpose—X-ray of the abdomen

    Informed Consent—No

    Pretest Nursing Care—Instruct patient on x-ray procedure

    Post-Test Nursing Care—None

42. Esophagogastroduodenoscopy

    Test Purpose—Examination of the esophagus, stomach, and duodenum with a lighted scope

    Informed Consent—Yes

    Pretest Nursing Care—NPO 8–12 hours; may be instructed to take PO medications at 6:00 AM; sedative and anticholinergic premedications; removal of dentures or partials; and oral assessment

    Post-Test Nursing Care—Vital signs; place client on one side; NPO until gag reflex returns; assess for signs of perforation: bleeding, fever, and dysphagia

CHAPTER 29: MANAGEMENT OF CLIENTS WITH MALNUTRITION

1. A clutter-free environment can stimulate appetite
2. Clients with adequate pain relief will eat more and are more mobile.
3. Stimulate appetite and make food taste better.
4. Eating is normally a social interaction.
5. Enhances swallowing and decreases risk of aspiration
6. Decreases risk of aspiration
7. Safety measure for clients at high risk for choking
8. Food lodged in a pocket can become dislodged later and cause aspiration
9. Safety measure for clients at high risk for choking
10. High Fowler's position for at least 30 minute helps reduce reflux and aspiration.
11. Elevation of HOB will help prevent aspiration
12. Residual volume may indicate delayed stomach emptying; the physician needs to be notified if this occurs.
13. Clients may develop dehydration with enteral feedings due to diarrhea, excessive protein intake, or osmotic diuresis.
14. Warm tap water is used to flush.
15. NS is isotonic and decreases electrolyte loss; water is hypotonic, which increases electrolyte loss through osmotic action.
16. Measuring pH confirms tube placement in the stomach.
17. Client will be breathing by mouth, causing the mouth to be dry; additionally, the absence of chewing prevents normal stimulation of salivary secretions adding to the dryness.
18. Clients on TPN are very susceptible to infection as the concentrated glucose solutions provide a good medium for bacterial growth in addition to the break in skin continuity caused by the central line placement.
19. Insures accuracy of rate and prevents giving the TPN too fast
20. The high concentration of glucose may overwhelm the body's ability to produce insulin.
21. During TPN administration insulin levels remain high, and if the TPN is stopped suddenly (therefore stopping the glucose source), the high insulin levels will result in hypoglycemia.
22. This will provide support and prevent purging.
23. People with bulimia and anorexia are prone to electrolyte imbalances, one of which, hypokalemia, can result in dysrhythmias.
24. B
25. B
26. A
27. B
28. B

29. A
30. B
31. C
32. B
33. C
34. A
35. A
36. A
37. A
38. A
39. B
40. High risk
41. Low risk
42. High risk
43. Low risk
44. Low risk

CHAPTER 30: MANAGEMENT OF CLIENTS WITH INGESTIVE DISORDERS

1. H
2. G
3. D
4. K
5. B
6. A
7. M
8. E
9. I
10. L
11. O
12. F
13. C
14. J
15. N
16. F
17. C
18. B
19. E
20. D
21. G
22. A
23. Carbohydrates stimulate bacterial acid production; when pH is 5.6 or below, decalcification of enamel occurs.
24. Removes plaque before it hardens to calculus, causing caries and periodontal disease
25. The alcohol content will cause increased pain.

26. Causes chronic irritation of oral mucous membranes, resulting in cell changes that may lead to cancer
27. Promotes venous and lymphatic drainage; prevents aspiration
28. To confirm placement of PEG tube in the stomach
29. Assists with food passage
30. Careful assessment of the oral cavity for early detection of oral infections, especially Candidiasis, and breakdown of mucous membranes
31. Increases LES pressures and prevents reflux
32. Increases LES pressure and rate of gastric emptying
33. Increases LES sphincter tone, improves esophageal peristalsis, and promotes gastric emptying
34. Suppresses secretion of gastric acid
35. Used for a person taking nonsteroidal anti-inflammatories to prevent ulcer formation
36. B   A hiatal hernia involves the herniation of part of the stomach into the thoracic cavity through a weakness in the diaphragm.
37. D   Small, frequent meals are better tolerated as the decreased volume of food results in feeling less fullness and pressure.
38. D   Keeping the drainage system below the level of the client's chest maintains gravity drainage and prevents air and fluid from going back into the pleural space.

CHAPTER 31: MANAGEMENT OF CLIENTS WITH DIGESTIVE DISORDERS

1. B, e
2. E, c
3. C, d
4. A, a
5. B, e
6. D, b
7. B
8. A
9. F
10. D
11. E
12. G
13. C
14. H
15. B
16. B
17. A
18. B

19. C
20. A
21. B
22. B
23. A
24. C
25. A, B
26. Physical and mental rest can help decrease gastric secretion and peristalsis.
27. These drugs can cause ulcers.
28. Abdomen rigidity can be a sign of perforation.
29. The parietal cells that produce intrinsic factor necessary for absorption of B_{12} are removed.
30. To treat *H. pylori* bacteria—the cause of 90% of duodenal ulcers and 70% of gastric ulcers. Omeprazole (Prilosec) suppresses gastric secretions.
31. Antacids will decrease the absorption of Zantac.
32. Can cause changes in mental status in older persons.
33. Will help protect the stomach from the ulcerogenic effects of these medications.
34. Because of the anticholinergic effects of decreasing peristalsis, relaxing smooth muscle (resulting in urinary retention), and the potential for stopping or slowing drainage of aqueous humor this drug is not recommended for persons with these pre-existing diseases.
35. In renal failure the kidneys are not excreting electrolytes appropriately; calcium and magnesium from the antacids will build up in the bloodstream and will have to be removed through dialysis.
36. Carafate acts by forming a viscid (sticky) gel that adheres to ulcer surface to form a protective barrier; the action aided by an empty stomach.
37. Helps delay gastric emptying
38. Helps delay gastric emptying
39. Helps delay gastric emptying
40. Helps delay gastric emptying
41. B   Gastric cooling, although somewhat controversial, if ordered should be done with cooled saline, not iced saline, to curtail hemorrhage. Iced saline is not used because it may lead to more mucosal damage by decreasing perfusion and it may cause a vagal response.
42. C   With perforation the person experiences sudden, sharp, severe pain beginning in the mid-epigastric region. The abdomen eventually becomes tender, hard, and rigid.
43. D   In the Billroth I procedure the surgeon removes a part of the distal portion of the stomach

including the antrum and the remainder of the stomach is anastomosed to the duodenum.
44. A   Vitamin B_{12} and folic acid deficiency are common nutritional problems after a gastrectomy. Intrinsic factor is necessary for B_{12} absorption and, as it is produced by stomach parietal cells which may be removed with a gastrectomy, the potential exists for pernicious anemia (B_{12} deficiency) to develop.
45. D   Increasing fat in the diet will help slow gastric emptying.

UNIT 7: ELIMINATION DISORDERS

1. Kidneys, ureters, bladder, urethra
2. Nephron, one
3. Filtration, reabsorption, secretion,
4. Kidneys, bladder
5. 400–500 mL, ureters, meatus
6. Wastes, electrolytes, blood pressure, hydrogen ions
7. I
8. D
9. C
10. A
11. H
12. F
13. B
14. G
15. E
16. D
17. F
18. E
19. A
20. C
21. B
22. C
23. A
24. D
25. B
26. Blood flow
27. Medications can alter the normal glomerular filtration rate by altering blood flow to the kidneys. Two drugs that can produce direct renal vasodilation are low levels of dopamine (a catecholamine) and glucagon (a protein produced by the islets of Langerhans). Norepinephrine bitartrate (Levophed), on the other hand, produces renal vasoconstriction and can drastically reduce the glomerular filtration rate.
28. The total glomerular filtration rate for a normal adult male of average size is estimated to be 125

mL per minute. During 24 hours this amounts to about 180 L. However, only about 1.0–1.5 L of glomerular filtrate per day is lost in the form of urine.

29. The combined volume of the adult pelvis and calices is approximately 8 mL; more than this can damage renal tissue. The normal adult bladder holds approximately 400–500 mL.

30. The number of nephrons decreases with age as does the amount of blood flow to the kidneys. Both factors decrease the glomerular filtration rate in this age group. Because of the impaired filtration rate, urea nitrogen, creatinine, uric acid, and drugs are excreted more slowly. Tubule cells have decreased reabsorption and selection abilities, causing a loss of water and electrolytes. In addition, the kidneys respond more slowly to the antidiuretic hormone and need more time to correct alkalosis, acidosis, and/or electrolyte disturbances.

CHAPTER 32: ASSESSMENT OF ELIMINATION

1. Gathering biographical and demographic data helps to identify risk populations for certain diseases.

2. Assessing the chief complaint requires conducting a symptom analysis. Components of this include questions about onset, duration, quality and characteristics, severity (rate the pain), location, precipitating factors (what makes it worse), relieving factors (what makes it better), and any associated manifestations.

3. Childhood and infectious disease helps to identify diseases that may have GI-related sequela.

4. Immunization information is for both health promotion to evaluate current immunization status and to help make recommendations.

5. Travelers exposed to enteropathogens and bacterial pathogens may have acute and chronic GI problems if not treated.

6. A thorough nutrition history is needed to identify factors in the dye that cause GI symptoms or GI symptoms that alter food and fluid intake.

7. Habits: Certain lifestyle habits may contribute to GI symptoms.

8. Family history: to identify familial disorders

9. A change of bowel habits can be one of the earliest signs of colon cancer. A change in color, size, and consistency needs follow-up.

10. GI-related symptoms are often side effects of some medications. OTC aspirin and nonsteroidal anti-inflammatories can cause gastric bleeding and/or gastritis. Identify any medications to treat constipation. Histamine antagonist, Tagamet, Zantac and Pepcid are prescription and OTC drugs. Identify nutrient supplement intake.

11. The abdomen is examined with auscultation following inspection because percussing or palpating before auscultating might alter the bowel sounds. During inspection assess the skin, shape of abdomen, and umbilicus. Assess for pulsations or peristaltic movement, and for *diastasis recti abdominis.* When auscultating, listen with the diaphragm of the stethoscope in all four quadrants and with the bell listen for vascular sounds. Percuss the four quadrants of the abdomen for comparison of sounds. Palpate in a circular motion, first using a light pressure and then a deeper pressure, noting for rigidity and guarding.

12. When assessing for bowel sounds, listen in all four quadrants with the diaphragm of the stethoscope. Listen for the frequency and character of the sounds (normal rate is 5–15 per minute; hypoactive would be 1 or fewer per minute) to determine an absence of bowel sounds. Listen for at least one minute in each quadrant.

13. Giving a complete bed bath, assisting to the bathroom or with using a bedpan, checking for an impaction, giving an enema, inserting a suppository.

14. Carcinoembryonic Antigen

Test Purpose—Blood test for glycoprotein not normally found after fetal life; may indicate presence of colorectal cancer

Informed Consent—No

Pretest Nursing Care—Explain purpose

Post-Test Nursing Care—None

15. Guaiac

Test Purpose—Examination of stool for hidden or occult blood

Informed Consent—No

Pretest Nursing Care—With orthotoluidine test, client may be instructed to eat high-fiber diet for 48–72 hours and avoid red meat, poultry, turnips, and horseradish; medications that may be withheld are iron preparations, bromides, rauwolfia derivatives, steroids, indomethacin, and colchicine

Post-Test Nursing Care—None

16. Stool for Ova and Parasites

Test Purpose—Procedural concerns are to collect the stool and immediately send it to the laboratory; stool needs to be fresh and warm.

Informed Consent—No

Pretest Nursing Care—Instruct client to avoid castor oil, mineral oil, and antidiarrheal medications; stool will be collected daily for 3 days

Post-Test Nursing Care—None

17. Flat Plate of the Abdomen

    Test Purpose—X-ray of the abdomen

    Informed Consent—No

    Pretest Nursing Care—Instruct patient on x-ray procedure

    Post-Test Nursing Care—None

18. Lower Gastrointestinal Series

    Test Purpose—Performed to visualize the position, movements, and filling of the colon. Barium (a radiopaque contrast medium) is given via a rectal catheter.

    Informed Consent—No

    Pretest Nursing Care—Low residue diet or clear liquids for 2 days; potent laxative 1 day before test; NPO; suppository or cleansing enema day of test

    Post-Test Nursing Care—Laxative or cleansing enema; instruct that stools may be white for 24–72 hours; increase liquids; report any pain, bloating, absence of stool, or bleeding to physician

19. Colonoscopy

    Test Purpose—Examination of the lining of the colon through a flexible lighted scope inserted into the colon

    Informed Consent—Yes

    Pretest Nursing Care—Clear liquids for 24 hours; cathartic the night before (policy could call for GoLYTELY or oral Fleet Phospho-Soda followed by 4 Dulcolax tablets 30 minutes later); cleansing enema the morning of test

    Post-Test Nursing Care—Assess for or teach client signs of perforation: abdominal pain, bleeding, or fever

20. B
21. J
22. I
23. A
24. G
25. E
26. H
27. D
28. C
29. F
30. E
31. D
32. H
33. A
34. G
35. F
36. I
37. B
38. J
39. C
40. B
41. E
42. C
43. A
44. D
45. C
46. A
47. B
48. E
49. F
50. D
51. **Health Perception–Health Management:** Risk factors for genetic disorders.
52. **Nutrition–Metabolic:** Risk for gout and kidney stones. Decreased fluid intake could increase the risk for urinary tract infections (UTIs).
53. **Elimination:** Major area to assess for urologic disorders.
54. **Health Perception–Health Management:** Client's past experiences with urinary tract disorders. Risk factors for renal disorders, such as radiation for reproductive cancers and sexually transmitted diseases.
55. **Health Perception–Health Management:** Assess for nephrotoxic effects of medications and medications that affect the amount and color of the urine.
56. **Sleep–Rest:** Change in voiding patterns that interrupt sleep should be investigated for possible causes.
57. **Cognitive–Perceptual:** Pain symptom analysis.
58. **Self-Perception–Self-Concept:** Chronic urologic problems affect every area of the client's life and place the client at risk for problems with self-worth and body image.
59. **Role–Relationship:** Assess for hazards in the work area that may increase the risk of developing urinary problems, such as exposure to nephrotoxic chemicals.
60. The specific gravity may be determined on a preoperative client to establish the client's general fluid status. It is important that the client scheduled for surgery be adequately hydrated. Adequate hydration decreases the possibility of postoperative complications.
61. Urine osmolality is a more precise measurement of the concentrating ability of the kidneys.
62. Proteinuria often denotes abnormal glomerular permeability, decreased tubular reabsorption, or an overflow of protein in the plasma. Some systemic diseases may cause proteinuria also.

63. The blood urea nitrogen (BUN) level helps to evaluate renal function. Urea is the end product of protein metabolism and is normally excreted from the body via the kidneys. Therefore, renal impairment causes an increase in the blood urea level.

64. N

65. A, normal is 4.5–8

66. N

67. N

68. A, 0–4 per field

69. A, 0–3 per field

70. No

71. Decrease risk contamination

72. Decrease risk contamination

73. Yes

74. Decrease anxiety

75. No restrictions post-test

76. Yes

77. Iodine-based dye is used for the test.

78. Increases excretion of the dye

79. High-serum creatinine indicates the kidneys are not excreting wastes. Injecting a dye that could not be excreted by the kidneys could cause more kidney damage.

80. Monitor excretion and kidney function

81. Yes, or per institution

82. Decreases anxiety and apprehension about the test

83. Yes

84. Decrease or minimize the risk of bladder trauma

85. Bladder, urethra trauma from the scope

CHAPTER 33: MANAGEMENT OF CLIENTS WITH INTESTINAL DISORDERS

1. F
2. D
3. E
4. B
5. A
6. C
7. E
8. C
9. D
10. B
11. A
12. G
13. D
14. F
15. B
16. C
17. I
18. J
19. E
20. A
21. H
22. B
23. C
24. A
25. A
26. A
27. B
28. B
29. A
30. A
31. A

32. Bacteria will multiply if GI motility is slowed (as the bacteria are retained).

33. May lead to rupture of the appendix and peritonitis

34. May indicate a ruptured appendix

35. Dark, dusky, or cyanotic tissue could indicate compromised blood supply

36. The alkaline content of the effluence is very irritating to the skin

37. Protects the skin with only 1/16" being exposed to the effluence.

38. Yearly digital rectal examinations will detect one-third of malignant tumors of the distal colon and rectum; stool guaiac tests will detect GI bleeding and diagnose some colon cancers; sigmoidoscopy every 3–5 years is effective in visualizing the colon and also allows for biopsy.

39. The perineal portion of the abdomino-perineal resection is completed in the lithotomy position, which is associated with an increase in phlebitis.

40. Normally 7–8 L of electrolyte fluid is secreted by the bowel and reabsorbed. With obstruction the fluid is partially retained within the bowel and partially eliminated by vomiting, resulting in hypotension, hypovolemic shock, and diminished renal and cerebral blood flow.

41. Distention with obstruction causes a temporary increase in peristalsis; within a few hours, the bowel becomes flaccid and bowel sounds become diminished or absent.

42. Severe intestinal distention may raise the diaphragm and inhibit respirations.

43. Imodium is superior to diphenoxylate hydrochloride (Lomotil) for controlling diarrhea with fewer side effects.

44. Steroids reduce the body's response to inflammation.

45. 6-MP is used for immunosuppression when other treatments fail.

46. Azulfidine prevents or controls infections and inflammation.

47. Neomycin decreases bacterial count in the colon, preventing infections during surgery.

48. This prevents spillage of effluence onto the skin.

49. Fiber and cellulose may absorb excessive moisture, leading to swelling and possibly constipation and even obstruction.

50. Due to shortened transit time in the intestines, poorly chewed food may pass through undigested.

51. This will prevent the bowel from becoming overdistended.

52. This will prevent the weight of the effluence from pulling the pouch off the skin or protective barrier.

53. These products will heal the skin or help prevent skin breakdown.

54. The person with a colostomy can become quickly dehydrated.

55. The rectal sphincters have been removed and there is no control over gas expulsion; therefore, diet has to be used to prevent unwanted flatus.

56. The incidence of diverticulosis is associated with a diet low in fiber. A high-fiber diet will help propel food through the colon and prevent constipation and complications.

57. A high-fiber diet will add bulk to the stool, will help prevent constipation and the necessity of straining with bowel movements, and will decrease the intra-abdominal pressure, which contribute to hemorrhoids.

58. This position impairs blood flow and puts pressure on the anal vessels.

59. C   Known risk factors for colon cancer include high-fat, low-residue diet, adenomatous polyps, being over age 40, and history of ulcerative colitis.

60. A   At least 50% of colon cancers occur in the rectal area.

61. D   The American Cancer Society's recommendations for early detection of colon cancer include yearly digital rectal examinations for people over age 40; sigmoidoscopic examinations at age 50, yearly for 2 years, then, after two negative tests, every 3–5 years; and annual guaiac tests after age 50.

62. B   A dusky or bluish stoma may mean decreased circulation and needs to be reported to the physician.

63. D   The pouch needs to be emptied when it is one-third to one-half full to avoid having a full pouch that might pull loose.

CHAPTER 34: MANAGEMENT OF CLIENTS WITH URINARY DISORDERS

1. F
2. B
3. C
4. D
5. E
6. A
7. C
8. B
9. A
10. D
11. E
12. G
13. F
14. I
15. H
16. B
17. A
18. C
19. D
20. E
21. F
22. G
23. H
24. E
25. D
26. B
27. C
28. A
29. B
30. C
31. A
32. E
33. F
34. G
35. H
36. I
37. D
38. Voiding after intercourse helps to flush organisms out of bladder and urethra.

39. Good perineal hygiene decreases the risk of organisms (especially *E. coli*) from the anus and rectum coming in contact with urethra.

40. Increased fluid intake helps to wash out bacteria and decreases pain and irritation to the bladder wall by diluting urine.

41. A decrease in urine output, especially in the first 24 hours, could be related to obstruction.

42. A change in color or size of the stoma could indicate decreased blood flow to the stoma.

43. High risk for uric acid and calcium stones

44. A urinary diversion is a high output/volume diversion. The high volume and urine pH can erode the karaya barrier.

45. Increased fluid intake hinders stone formation by diluting the urine and helps to wash out stones.

46. Strain urine to recover stones for lab analysis and treatment.

47. Modified diet decreases the risk of stone formation.

48. Ambulation enhances stone excretion.

49. Good care of catheter decreases the risk of complications.

50. Possible allergic reaction

51. Works best in an alkaline environment

52. Contraindicated in client with narrow-angle glaucoma because it inhibits the effects of acetylcholine, which could increase intraocular pressure

53. Works against the medical treatment for myasthenia gravis

54. Turns the urine dark-brown to red, which can be mistaken for blood

55. Optimize drug action and decrease the risk of crystal formation.

56. Optimize drug action and minimize side effects.

57. Because it is poorly absorbed in acidic urine and may crystallize in the renal tubules

58. Urine output, stoma, patency of appliance, abdomen

59. Continue to monitor client (bowel sounds would not be expected 12 hours after surgery). Closely monitor the rigid abdomen and correlate with other assessments because it may indicate an obstruction or bleeding into the abdomen.

60. Document the assessments, check the appliance for proper fit, and notify the physician.

61. Opiates, antispasmodics, and beta blockers can cause urinary retention.

62. Obstruction of the urinary tract causes retention of urine. The retained urine increases hydrostatic pressure against the bladder wall causing hypertrophy of the detrusor muscle. Because the peristalsis in the ureteral musculature increases against the pressure of the accumulating urine, the ureter becomes elongated, tortuous, and fibrotic. There is also increased pressure in the renal pelvis and calices. This increase in pressure causes hydronephrosis. If the obstruction is not removed, ischemia of renal tissue occurs and renal failure results.

63. Catheterizing the client for residual urine

64. D   The motion during coitus "milks" the organisms up the urethra and into the bladder.

65. A   Voiding immediately after intercourse helps to flush the organism out of the bladder and urethra.

66. B   The medication causes gastric irritation and should be taken with meals.

67. C   Fish, poultry, cheese, eggs, cereals, and cranberries, prunes, plums and their juices are allowed. All milk and milk products and all vegetables except corn and lentils are prohibited.

CHAPTER 35: MANAGEMENT OF CLIENTS WITH RENAL DISORDERS

1. E

2. G

3. D

4. F

5. C

6. B

7. A

8. High-calorie diet prevents protein catabolism. Low-protein diet allows the kidneys to rest because they handle less protein molecules and metabolites.

9. Indicator of fluid retention/edema and kidney function

10. Total fluid intake is reduced; hard candy or lemon may help to relieve thirst.

11. Edema causes tissue damage.

12. Evaluate fluid retention.

13. Prevent further protein loss in urine

14. Decrease the chance of infection

15. The client's fluid intake should be high enough to ensure 2500–3000 mL of urine output daily.

16. Maintain a consistent urine output

17. Stage I: tumor within capsule

    Stage II: tumor invades perirenal fat

    Stage III: tumor extends into renal vein or regional lymphatics

    Stage IV: metastasis to other parts of the body

18. Continue to monitor intake and output and renal function; encourage high fluid intake to dilute the medication in the urine. Insure that a gentamicin peak and trough are drawn.

19. Did she have a follow-up urine culture? Does she take tub baths? How much fluid intake?

20. Three liters or more per day

21. The urine must be strained so that any stones or sediment can be saved and analyzed. The stone

analysis will help determine treatment measures to prevent recurrence.

22. Gather more data because the tube may be obstructed with a stone fragment or may be kinked. Check output records. Notify the physician.

23. Gather more data to determine the reason for the client not wanting to care for his conduit. Allow time for the client to vent his feelings and fears about a possible recurrence of the cancer. Consult with the enterostomal therapist concerning the skin irritation.

24. B

25. C

26. C

CHAPTER 36: MANAGEMENT OF CLIENTS WITH RENAL FAILURE

1. E
2. I
3. D
4. F
5. A
6. C
7. G
8. B
9. H
10. K
11. C
12. D
13. A
14. B
15. I
16. F
17. G
18. E
19. J
20. H
21. Accurate intake and output measurements guide fluid replacement.
22. Improve circulation and prevent skin breakdown
23. The client with ARF is susceptible to secondary infection.
24. Manifestations of fluid overload
25. Removal of the end products of protein metabolism, such as urea and creatinine, from the blood; maintenance of safe concentration of serum electrolytes; correction of acidosis and replenishment of the blood's bicarbonate buffer system; and removal of excess fluid from the blood

26. Peritonitis and obstruction of the catheter

27. The external arteriovenous shunt requires the surgical placement of two Silastic cannulas into the forearm or leg. The two cannulas are connected to form a U shape. The internal arteriovenous fistula is the access of choice for chronic dialysis patients. The fistula is created through a surgical procedure where the vein and artery are anastomosed.

28. Low-protein diets are typically deficient in water-soluble vitamins. The dialysis may deplete water-soluble vitamins.

29. To treat hyperkalemia

30. Explain in terms that she can understand that anemia is a problem for clients with chronic renal failure because of a decrease in erythropoietin.

31. Explain in terms that she can understand the reason for the dry skin, itching, and rash. Tell her to avoid skin products that contain alcohol or perfumes because they have a drying effect on the skin.

32. Clinical manifestations of renal transplant rejections are fever, graft tenderness at the site of the transplanted kidney, anemia, and malaise.

33. Causes of renal failure:
    - Prerenal: decreased blood flow to the kidneys
    - Renal: problem within the kidney, such as infections, genetic disorder, acute tubular necrosis
    - Postrenal: the kidneys, such as obstruction, spinal cord injury, or pelvic trauma

34. A
35. B
36. A
37. D

UNIT 8: SEXUALITY AND REPRODUCTIVE DISORDERS

1. G
2. D
3. F
4. A
5. C
6. E
7. H
8. B
9. See Figure U8-1B.
10. See Figure U8-4.
11. See Figure U8-2.
12. Because the largest amount of breast tissue is there
13. The breast is fixed to the overlying skin and underlying pectoral fascia by the ligaments.

14. Estrogen is responsible for the growth of the breast and the periductal stroma.

15. With loss of estrogen there is involution of breast tissue with loss of glandular elements and tissue atrophy.

16. FSH influences development of the follicular cells. LH and FSH stimulate further production of estrogen. LH takes over stimulating the maturation of the follicle and eventually to produce ovulation. Estrogen begins creating a new endometrial surface layer, restoring the uterine epithelium, and stimulating the growth of glands and stromata. The luteal cells produce progesterone. Progesterone and estrogen promote the endometrium's secretory activity in preparation for the fertilized egg. If the fertilized egg does not implant, progesterone and estrogen production drop causing endometrial retraction and degeneration resulting in menstruation.

17. Positive nitrogen balance; calcium and phosphorous metabolism and calcium retention in bones; sodium chloride retention and, hence, sodium and water balance; control of blood proteins and lipids; the vascular and skeletal systems; and thyroid function, insulin production, and adrenal function.

18. The prostate secretes a milky fluid that forms part of the semen, which aids the passage of sperm and helps keep them alive.

19. They produce testosterone and sperm.

20. Development of male genitalia, modulates the secretion of Gn-RH, LH, and FSH, and stimulates Sertoli's cells and germinal cells to start and complete spermatogenesis.

CHAPTER 37: ASSESSMENT OF THE REPRODUCTIVE SYSTEM

1. B
2. I
3. G
4. A
5. D
6. H
7. E
8. F
9. C
10. B
11. H
12. A
13. C
14. G
15. J
16. I
17. E
18. D
19. F
20. C
21. A
22. E
23. B
24. D

25. Rubella in the first trimester of pregnancy can cause birth defects. A woman contemplating pregnancy should have a rubella titer to determine immunity; if negative, the woman is encouraged to receive immunization.

26. Excess alcohol consumption and use of illegal drugs may be suggestive of behaviors that put a woman at risk for sexually transmitted diseases (STDs).

27. Condoms and diaphragms are also made of these products. Additionally, it will be necessary to complete the examination using vinyl gloves.

28. Delaying the breast examination until after "hands on" examinations of the heart and lungs shows sensitivity to a woman's potential discomfort with the breast examination and allows a little more time to develop rapport between the examiner and the client.

29. This maneuver results in contraction of the pectoral muscles and will emphasize any retractions or skin flattening.

30. These activities may interfere with the accuracy of the Pap smear.

31. A history of mumps may be an indication of sterility.

32. Certain antihypertensives may cause impotence.

33. Concerns about behaviors that may place the client at risk for AIDS or other STDs or the client's need to discuss sexual concerns may be identified with this intervention.

34. The breasts may be firmer, more cystic, and painful during the luteal phase of menstruation; therefore, at 7–10 days after onset of menses the breasts will be easier to examine.

35. Test—Papanicolaou smear

    Informed Consent—No

    Pretest Nursing Care—Explain procedure

    Instruct client not to douche, have intercourse, use vaginal products (for 2–3 days), or take a tub bath before procedure.

    Client should not be menstruating.

    Empty bladder and bowel.

Disrobe from waist down.

Assist client to relax during procedure.

Maintain privacy.

Lithotomy position

Post-Test Nursing Care—Assist out of stirrups

Instruct to stand slowly.

Provide material for client to clean off lubricant.

36. Test—Ultrasound

Informed Consent—No

Pretest Nursing Care—Explain procedure, particularly aspects of use of vaginal probe when needed.

Full bladder if not using vaginal probe

Post-Test Nursing Care—None

37. Test—Endometrial biopsy

Informed Consent—Yes

Pretest Nursing Care—Explain procedure

Lithotomy position

Post-Test Nursing Care—May require pain medication for cramping

38. Test—Cervical biopsy

Informed Consent—Yes

Pretest Nursing Care—Explain procedure.

Client cannot be menstruating.

Lithotomy position

Biopsy causes discomfort.

Post-Test Nursing Care—Rest before leaving clinic.

Avoid activity for 24 hours.

Report excessive bleeding.

Abstain from sexual intercourse, use of tampons, and douching for several days.

39. Test—Laparoscopy

Informed Consent—Yes

Pretest Nursing Care—Explain procedure.

Plan for another person to drive the client home after the procedure.

NPO

Cathartic or enema per physician preference

Post-Test Nursing Care—Assess vital signs.

With local anesthesia client can have fluids and light snack as desired.

Explain potential feeling of "bloatedness."

Wound care instruction

Sexual intercourse can be resumed in a week.

40. Test—Mammography

Informed Consent—No

Pretest Nursing Care—Explain procedure.

Instruct client not to wear any deodorant, body powder, or creams on torso the day of the procedure.

Client will be disrobed from waist up.

Post-Test Nursing Care—Client should receive results in 1 day to 3 weeks.

41. Test—Prostatic biopsy

Informed Consent—Yes

Pretest Nursing Care—Explain procedure.

Know which approach is planned in order to give the correct instruction.

Enemas with transrectal or perineal approach

Have client empty bladder.

With transurethral approach client will be in the lithotomy position.

With transrectal approach, the Sims' position will be used.

Post-Test Nursing Care—Assess vital signs.

Report frank bleeding from urethra.

Assess client's ability to void.

Assess perineal approach for bleeding.

Assess transrectal approach for bleeding and infection.

42. Test—Cystoscopy

Informed Consent—Yes

Pretest Nursing Care—Explain procedure.

May be completed with local or general anesthesia

May have enema orders

NPO with general anesthesia

Oral or IV fluid to fill bladder

Lithotomy position

Assist client during procedure with relaxation measures.

Post-Test Nursing Care—Assess vital signs.

Assess urine for excess blood.

Bed rest for short time

Client may expect some back pain, bladder spasms, burning with urination.

Assess ability to void.

Hot sitz or tub baths may relieve spasms or urinary retention.

43. The prostate is normally 4 cm long and 5 cm wide; it is doughnut-shaped and wraps around the neck of the urethra. Only the posterior and lateral lobes can be felt through the rectal wall. The lateral lobes should be symmetrical and feel smooth, rubbery, and firm. With benign prostatic hypertrophy, the prostate feels larger than normal with firmer consistency. Tenderness and bogginess may indicate acute or chronic prostatitis. A carcinoma feels "stony hard," like a hard nodule; that is, a circumscribed area of induration.

44. The pectoral (anterior), midaxillary (central), subscapular (posterior), brachial (lateral), and infraclavicular nodes.

45. BSE should be performed monthly for women over age 20. A mammogram is recommended every year for women 40 years of age and older. A Pap smear should be given to women who are 18, or sexually active, annually; after three or more consecutive normal results, the Pap smear may be given less often (at the discretion of the health care provider).

CHAPTER 38: MANAGEMENT OF MEN WITH REPRODUCTIVE DISORDERS

1. F
2. L
3. D
4. C
5. I
6. J
7. M
8. N
9. A
10. G
11. O
12. B
13. P
14. K
15. H
16. E
17. Forcing a catheter can cause trauma to the urethra. If you cannot insert the catheter, the urologist needs to be notified as special instruments may be required.
18. A blocked catheter may lead to such complications as infection, bladder distention, and painful bladder spasms. Overdistention of the bladder could also cause hemorrhage by placing strain on recently coagulated vessels.
19. These drugs can cause urinary retention.
20. Bladder spasms are common after prostatic surgery due to irritation from the catheter, manipulation during surgery, or overdistention of the bladder. They are very painful and need to be treated.
21. Exposure to occupational and environmental agents can cause infertility. Occupational and environmental agents that may affect the male reproductive system include pesticides dibromochloropropane (DBCP), ethylene dibromide, and chlordecone; anesthetic agents, carbon disulfide, estrogen, inorganic lead and mercury, microwaves, neurotoxins from the

manufacture of polyurethane, ionizing radiation, gamma-emitting radioisotopes, Urolene diamine, and wastewater from petroleum refineries.

22. Numerous drugs can have major sexual and reproductive effects.
23. History of STDs may affect fertility.
24. Prolonged sitting increases intra-abdominal pressure and may precipitate bleeding.
25. Straining can lead to bleeding from the operative site for up to 6 weeks after surgery.
26. Dribbling after prostate surgery is common and the perineal exercises help the client regain urinary sphincter control.
27. One can screen for colon cancer and prostate cancer at the same time.
28. Endocrine therapy is used based on an observation that prostatic epithelial cells atrophy if they are deprived of androgens. The use of estrogen suppresses the release of pituitary gonadotropin and reduces serum testosterone levels.
29. B   BPH is caused by an abnormal increase in the number of cells (hyperplasia) that, with aging, grows and compresses surrounding normal prostatic tissue, pushing it toward the gland periphery forming a false or surgical capsule.
30. D   The TURP is performed by inserting a resectoscope through the urethra. The most common resectoscope is a hot-wire scope with a movable loop wire that cuts tissue with a high-frequency current.
31. A   Pink-tinged urine is normal for several days postoperatively.
32. C   When the bladder is distended, manipulated, or irritated by the indwelling catheter it will spasm and cause pain.
33. C   Assessing patency would be the first step to determine if the catheter was plugged or kinked.
34. B   Irrigating the catheter would be the second step based on the findings in the assessment. If the urine output increased, no further action would be necessary.
35. D   If the catheter was neither kinked or plugged, D would be the second step.
36. A   The physician would likely have to be notified of the decreased urine output and would need data about the intake and output.

CHAPTER 39: MANAGEMENT OF WOMEN WITH REPRODUCTIVE DISORDERS

1. B
2. E
3. O

4. P
5. H
6. A
7. Q
8. S
9. F
10. J
11. U
12. R
13. G
14. M
15. L
16. C
17. D
18. T
19. N
20. I
21. K

22. HRT is used to manage menopausal effects of atrophic vaginitis, hot flashes, and urinary tract changes. HRT also decreases the risk for developing osteoporosis and possibly has cardioprotective effects.

23. HRT is contraindicated in clients with breast or uterine cancer or with any estrogen-dependent neoplasia, undiagnosed abnormal uterine bleeding, previous or present thrombophlebitis, or acute liver or cerebrovascular disease.

24. Postoperative gas is a major cause of pain and discomfort after a hysterectomy. Ambulation and enema may increase peristalsis resulting in relief from the gas and discomfort.

25. Due to the proximity of the bladder and the vagina, the Foley is inserted to prevent bladder distention and potential injury during surgery.

26. DES was a drug used until 1960 to prevent miscarriage. Maternal ingestion of DES is associated with increased risk of vaginal cancer in the daughters of these women.

27. These drugs are prostaglandin synthesis inhibitors and they are effective because it is believed that dysmenorrhea is caused by either an excess of prostaglandins or increased sensitivity to prostaglandins.

28. Spironolactone (Aldactone) is a synthetic steroid aldosterone antagonist that inhibits the physiologic effect of aldosterone on the distal renal tubules resulting in diuresis.

29. Progesterone and oral contraceptives are used with endometriosis to cause the ectopic endometrium to slough off resulting in this tissue no longer functioning in abnormal sites. This treatment is not successful in all women.

30. Important modifiable risk factors include early age of first intercourse, frequent intercourse with multiple sex partners, infection with human papillomavirus, sexually transmitted diseases (STDs), and untreated chronic cervicitis.

31. Risk factors for endometrial cancer include exogenous estrogen replacement therapy without concomitant progesterone therapy, history of pelvic radiation, early menarche, late menopause, dysfunctional uterine bleeding, delayed onset of ovulation, increasing age, other reproductive cancer, infertility or habitual abortion, family history of endometrial cancer, Caucasian race, and postmenopausal bleeding.

32. Exercise is recommended because it increases blood levels of beta-endorphins, the body's natural opiates, making them available for pain relief.

33. Hormone replacement therapy and estrogen replacement therapy decrease the risk of developing osteoporosis. However, estrogen replacement therapy alone may increase a woman's risk for endometrial cancer.

34. Items to include in teaching (as situation warrants): avoid unprotected intercourse, avoid multiple partners, avoid use of intrauterine contraceptive device (IUD) if having more than one sexual partner, discourage douching, risk of sterility with infections, general hygiene measures such as washing the perineal area with soap and water, wiping from front to back, hand-washing, and frequent (at least four times a day) changing of tampons or pads.

35. Begin abdominal strengthening exercises 2 months after surgery; avoid heavy lifting for 2 months; avoid activities that will increase pelvic congestion such as dancing, prolonged standing, and horseback riding; and resume intercourse and douching per physician instructions, usually at about 6 weeks postoperatively.

36. Nursing interventions and suggestions for women having hot flashes include dressing in layers; avoiding hot environments; avoiding getting excited; avoiding highly seasoned, spicy foods, coffee, tea and alcohol (triggers may vary from person to person); keeping a diary of when hot flashes are experienced to identify triggering events; learning to control reactions to hot flashes; and using cooling techniques.

37. The most obvious benefit is that a Pap smear will detect early cervical cancer, when it is 100% curable. The death rate from cervical cancer has dropped 50% in the past 20 years—directly due to

women having Pap smears. The Pap smear has a role in identifying endometrial cancer; however, it is only 50% effective.

38. C   Pap smear is the primary test for cervical cancer; it can be used to detect uterine cancer but it is not nearly as effective as for detecting cervical cancer.

39. A   Early treatment of cervical infections helps prevent chronic cervicitis, which is believed to lead to cervical dysplasia, an early premalignant cell change.

40. D   Treatment for cancer in situ results in 100% cure.

41. A   Ms. I. should avoid baths or sitz baths in order to prevent infections at the surgical site. She should instead take showers to maintain hygiene.

CHAPTER 40: MANAGEMENT OF CLIENTS WITH BREAST DISORDERS

1. B
2. D
3. H
4. A
5. G
6. C
7. E
8. F
9. F
10. D
11. H
12. A
13. G
14. J
15. B
16. E
17. I
18. C
19. E
20. D
21. H
22. A
23. I
24. B
25. F
26. G
27. C
28. A
29. B
30. A

31. B
32. A
33. B
34. B
35. A
36. A
37. The woman is at risk for arm edema and taking blood pressures on the arm of the operated side could increase edema.

38. Reach to Recovery is an American Cancer Society volunteer group of breast cancer survivors. These volunteers are trained to help women with common psychosocial, physical, and cosmetic needs. They bring information about exercises, brassiere comfort, prostheses, and exercise equipment as well as answer questions for clients newly diagnosed with breast cancer.

39. Used with women who have estrogen receptor-positive breast tumors. It has an anti-estrogen, antitumor effect.

40. Exercise helps maintain and/or restore hand, arm, and shoulder strength and range of motion.

41. The woman who has had a lymph node resection is at risk for edema and infection. Prevention of infection in the hand and arm on the operative side is very important.

42. Major risk factors include gender, over age 55, family history of breast cancer, especially if they are carriers of the BRCA-1 gene. Other risk factors include previous breast cancer, being over age 30 at time of first pregnancy, nulliparity post-menopausal obesity, history of cancer of the uterus, ovary, or colon, and early menarche and late menopause.

43. Side effects of external beam radiation to the breast include temporary skin changes (itchy, dry, tender, red, swollen, or dry desquamation), fatigue, dry throat (rare), pneumonitis (rare), arm edema (rare), and increased susceptibility to rib fracture in the irradiated field. To care for the skin changes women should check with their radiation facility for their specific protocol. Fatigue needs to be addressed by careful planning of activities with periods of rest and having their families reallocate household duties.

44. Discharge teaching should include wound and drain management, arm exercises, arm precautions (trauma, infection, edema), grieving and support systems, temporary prosthesis, permanent prosthesis/reconstruction, breast self-examination, and follow-up medical care.

45. Provide opportunity for the client and family to ask questions, encourage the woman to discuss her

feelings and provide supportive, nonjudgmental listening; assist to understand treatment options, provide written as well as verbal instruction, and repeat information as needed.

46. C Typical symptoms include a fixed, irregular mass. Additionally, the mass is usually unilateral, single, painless, nontender, and hard. It can also appear as a thickening of tissue.

47. C In a modified radical mastectomy, the breast and overlying skin are removed.

48. D Tamoxifen may be used when tumors are estrogen receptor-positive for the antitumor, anti-estrogen effect.

49. B Elbow flexion and extension exercises can begin almost immediately postmastectomy. Shoulder abduction and rotation exercises should begin after wound healing is well established.

50. A After lymph node removal, there is an increased chance of infection on the operated side; therefore, women are taught infection precautions.

CHAPTER 41: MANAGEMENT OF CLIENTS WITH SEXUALLY TRANSMITTED DISEASES

1. I
2. E
3. J
4. B
5. L
6. A
7. G
8. H
9. F
10. D
11. K
12. M
13. C
14. Because gonorrhea and Chlamydia commonly coexist, with the diagnosis of gonorrhea, doxycycline is added for Chlamydial treatment.
15. Intake of alcohol will cause nausea, vomiting, and headaches.
16. To increase absorption and efficacy
17. HPV infections are strongly associated with cancer of the cervix or vulva in women.
18. Chlamydia is known as the "great sterilizer" and is the most common bacterial STD. Untreated, it causes an inflammation leading to scarring and ulceration of the involved tissue that may result in sterility.
19. For these diseases, clients should be instructed to avoid sexual contact for 30 days.

20. Infection with an STD does not provide immunity to reinfection.
21. STD rates are highest for adolescents and young adults.
22. D Incidence of genital warts, caused by the human papillomavirus (HPV), has been associated with genital cancer in women.
23. A The surest way to prevent STDs is abstinence. Other forms of prevention carry some risk.
24. C Sexual contact investigation is essential for the prevention and control of gonorrhea.
25. B Taking Flagyl with alcohol may result in nausea, vomiting, and headaches.
26. B Condoms are fragile and multiple use can result in damage to the condom which results in condom failure.

UNIT 9: METABOLIC DISORDERS

1. (a) pineal, (b) pituitary, (c) parathyroids, (d) thyroid, (e) thymus, (f) adrenals, (g) pancreas, (h) ovaries, (i) testes
2. E
3. D
4. B
5. G
6. F
7. D
8. H
9. G
10. A
11. G
12. G
13. E
14. C
15. I
16. G
17. Aldosterone, glucocorticoids (cortisol, cortisone, hydrocortisone)
18. Metabolism, glucagon
19. Thyroid-stimulating hormone (TSH) and adreno-corticotropic hormone (ACTH)
20. Retention
21. Parathyroid [which secretes parathormone (PTH), which increases serum calcium levels and decreases serum phosphate levels. (The thyroid gland secretes thyrocalcitonin, which decreases serum calcium levels and increases serum phosphate levels.)]
22. Hypothalamus
23. M

24. G
25. H
26. I
27. J
28. P
29. L
30. C
31. K
32. A
33. O
34. B
35. N
36. E
37. D
38. F
39. The ribs and peritoneum
40. Superior mesenteric, inferior mesenteric, splenic
41. The veins become engorged.
42. Portal
43. Liver engorgement
44. (1) Emulsifying or detergent function: decreasing the surface tension of fat particles in food allowing the agitation of the intestine to break the fat globules into a smaller size, and (2) assisting in the absorption of fatty acids, monoglycerides, cholesterol, and other lipids.
45. (1) Oxidation of fatty acids for energy, (2) formation of most lipoproteins, (3) synthesis of cholesterol and phospholipids, and (4) synthesis of fat from proteins and carbohydrates.
46. Glucogenesis, glycogenolysis, gluconeogenesis, conversion of galactose and fructose to glucose, storage of glycogen
47. Ammonia, urea
48. Prothrombin, fibrinogen, V, VI, VII, IX, X
49. Ammonia
50. Hormones, drugs, other chemicals
51. Blood
52. The bile ducts act as reservoirs and body processes proceed normally, but the ability to excrete large quantities of bile after ingestion of a fatty meal is lost.
53. Insulin, glucagon
54. Amylase, lipase, trypsin
55. A special trypsin inhibitor in the pancreas prevents activation of the enzymes.
56. The bicarbonate ions neutralize the acid chyme from the stomach present in the duodenum.

CHAPTER 42: ASSESSMENT OF THE ENDOCRINE AND METABOLIC SYSTEMS

1. C
2. A
3. D
4. B
5. B
6. G
7. A
8. C
9. D
10. E
11. F
12. A
13. C
14. D
15. H
16. I
17. F
18. B
19. E
20. G
21. Exhalation moves the diaphragm up, so this will help prevent it from being punctured.
22. This decreases the risk of hemorrhage and bile leakage.
23. The liver is a vascular organ; there is a danger of penetration of the arterial tree or distended veins.
24. Monitor vital signs for 8–12 hours. Assess for increase in pulse and decrease in blood pressure. Observe for pain in right upper quadrant or right shoulder. Maintain bed rest for 24 hours. Maintain right-side lying position 1–2 hours postprocedure. Administer vitamin K as ordered. Assess for signs of dyspnea.
25. Alcoholism may accompany liver and pancreatic disease.
26. Begin at the RMCL superior or inferior to the estimated liver borders. Superiorly, begin at the third intercostal space over lung resonance and percuss down until the sound changes to dull. Mark this level with a pen. Inferiorly, start over a tympanic area and percuss upward until the sound changes to dull. Mark this line with a pen. At the midsternal line, percuss upward from above the umbilicus from tympany to dull and mark. Superiorly, percuss down to the sternum until the sound changes and mark.
27. The spleen should not be palpated as there is a risk of rupture.

28. Ask about allergies to iodine, Betadine, or seafood, or difficulty with previous diagnostic tests when a contrast medium was injected.

29. A hypersensitivity reaction to iodine might produce symptoms of nausea and vomiting, diarrhea, abdominal pain, rash, and anaphylaxis.

30. Key drugs to inquire about include alcohol, gold compounds, mercury, phosphorus, anabolic steroids, acetaminophen, isoniazid, halothane, sulfonamides, arsenic, thiazide diuretics, zidovudine (azidothymidine or AZT), anticancer drugs such as methotrexate, oral contraceptives, anesthetic agents, and antipsychotics. These drugs may be hepatotoxic.

31. Ultrasonography
Informed Consent—No
Pretest Nursing Care—Explanation of test
Post-Test Nursing Care—None

32. Oral cholecystography
Informed Consent—No
Pretest Nursing Care—Assess client for allergy to iodine or seafood.
With regular or low-fat dinner, give ipodate sodium (Oragrafin sodium)
With high-fat diet, give iopanoic acid (Telepaque)
Post-Test Nursing Care—Encourage fluids.

33. Cholangiography
Informed Consent—Yes
Pretest Nursing Care—Assess for allergy to iodine or seafood.
Post-Test Nursing Care—Monitor for 24 hours for allergic reaction.
Encourage fluids (IV if client unable to take oral fluids).

34. Angiography
Informed Consent—Yes
Pretest Nursing Care—Explain procedure
NPO for 6–8 hours
NSAIDs or anticoagulants are usually avoided for one week prior to procedure.
Client will need to lie still during procedure.
There will be sensation of pressure during catheter placement.
Assess pulses distal to insertion site before procedure.
Post-Test Nursing Care—Assess insertion site for bleeding.
Assess pulses distal to insertion site.

35. Radionuclide scanning
Informed Consent—Not usually
Pretest Nursing Care—Explanation of test

Pregnancy and breast-feeding may be contraindications.
Post-Test Nursing Care—Monitor injection site
Avoid prolonged contact with client for 24–48 hours

36. Paracentesis
Informed Consent—Yes
Pretest Nursing Care—Explanation of test
Have client void prior to procedure.
Position client upright on side of bed with feet resting on a stool and back supported
Post-Test Nursing Care—Assess vital signs and peripheral circulation.
Observe for hypovolemic shock.
Assess for abdominal pain.
Assess insertion site.

37. Peritoneoscopy
Informed Consent—Yes
Pretest Nursing Care—Explanation of test
Assess for drug allergies.
Assess clotting lab values.
NPO
Empty bowel and bladder prior to procedure.
Assess client's ability to follow directions during procedure.
Explain that it may be difficult to breathe when air is placed in abdominal cavity.
Instruct client to hold breath at appropriate time.
Post-Test Nursing Care—Resume activities following recovery from medication effects.
Assess abdominal stab wound site.

38. Liver biopsy
Informed Consent—Yes
Pretest Nursing Care—Explanation of test
Check coagulation lab values.
Give presedation medication as ordered.
Instruct client to avoid anticoagulants, aspirin, or NSAIDs for 2 weeks prior to procedure.
NPO for 6 hours
Post-Test Nursing Care—Assess vital signs.
Assess puncture site.
Assess for pain in right upper quadrant of abdomen or right shoulder.
Right-side lying position for 2 hours.
At 2 hours postprocedure elevate head of bed (HOB) 30 degrees.
At 4 hours postprocedure raise HOB to 45 degrees.
Vitamin K as ordered
Assess respiratory status.

39. B

40. B
41. E
42. A or C
43. C
44. B
45. C
46. A
47. B
48. A
49.-54. Yes

CHAPTER 43: MANAGEMENT OF CLIENTS WITH THYROID AND PARATHYROID DISORDERS

1. Hypo
2. Hyper
3. Hyper
4. Hyper
5. Hyper
6. Hyper
7. Hyper
8. Hypo
9. Hypo
10. Hypo
11. Hyper
12. Hyper
13. Hyper
14. Hyper
15. If a person's diet lacks sufficient amounts of iodine or if the production of the thyroid hormone is suppressed, the thyroid gland enlarges to compensate for hormonal deficiency. Goiter with Graves' disease is due to hyperplasia and hypertrophy of the thyroid cells.
16. With hypothyroidism there is decreased heart rate and decreased stroke volume producing decreased cardiac output. Hyperlipidemia and hypercholesterolemia (present with hypothyroidism) can cause cardiac damage. With hyperthyroidism there is increased heart rate and stroke volume initially increasing cardiac output; however, congestive heart failure and hypertension (present with hyperthyroidism) can produce cardiac damage.
17. Nutrition, altered: More than body requirements R/T slowed metabolic rate. Provide a low- calorie nutritious diet. Hypothermia R/T slowed metabolic rate. Provide the client with a comfortable, warm environment and supply extra blankets if necessary.
18. Altered nutrition: Less than body requirements related to accelerated metabolic rate. Provide a well-balanced, high-calorie diet with supplemental vitamins, particularly B complex. Activity intolerance related to exhaustion secondary to accelerated metabolic rate. Provide a restful environment.
19. Normal saline, furosemide (Lasix)
20. C   Because she has an increased metabolic rate, she has an intolerance to activity and could become exhausted. It is a challenge to help hyperthyroid clients to relax. Preferably, she will need a private room.
21. B   If her exophthalmos was severe, she may need to have her eyes patched. Antibiotics are not indicated as this is not an infection.
22. A   An increased metabolic rate will increase pulse rate. In fact, one method of assessing the patient's response to therapy is to take a sleeping pulse rate. She will most likely be anxious about her surgery, but usually this will not cause a sustained tachycardia. Her thyroxine level will be increased but this will result in an increased B/P. Her increased metabolic rate and subsequent heat intolerance will cause her to drink more water.
23. D   Saturated solution of potassium iodide (SSKI) is given for about 10 days prior to surgery to reduce the size and vascularity of the thyroid gland to diminish the chance of hemorrhage.
24. C   All the other signs and symptoms are characteristic of hypothyroidism.
25. B   Oral suction is needed at first, as it may be difficult for her to swallow secretions. She will not have a nasogastric tube or a tracheostomy. She will have a neck dressing, but will not need a collar.
26. A   Because her parathyroid glands could have been removed during the surgery, she may develop tetany as a result of low serum calcium levels. Check for tingling around her mouth and in her fingertips, a hyperactive knee reflex, or positive Chvostek's or Trousseau's signs.

CHAPTER 44: MANAGEMENT OF CLIENTS WITH ADRENAL AND PITUITARY DISORDERS

1. Obtain identification bracelet, wallet card, and emergency kit for Ms. B. and impress on her that she must wear her bracelet and have the card and emergency kit with her at all times. The card should state that she takes hydrocortisone 30 mg, PO daily and that during an emergency, the drug must be given by injection. The kit should contain an injectable steroid in a prepared syringe with sterile alcohol wipes; written information that she has Addison's disease; takes hydrocortisone 30 mg, PO daily; who to notify in an emergency; and her physician's name and phone number. If her current

work-up results in a change in her medication, then this change would be made in her emergency kit.

2. sensitivity to cold, fatigue, weight gain

3. decreased sex drive

4. excessive thirst

5. constant swallowing, increased nasal congestion

6. stiff neck, persistent headache

Chapter 45: Management of Clients with Diabetes Mellitus

1. Check your food choices; percent of carbohydrates, protein, and fat; and total calories by referring to guidelines and nutrition text.

2.-21. You may ask your clinical instructor to check your answers while you are both with the client.

22. Insulin is destroyed by the gastric juices if given orally.

23. Only regular insulin

24. Decreases the amount of insulin that is needed

25. Yes; increases the need for insulin as stress increases the release of glucocorticosteroids, which raise blood glucose levels

26. Midmorning

27. Midmorning when the regular insulin peaks and then again midafternoon when the NPH insulin peaks

28. In the refrigerator except for the vials being used, which can be kept at room temperature for one month

29. No; because the regular insulin will peak about midmorning

30. U-100 syringe for U-100 insulin is most often used. If the client is resistant to insulin, then higher dosages will be required and U-500 syringe and U-500 insulin will be needed.

31. Intramuscularly

32. Glucagon raises blood glucose levels by stimulating glycogenolysis in the liver (converting glycogen to glucose).

33. They lower blood glucose levels by stimulating the beta cells in the pancreas to release insulin and by increasing the number of receptor sites for insulin in the tissues throughout the body. Some oral hypoglycemics also decrease glucose production in the liver (gluconeogenesis).

34. If regular insulin is given before breakfast at 7:30 AM, it will peak midmorning or about 10:00 AM and its duration will end by 1:30 PM. The NPH, given at 7:30 AM along with the regular insulin, will peak about midafternoon or about 3:30 PM and its

duration will end by about 11:30 PM. See Table 45-5 in the text.

Chapter 46: Management of Clients with Exocrine Pancreatic and Biliary Disorders

1. C

2. A

3. K

4. L

5. D

6. E

7. I

8. G

9. B

10. F

11. N

12. J

13. H

14. M

15. The location of the incision makes it painful to take deep breaths. Therefore, clients tend to "guard" and not take deep breaths, which increases the risk of lung congestion.

16. With the client who is NPO there is increased dryness of mucous membranes, decreased moisture, and increased risk of tissue breakdown.

17. Removes gastric juices that otherwise would stimulate cholecystokinin which stimulates the gallbladder to release bile. This stimulation will cause pain.

18. To ensure that the local anesthesia used on the back of the throat for insertion of the scope has worn off. Without a functioning gag reflex, fluids could cause choking and aspiration.

19. Fatty foods may precipitate an attack, as bile is needed for fat digestion, and the gallbladder's attempt to release it may result in painful colic.

20. Edematous distention of pancreatic capsule; local peritonitis due to enzyme release into peritoneum; and ductal spasm or pancreatic autodigestion stimulated by increased enzyme secretion while eating

21. Loss of fluid into the retroperitoneal space and decreased preload into the heart; release of kinins causes peripheral vasodilation and increased vascular permeability and toxemia

22. Decreases pancreatic stimulation and release of enzymes that will help decrease pain

23. Abdominal distention or ascites can cause restricted lung expansion.

24. These may stimulate pancreatic secretions and produce attacks of pancreatitis.

25. In a large percent of pancreatitis cases, the cause is related to alcohol intake.

26. The islet cells that produce insulin may be damaged.

27. The cells producing pancreatic enzymes may be damaged; therefore, exogenous enzymes may be necessary.

28. Contraindicated in pregnancy as it may be toxic to the fetal liver

29. B   Risk factors include aging, hormone replacement with estrogens, obesity, as well as being female and having multiple births.

30. C   As Ms. D. is having an exploration of the common bile duct, it is likely that she will have a T-tube.

31. A   A stone blocking the common bile duct will be the most likely cause of jaundice with gallbladder disease, as bile will not be able to be released in the duodenum, yet production and stimulation for release will continue.

32. C   Morphine may cause spasms of the sphincter of Oddi, which could increase pain rather than decrease it.

33. D   T-tube drainage should be measured and color noted every 8 hours. Additionally, care should be taken not to put tension on the tubing, and the tubing and drainage bag should be kept on the bed. The first day's volume would be expected to be 300–500 cc.

CHAPTER 47: MANAGEMENT OF CLIENTS WITH HEPATIC DISORDERS

1. H
2. E
3. D
4. B
5. J
6. C
7. K
8. A
9. I
10. F
11. G
12. L
13. D
14. C
15. A
16. E

17. B
18. B
19. C, possibly D and E
20. D, possibly E
21. A
22. C
23. D, possibly E
24. C, F
25. D
26. A
27. B, C, D
28. A, B, C, D
29. A
30. B
31. F
32. B, C, D
33. A
34. E
35. C, b, c
36. A, a, b, c
37. B, a, c, b (may be elevated or normal)

38. Tepid water, emollient baths, avoid alkaline soap, frequent applications of lotion, recommending loose-fitting clothing; per physician orders may administer antihistamines and/or cholestyramine.

39. The cause of portal hypertension is that damaged liver structure causes an obstruction to blood flow. The blood congests in the portal vein resulting in an increase in the portal vein pressure. The outcome of portal hypertension is esophageal varices with the potential for rupture and hemorrhage, enlarged spleen, internal hemorrhoids, and ascites.

40. Assess for bleeding gums, purpura, melena, hematuria, hematemesis, decreased blood pressure, increased pulse, decreased urine output, and changes in level of consciousness. Protect the client from falls and abrasions, give injections only if absolutely necessary, and use a small-gauge needle. Instruct the client to avoid vigorous blowing of nose, use a soft-bristle toothbrush and refrain from flossing, avoid straining with bowel movements, and avoid eating rough foods.

41. The three main causes of ascites are (1) portal hypertension; (2) decreased production of albumin to maintain plasma oncotic pressure; and (3) decreased circulating volume leads to increased release of aldosterone. Aldosterone increases sodium and water retention, which increases the fluid in the peritoneal cavity. The pathophysiologic bases are (1) portal hypertension is caused by

obstruction in the liver, causing increased hydrostatic pressure in the portal vein that leads to leakage of fluid into the peritoneal cavity; (2) the damaged liver is unable to synthesize normal amounts of albumin; and (3) with hepatocellular damage, aldosterone is not inactivated, thus sodium and water retention continue.

42. Ascites is assessed through daily weights, measuring abdominal girth, percussing dependent portions of the abdomen for dullness, and checking for fluid wave.

43. Hepatic encephalopathy is caused by the liver cells' inability to convert ammonia to glutamine and later urea for excretion. Ammonia levels in the blood rise. Ammonia is toxic to the CNS and affects CNS metabolism and function. Any process that increases protein in the GI tract (dietary or GI bleeding) can increase ammonia levels. Surgical procedures to reduce portal hypertension can also contribute to risk for hepatic encephalopathy.

44. Assess for hepatic encephalopathy by checking client's level of consciousness and orientation, having client write his or her name daily, assessing for development of asterixis, monitoring ammonia levels, and checking for GI bleeding.

45. Methods for reducing protein and bacteria, which support the breakdown of protein include reduce protein in the intestine, prevent GI bleeding, give neomycin and lactulose to reduce bacterial production of ammonia, eliminate fluid and electrolyte imbalances, prevent infection, and remove drugs that are hepatotoxic.

46. Care would include elevating the head of bed to high Fowler's position, closely monitoring respirations, turn, cough and deep breathe, and incentive spirometry or ultrasonic treatments as ordered.

47. Assess the client for increased enzymes; abnormal bilirubin, albumin, and clotting factors; increased temperature; tachycardia; malaise; hypertension; fluid retention; enlargement of the liver; and tenderness over the transplant site.

48. B If Mr. G. is in the active phase of hepatitis B, his serum will have HBsAg.

49. D Blood and body fluid precaution guidelines require that blood being sent to the lab for analysis be marked with special brightly colored labels noting blood and body fluid precautions.

50. B Current recommendations are for normal protein for tissue repair, high carbohydrates for energy and protein sparing, and low fat.

51. B Mr. G.'s activity would generally be "as tolerated," without becoming fatigued. Occasionally clients will push themselves too hard and activity precautions will be necessary.

52. B Verify the order with the physician as Compazine is a phenothiazine and is not recommended when the liver is inflamed or infected.

53. C It is very important to caution Mr. G. about alcohol and aspirin use because these are toxic to the liver.

UNIT 10: INTEGUMENTARY DISORDERS

1. Capillary
2. Sebaceous gland
3. Nerve endings
4. Hair follicle
5. Dermal papilla
6. Sweat gland
7. Fat
8. Blood vessels
9. As extension of blood vessels, provides metabolic skin requirements, thermoregulation
10. Production of sebum, disintegration of cells
11. Perception of heat and cold, pain, itching
12. Protection, cosmetic adornment
13. Connects dermis with epidermis, blood supply with a loop of capillary within papilla
14. Thermoregulation by perspiration
15. Energy storage and balance, trauma absorption
16. Provide metabolic skin requirements, thermoregulation

CHAPTER 48: ASSESSMENT OF THE INTEGUMENTARY SYSTEM

1. N
2. A
3. C
4. M
5. D
6. O
7. H
8. I
9. L
10. P
11. E
12. G
13. J
14. F
15. K
16. B
17. In a dark room, a light is used to look at skin.

18. The physician uses a scalpel to completely remove skin lesion or "sore"—a local anesthetic is given.

Chapter 49: Management of Clients with Integumentary Disorders

1. This will reduce discomfort and there will be no side effects.

2. Use of the medication needs to be discontinued if irritation occurs or inflammatory condition worsens or does not improve.

3. Use glove to avoid autoinoculation; wash after applying.

4. To be effective treatment must be started early, during prodromal stage.

5. Apply only to involved area; can produce irritation and erythema in normal skin.

6. To protect surfaces surrounding area to be treated and keep medicine in contact with skin to be treated. Also, a layer of petrolatum on the surrounding area will help protect that normal tissue.

7. Corticosteroids should be used in smallest amounts and lowest potency that is effective to avoid side effects.

8. The steroids can be absorbed systemically and side effects may result. As the skin disorder improves, the frequency of use may be changed or a less potent topical corticosteroid prescribed.

9. Intertriginous areas are erythematous skin eruptions occurring on opposed surfaces of the skin, such as the creases of the neck, folds of the groin and armpit, and beneath pendulous breasts. They are caused by moisture, warmth, friction, sweat retention, and infectious agents. Treatment consists of keeping the areas clean, dry, and separated if possible. Emollients are contraindicated as this would keep the areas moist.

10. Reapplication is necessary for continued protection.

11. Tar preparations have photosensitizing properties, making the person more likely to be sunburned with sun exposure.

12. Tar preparations cause staining.

13. Pruritus following treatment may be due to delayed hypersensitivity or may indicate treatment failure.

14. These can be highly toxic drugs if used excessively as they can be absorbed systemically; for example, they could cause aplastic anemia.

15. People with fair skin; sunburns easily; brown, red, or blond hair and gray/green or blue eyes; people with atypical nevi (dysplastic nevus syndrome); and those who have sustained major sunburns are at risk for developing skin cancer.

16. Clients who score between 12 and 16 on the Braden risk assessment scale are considered at risk. A score of 12 or less puts a client at high risk. The Braden scale considers sensory perception, moisture, activity, mobility, nutrition, and friction and shear. See Figure 49-9 in Chapter 49 of the text. Quadriplegic clients, elderly persons with femoral fractures, and clients in critical care have a higher prevalence.

17. Stasis dermatitis is the development of areas of very dry skin and sometimes shallow ulcers on the lower legs primarily due to venous insufficiency.

18. The elderly and clients with lowered resistance from diabetes, malnutrition, steroid therapy, and the presence of wounds and ulcers are at increased risk.

19. Predisposing factors include pregnancy; systemic use of antibiotics, birth control pills, or corticosteroids; malnutrition; diabetes; immunosuppressed conditions; and local environment of warmth and moisture.

20. Apply occlusives such as petrolatum or petrolatum with mineral oil or emollients evenly and smoothly immediately after bathing. Reapply when product has been absorbed or has worn off. Eliminate irritating or drying compounds such as soaps and solvents, and cleansing agents and moisturizers.

21. Tretinoin (Retin-A) has been found to be one of the most effective comedolytic agents; it reduces the size and number of comedones present and may inhibit sebum secretion.

22. The most common skin lesion in the elderly is actinic keratosis, which is also known as solar keratosis, and is an epithelial precancerous lesion. *Solar* and *actinic* refer to the induction of these lesions by sunlight. *Keratosis* means that the lesions often have excess keratin scale or horn on their surface.

23. The appearance of skin lesions may make the client feel "dirty" or untouchable. In addition, the smell of the tar preparations and their stains may add to the psychological reaction.

24. Herpes zoster, or shingles, is an infection caused by reactivation of the varicella virus in clients who have had chicken pox. Antiviral therapy (acyclovir or Zovirax) given in a large dose orally, or smaller doses IV five times a day, early in the course of the disease reduces acute pain and accelerates healing.

25. Stage III (See Figure 49-7 in Chapter 49 the text.)

26. Reposition client at least every 1 1/2 to 2 hours and never on the ulcer.

27. *Streptococcus pyogenes* is the usual cause of this infection; however, other pathogens may be responsible.

28. Lymphangitis may occur; if cellulitis is untreated, gangrene, metastatic abscesses, and sepsis result.

29. Malignant melanoma; basal cell carcinoma

30. Expectations should be realistic. Aesthetic surgery will improve appearance, but will not make someone "perfect." Reconstructive surgery will help make the abnormal part more normal in appearance and function, but may not make the part completely "normal."

31. Blisters (small blebs of serum) can shear the skin graft from the underlying wound and the blisters may need to be drained.

32. To support the client who has a changed body image (See Box 49-3 in Chapter 49 of the text for additional interventions.)

33. To minimize edema

34. Any sign of decreased vascularity (change in color or temperature, size, or tightness) must be reported immediately; therefore, the nurse needs to be able to observe the flap at all times. The flap should be relaxed and elevated because gravity promotes edema and venous congestion that impedes blood flow and oxygenation.

35. To avoid moving the pectoralis muscle and irritating the surgical site

36. Although complications following blepharoplasty (surgical removal of excessive tissue from the upper or lower eyelid) are rare, bleeding behind the eye may occur. The earliest indications are increasing eye pain and diminishing vision caused by increasing intraorbital pressure. Mannitol may be ordered to increase blood osmolarity and draw fluid from the eye.

37. Abdominoplasty is an abdominal operation in which repairs are made on separated rectus abdominis muscles, for example, umbilical hernia, and is therefore uncomfortable. Adequate analgesia and other pain-relieving measures are needed.

38. The blink reflex may be slower for a few days and the cornea needs to be kept moist.

39. These baseline data are critical to assess postoperative changes. An ophthalmologist may need to examine the client before surgery if vision problems are noted in the preoperative assessment.

40. Clients with autoimmune disorders are not candidates for collagen injection and some clients have induration (swelling, hardness) at the injection site.

41. Digits will remain viable if oxygen saturation remains above 95%.

42. Postoperatively, the nurse needs to assess for bleeding. While the client is sleepy from the anesthetic, excessive swallowing may be the only sign of bleeding. Examine the back of the throat with a flashlight to look for blood. Some bleeding is normal down the back of the throat and on the nasal packs and dressings.

43. To prevent disruption/dislocation of repaired nasal bones and cartilage

44. If airway problems develop that cannot be managed by suction, cut two wires on each side of the mouth to free the upper and lower jaws.

45. Moisture allows bacteria to enter the wound along the sutures. Infected incisions tend to produce more scar tissue.

46. To reduce blood-clotting tendencies

47. A woman with a subpectoral implant does not wear a bra immediately postoperatively because the implant needs to move into the pocket created in the chest wall.

48. Oral care aids in healing oral wounds, prevents infection and destruction of teeth and gums, increases comfort, and enhances self-esteem.

49. A reimplanted part may have blocked arterial or venous blood flow, which, if it is not immediately corrected surgically, will cause the part to die.

CHAPTER 50: MANAGEMENT OF CLIENTS WITH BURN INJURY

1. (1) Thermal burns caused by flame, hot liquids, steam, or hot substances or objects; (2) chemical burns caused by strong acids, alkalis, or organic compounds; (3) electrical burns caused by electrical energy; and (4) radiation burns caused by a radioactive source.

2. Teach residential burn injury prevention (see Box 50-1 in the text).

3. Burn depth, burn size, burn location, age, general health, and mechanism of injury

4. Partial-thickness burn, first degree: epidermis remains intact and without blisters, skin is erythematous and blanches with pressure; Partial-thickness burn, second degree: surface is wet, shiny, and weeping with blisters and blanches with pressure; Full-thickness burn, third degree: surface is dry with thrombosed vessels, color is variable and there is no blanching; Full-thickness burn, fourth degree: charring in deepest areas with variable color and if the extremity is the burned part extremity movement is limited

5. Partial-thickness burn, first degree: painful; Partial-thickness burn, second degree: painful and very sensitive to touch and air currents; Full-thickness burn, third degree: decreased pinprick sensation and not painful; Full-thickness burn, fourth degree: no sensation (Remember that one burn injury may

have varying degrees of injury depth, so sensation may vary accordingly.)

6. (1) Superficial burns: within 3–7 days the injured epithelial cell layers peel away, exposing new epithelium; (2) uncomplicated superficial partial-thickness burns: heal within 14–21 days with minimal scarring; deep partial-thickness burns: may take 3–4 weeks to heal with resulting epithelium easy to injure; (3) full-thickness burns: require excision and autografting for healing; (4) fourth-degree burns: amputation of injured extremity often necessary.

7. Any finding indicative of poor perfusion needs to be reported to the physician. An escharotomy may be necessary to alleviate circulatory compromise due to circumferential burns, which is more likely to occur during the resuscitation period when fluid shifts into the interstitial tissues. Check the unburned skin that is close to the burned area by palpation.

8. Burns of the head, neck, and chest

9. Burns of the ears and perineal area

10. Children younger than 4 years and clients older than 65 years

11. In electrical burn injuries, heat is generated as the electricity travels through the body, resulting in internal tissue damage. The risk of renal failure is increased as myoglobin from injured muscle tissue precipitates in the renal tubules. Alternating current (AC) injuries are often associated with cardiopulmonary arrest, ventricular fibrillation, tetanic muscle contractures, and long-bone or vertebral compression fractures.

12. (1) Stop the burning; (2) assess airway, breathing, and circulation and begin cardiopulmonary resuscitation if necessary; (3) conserve body heat; (4) minimize wound contamination; (5) transport the person quickly

13. To facilitate immediate treatment

14. Restlessness and/or excitement, altered level of consciousness, decreased blood pressure, increased pulse, cyanosis, and oliguria

15. Immediate fluid resuscitation to obtain urine output of 30–50 ml per hour, clear sensorium, pulse rate < 120 per minute without dysrhythmias, and blood pressure within expected range for age and medical history

16. An escharotomy is a lengthwise incision through eschar (dead tissue resulting from coagulation necrosis). This is done to relieve the constriction in circulation in an area with a circumferential burn.

17. Control localized infection with vigilant monitoring for clinical manifestations of impending sepsis, maintain a clean environment to reduce the reservoir of microorganisms, use aseptic techniques for all invasive procedures and wound care, and administer prescribed antimicrobial agents in a timely fashion, and use universal precautions and specific infection-control practices for burned clients (use of gloves, caps, masks, shoe covers, scrub clothes, and plastic aprons, as needed). Strict hand-washing is essential! Assigning one team to care for one group of patients throughout the care period has decreased infection rates.

18. While the client is acutely ill, all medications, except tetanus toxoid, are administered IV to avoid the medication pooling in the tissues when capillaries are damaged and permeability is increased, because later this medication could flood the vascular system with the return of capillary integrity. As the client recovers, pain medication may be given orally.

19. In burned clients the basal metabolic rates may be 40–100% higher than normal levels, depending on the extent of the burn. Glucose metabolism is altered resulting in hyperglycemia. See Table 50-4 in the text for energy calculation formulas used for the burn-injured adult.

20. Usually 12–18 months continuously except during bathing

21. Using the Rule of Nines: 9% for each upper extremity and 5% for face = 23%. Using the chart: 7% partial-thickness burn for the face, 4% partial-thickness burn for each upper arm, 3% partial-thickness burn for each lower arm, and 2 1/2% full-thickness burn for each hand = 26%.

22. B   The primary goal during the emergent phase is to prevent hypovolemic shock and to preserve vital organ functioning.

23. A   The cream should be applied using a gloved hand at a thickness of 1/16 of an inch (approximately the width of a nickel) or using mesh gauze impregnated with the prescribed cream.

24. C   The fine-mesh gauze is allowed to dry often assisted by radiant heat lamps. Once new epithelium forms beneath the gauze, the gauze is gently lifted and trimmed away. Other types of dressings may be covered with compression dressings usually left in place for 48 hours.

25. B   The hemoglobin will be decreased due to hemolysis. The other lab values will be increased: the hematocrit due to fluid shifts from the intravascular space, the serum potassium due to cell lysis and fluid shifts into the interstitial spaces, and the BUN due to the hypovolemic state.

26. B   The pain medication needs to be given 30 minutes before the procedure so the client will have analgesia during the procedure (which could be painful).

UNIT 11: CIRCULATORY DISORDERS

1. Away from
2. Artery intima
3. Venous
4. Capillaries
5. Interstitial; fat
6. Tonsils
7. Thoracic
8. H
9. D
10. C
11. B
12. G
13. E
14. F
15. A
16. B
17. A
18. B
19. A
20. A
21. B
22. A
23. B
24. A
25. D
26. I
27. D
28. I
29. D
30. I
31. I
32. D
33. D
34. *Arteriosclerosis* is characterized by loss of elasticity, thickening, and calcification of arterial walls. *Atherosclerosis* is characterized by fatty plaque deposits in the artery that decrease its diameter.
35. Both are processes that develop over time and affect every body system.
36. Vasodilators decrease blood pressure and vasoconstrictors increase blood pressure.

CHAPTER 51: ASSESSMENT OF THE VASCULAR SYSTEM

1. J
2. C
3. D

4. F
5. E
6. G
7. I
8. A
9. B
10. H
11. B
12. B
13. A
14. B
15. A
16. B
17. B
18. B
19. A
20. Purpose: diagnose and evaluate deep vein thrombosis (DVT). Explain purpose of test. Explain the procedure and the possibility of minimal discomfort during cuff inflation.
21. Evaluate patency of peripheral arteries. Invasive test, informed consent required. Similar to heart cath. Performed in cath lab. Explain procedure. Obtain signature on informed consent. NPO. Iodine allergies. Baseline peripheral vascular checks. Monitor renal function.
22. Similar to heart cath. Monitor pressure dressing. Bed rest for two hours. Vital signs q15 X 1h then qh X 8. Peripheral vascular checks as indicated. Hydration to excrete dye. Monitor intake and output.
23. Past medical history, current medications, family history
24. Type of diet, weight
25. No pertinent data
26. Exercise pattern, occupation, daily activities, how the illness has affected ADLs
27. Changes in sleep patterns
28. Pain analysis
29. How the illness or condition affects how the person feels about him- or herself
30. Occupation: for risk factors
31. Obstetric history (if applies), problems with sexual functioning
32. Normal coping patterns
33. Any religious belief or practice that could affect disorder or treatment
34. Peripheral vascular disorders often present with very specific pain patterns

35. Arterial disorders reveal changes in quality of the pulses and circulation. Venous disorders, unless edema is present, do not alter the pulses.

36. Arterial disorders will appear pale with dependent cyanosis. Venous disorders will have brown discoloration and dependent cyanosis.

37. Arterial disorders will have cool skin. Venous disorders: no change or warm

38. Arterial: decreased sensations and numbness and tingling. Venous: no change

39. Can be affected by either disorder. Usually arterial causes the most changes

40. Arterial: no changes. Venous: causes edema.

41. Slow capillary refill, nail changes, and trauma correlate with arterial disorders.

CHAPTER 52: CLIENTS WITH HYPERTENSIVE DISORDERS: PROMOTING POSITIVE OUTCOMES

1. D
2. B
3. B
4. C
5. D
6. C
7. C
8. A
9. Monitor fluid loss.
10. Diuretics can cause rapid fluid loss.
11. Frequent trips to bathroom would interfere with sleep.
12. Sodium and potassium are excreted in urine.
13. Beta blockers decrease pulse.
14. Normal CNS stimulation to dilate bronchioles is blocked.
15. CNS stimulation is similar to the clinical manifestations of hypoglycemia. Beta blockers block the mechanism to increase the blood glucose.
16. The normal decrease in B/P upon arising is potentiated.
17. May exacerbate myocardial ischemia.
18. Detects renal damage.
19. Side effect of the medication that may alter eating habits.
20. Rapid onset of the medication.
21. Drug action is potentiated by alcohol, sedatives, digitalis, and propranolol.
22. Decreases the effect of insulin.
23. The client has isolated systolic hypertension. His systolic reading is more than 140 mm Hg and his diastolic is less than 90 mm Hg.

24. His classification according to Table 52-2 would be systolic hypertension stage 3 (severe).
25. Risk factors: age 72 years; race: black; overweight.
26. Recheck within 2 months
27. Step 1 is lifestyle modifications: weight reduction, moderation of alcohol intake, regular physical activity, reduction of sodium intake, and cessation of smoking.

CHAPTER 53: MANAGEMENT OF CLIENTS WITH VASCULAR DISORDERS

1. F
2. G
3. A
4. E
5. D
6. B
7. A
8. D
9. H
10. B
11. F
12. E
13. C
14. G
15. D
16. C
17. C
18. B
19. A
20. B
21. A
22. C
23. B
24. Decrease risk of increasing size, reduce the risk of dislodging, and allow normal body phagocytosis to eliminate the DVT.
25. Reduce venous congestion.
26. Decrease pain, increase blood supply to area.
27. Prevent future thrombus formation.
28. Passive debridement
29. Permeable dressing that contains medications to enhance healing and provides compression to reduce venous congestion
30. B
31. A
32. B
33. A

34. B
35. B
36. A
37. B
38. B
39. B
40. A
41. A
42. I
43. D
44. I
45. D
46. D
47. I
48. At risk for hemorrhage: Large vessels are severed and sutured closed.
49. Reduces edema
50. Increases risk of hip contracture
51. Prevent hip contracture, stimulate circulation to stump.
52. Prevents contracture
53. Pain or sensations in the amputated limb thought to be related to severing the nerve endings in the amputated limb. These are normal sensations and can occur for up to 2 years.
54. Signs of infection
55. Monitor for infection or skin lesions.
56. Dries the skin
57. Prevents stump edema
58. Moisture damages prosthesis
59. Arterial insufficiency is inadequate blood flow in the peripheral arteries caused by atherosclerosis, emboli, aneurysms, or hypercoagulability states. Venous insufficiency is a decreased blood return to the heart from the legs.
60. Raynaud's syndrome is a condition in which the small arteries and arterioles constrict in response to various stimuli.
61. Fibrinolytic medications dissolve thrombi by stimulating the conversion of plasminogen to plasmin, an enzyme that decomposes fibrin.
62. Primary lymphedema is classified according to age at onset. Lymphedema praecox (onset before age 35) is the most common form. The cause is unknown. Secondary lymphedema occurs because of some damage or obstruction to the lymph system.
63. Ms. N. was susceptible for the development of deep vein thrombosis for several reasons. She had been without fluids since 10 PM; dehydration can precipitate hypercoagulability. She was immobile

with a long leg cast, and the leg cuff during surgery impeded circulation and could have traumatized the vein.
64. D
65. C
66. 7.5 mL per hour
67. No
68. 1000 units of heparin
69. B
70. D
71. A dissecting aneurysm is a bilateral pouching of the aorta. The layers of the vessel wall separate. The 7 cm refers to the diameter of the aneurysm. An abdominal aortic aneurysm measuring 6 cm or more has a 20% chance of rupturing in one year.
72. Hypertension and atherosclerosis
73. Symptomatic, CT revealed a 7-cm aneurysm
74. Vital signs stable, dressing dry, minimal drainage, hemoglobin and hematocrit stable, urine output greater than 30 mL/hour, and hemodynamic parameters within normal limits.
75. Pulse oximeter greater than 95%, effective cough, lung sounds clear bilaterally, respirations 12–20 per minute, color pink.
76. The "8 Ps" of peripheral vascular circulation: pedal pulses strong, color pink, capillary refill less than 5 seconds, skin warm, no edema, absence of numbness and tingling and pain in extremities
77. Bowel sounds present, no abdominal distention, no diarrhea or sudden abdominal pain, and no sudden increase in white blood cell count.
78. Verbalizes less pain, use of decreasing amounts of pain medication, and ambulating and coughing without complaints of extreme pain.
79. Increased blood pressure causes increased pressure on the graft site, which could cause bleeding or rupture at the graft site.

UNIT 12: CARDIAC DISORDERS

1. B
2. C
3. A
4. Epicardium
5. Myocardium
6. Endocardium
7. Pericardium
8. Oxygenated, lungs, systemic
9. Deoxygenated, body, lungs, pulmonary arteries
10. Semilunar (aortic and pulmonic)
11. Atrioventricular (A/V) (mitral and tricuspid)

12. Systole, diastole
13. H
14. C
15. A
16. B
17. D
18. E
19. G
20. F
21. H
22. J
23. I
24. G
25. F
26. A
27. C
28. B
29. D
30. E
31. I
32. I
33. I
34. D
35. D
36. D
37. D
38. I
39. Carry oxygenated blood and nutrients to the cells and to collect deoxygenated blood and waste products from the cells
40. Heart rate, blood volume
41. The more the left ventricle fills and stretches the greater the contraction of the left ventricle
42. Arteries lose their elasticity. Coronary arteries become rigid, thick, and the heart enlarges and chambers dilate and have less contractility. Heart valves become thickened. The conduction system loses pacemaker cells, and conduction abnormalities can occur.
43. Refer to Figure U12-2.

CHAPTER 54: ASSESSMENT OF THE CARDIAC SYSTEM

1. Health Perception–Health Management
   Chief complaint, past medical history, risk factors for coronary artery disease, family history of cardiovascular disorders, current medications, health promotion activities, smoking
2. Nutrition–Metabolic
   Diet history: high sodium, high fat, high calorie, changes in eating habits or digestion, ability to purchase and prepare food
3. Elimination
   Normal elimination, changes in patterns
4. Activity–Exercise
   Typical activities, any activity intolerance, fatigue, type of work, any chest pain, shortness of breath, palpitations
5. Sleep–Rest
   Changes in sleep patterns, how many pillows, any awakenings during the night
6. Cognitive–Perceptual
   Chest pain symptom analysis
7. Self-Perception–Self-Concept
   Body image: risk for depression
8. Role–Relationship
   Roles and responsibilities, possible sources of stress
9. Sexuality–Reproductive
   Sexual activity
10. Coping–Stress Tolerance
    Any stressful life events in past 6 months, normal coping pattern
11. Values–Beliefs
    Any religious or cultural practices that influence health practices
12. Signs of significant cyanosis or pallor, the client's ability to answer questions without fatigue or dyspnea, mental functioning/adequacy of cerebral perfusion
13. Changes in cardiac output
14. Changes in rate, rhythm, amplitude
15. Signs and symptoms of congestive heart failure
16. Signs and symptoms of right congestive heart failure
17. Signs and symptoms of right congestive heart failure
18. Displaced PMI indicates enlarged heart
19. Yields information about normal and abnormal heart rate, ventricular filling, and blood flow across the heart valves
20. Signs and symptoms of right congestive heart failure
21. Signs and symptoms of right congestive heart failure
22. Erythrocytes decrease in rheumatic fever and infective endocarditis and increase in heart disease characterized by inadequate oxygenation. Hematocrit increases in hypovolemia and decreases in blood loss and anemia.

White blood cell count (WBC) is elevated with infections, inflammatory disease, and myocardial infarction

23. <u>CK</u>: Increase indicates myocardial tissue damage, especially myocardial infarction.
    <u>CK-MB</u>: specific CK isoenzyme indicates myocardial tissue damage.
    <u>LDH_1 and LDH_2</u> are cardiac cardiac-specific isoenzyme of LDH. LDH_1 is normally higher than LDH_2. A "flipped" LDH_1 and LDH_2 means the LDH_2 is higher than LDH_1 indicating myocardial necrosis.
    <u>Troponin I & T</u> elevations are very specific indicators of myocardial damage.

24. Examines the blood's ability to clot.

25. Serum lipids play a major role in the development of atherosclerosis.

26. Cardiac effects with changes in potassium, calcium, magnesium levels; sodium reflects water balance; blood urea nitrogen (BUN) tests renal function

27. Diabetes mellitus is a major risk factor in the development of atherosclerosis.

28. No; skin irritation

29. No; monitors heart rhythm for 24 hours while the client is engaging in normal activities of daily living (ADLs); keeping a diary will help to correlate signs and symptoms, activity, and cardiac rhythm.

30. Yes; to compare any changes that occur during the test; exercise causes an increased demand on the heart that could cause angina or a myocardial infarction.

31. Yes; decrease the risk of dislodging the clot formation at the puncture site

32. Yes; iodine-based contrast dye is used to establish a baseline for postprocedure neurovascular checks, possible delayed allergic reaction to the dye.

33. Magnetic force would attract any metal object, the part of the body containing metal could be damaged; eyeglasses or clothing could be damaged

34. B/P: I, D, D
    Pulse: D, I, I

35. Postural hypotension: a drop of more than 10–15 mm Hg systolic and more than 10 mm Hg diastolic. Typically there is a 10–20% increase in heart rate.

36. H
37. A
38. C
39. G
40. F

41. E
42. D
43. B
44. B
45. A
46. A
47. B
48. A
49. B
50. Chest pain, shortness of breath, syncope, fatigue
51. Symptom analysis of the chest pain: onset, location, duration, characteristics, aggravating factors, associated factors, alleviating factors
52. Smoking, lack of exercise, high-fat diet
53. Fluid overload or increased pressure and volume in the right atrium
54. *Timing:* where it occurs in the cardiac cycle
    Quality: describe the sound
    Pitch: high pitch—best heard with diaphragm, or low pitch—best heard with bell
    Location: where it is heard the loudest
    Radiation: Is the sound transmitted in the direction of the blood flow?
    Upstream equals regurgitant murmurs, downstream equals stenotic murmurs
    Configuration: the shape of the sound
    Intensity: the loudness of the murmur on a scale of 1–6
55. I
56. D
57. D
58. I
59. I
60. I
61. D
62. I

CHAPTER 55: MANAGEMENT OF CLIENTS WITH STRUCTURAL CARDIAC DISORDERS

1. A
2. B
3. A
4. B
5. A
6. B
7. B
8. A
9. B

10. A

11. B

12. A

13. A

14. C

15. A

16. B

17. C

18. A

19. B

20. C

21. C

22. C

23. A

24. A

25. E

26. C

27. A

28. B

29. C

30. A

31. E

32. D

33. B

34. B

35. A

36. B

37. A

38. Risk for peripheral emboli

39. Indicator of cardiac output

40. Monitor fluid volume status.

41. Hypothermia decreases drug metabolism and excretion. Medications will stay in circulation longer than normal.

42. Improves orientation

43. Stimulates circulation and decreases the risk of deep vein thrombosis

44. Universal precautions: decreases the spread of infection

45. Monitor changes in heart rate and rhythm.

46. Indicator of cardiac output: a decrease in B/P decreases tissue perfusion, an increase will increase the cardiac workload and possibly damage the surgery.

47. Cardiac output: a gallop indicates hypervolemia, a new murmur indicates myocardial ischemia, hypervolemia, and problems with the valves.

Distant or muffled heart sounds could indicate cardiac tamponade.

48. Monitor for hemorrhage. There should be a progressive decrease in the amount of blood (100 ml first hour; 500 ml first 24 hours) and change in color (dark-red to serous).

49. A

50. A

51. *Risk for Decreased Cardiac Output:* Vital signs stable and within normal limits for client, urine output > 30 mL/h, heart sounds regular, lung sounds clear, alert and oriented

52. *Risk for Cardiac Tamponade:* Heart sounds audible, regular rate and rhythm, progressive decrease in chest tube drainage, no water-hammer peripheral pulses, hemodynamic pressures within normal limits

53. *Risk for Paralytic Ileus:* Bowel sounds 3–35 per minute in all four quadrants, passing flatus via rectum, no complaints of nausea or vomiting, abdomen soft

54. *Pain:* Verbalizes a decrease in pain, progressive decrease in amount of pain medication, progressive increase in the time between pain medication, vital signs stable and within normal limits for client, ambulates and performs ADLs

55. The predisposing factors that are present in this situation are crowded living conditions, urban slum, and the client's age.

56. The major clinical manifestations are polyarthritis and subcutaneous nodules. The minor clinical manifestations are fever, arthralgia, and leukocytosis.

57. Bed rest is prescribed for the client with rheumatic fever in an attempt to reduce cardiac workload until evident that the inflammation has subsided.

58. Eight-year-olds enjoy simple games, toys, coloring, and puzzles. Complete an assessment of the child's play habits. Provide simple books from the library. Provide cards, simple games, playing cards, and coloring books.

59. Inflammation has subsided. No cardiovascular symptoms: resting HR > 90, no complaints of chest pain, no ECG changes.

60. Antibiotics are prescribed to eradicate the streptococcal infection that usually exists in clients with acute rheumatic fever. The steroids are used to treat existing carditis.

61. Activity intolerance

62. Valvular disease, cardiomegaly, and congestive heart failure

CHAPTER 56: MANAGEMENT OF CLIENTS WITH FUNCTIONAL CARDIAC DISORDERS

1. N
2. N
3. N
4. CF
5. M
6. N
7. M
8. M
9. M
10. CF
11. CF
12. 4
13. 1
14. 6
15. 3
16. 2
17. 7
18. 5
19. Class III
20. A
21. B
22. B
23. A
24. B
25. B
26. A
27. B
28. Digoxin decreases the heart rate and is contraindicated if the apical heart rate is less than 60.
29. Low potassium levels increase myocardial sensitivity to digoxin. The digoxin level must be within therapeutic range or below.
30. Signs and symptoms of digoxin toxicity
31. Usually first the sign and symptom of digoxin toxicity
32. Lasix is a loop diuretic that depletes potassium.
33. To evaluate the effectiveness of the drug—clients gain water weight with congestive heart failure.
34. C
35. A
36. B
37. B
38. B, C
39. A
40. B
41. B
42. D
43. B
44. D
45. C
46. A
47. B
48. C

CHAPTER 57: MANAGEMENT OF CLIENTS WITH DYSRHYTHMIAS ANSWERS

1. 60–100 BPM
2. 40–60 BPM
3. 20–40 BPM
4. 8
5. 2
6. 1
7. 4
8. 3
9. 6
10. 5
11. 7
12. A
13. B
14. C
15. F
16. D
17. E
18. B
19. C
20. A
21. B
22. C
23. A
24. B
25. F
26. A
27. C
28. E
29. H
30. G
31. D
32. B
33. C
34. D
35. A
36. D
37. G

38. B
39. C
40. A
41. E
42. F
43. Signs and symptoms of infection
44. Monitor pacemaker set rate.
45. In case of emergency
46. Pacemaker will trigger alarm.
47. Displace pacemaker wires.
48. Damage the pacemaker or the wires, displace the pacer wires.
49. Compare to a standard and client's baseline.
50. No signs and symptoms of alterations in cardiac output, compare evaluation criteria to standard (therapeutic effect) for type of medication (if indicated).
51. Temperature within normal limits for client, lungs sound clear, regular heart sounds, no S_3 or S_4, vital signs stable
52. Compare laboratory values to baseline values and a standard.
53. Monitor intake and output, diet consumption, consult with dietitian as indicated.
54. Monitor intake and output, voiding and bowel movement patterns.
55. Monitor progression of activities and compare with ADLs prior to admission.
56. Daily mental status screening. Compare with admission baseline data. Consult with family members for normal mental status for client.
57. Consult with client, family, physician, case manager, and/or social worker to determine what type of services are needed; delegate the actual referral to appropriate members of health care team.
58. Client and family's verbal response and/or return demonstration
59. Interview with client's family or significant others and monitor appropriateness of nonverbal communication.
60. Normal sinus rhythm (NSR)
61. Ventricular tachycardia (VT)
62. Controlled atrial fibrillation (CAF)
63. Sinus rhythm (SR) with premature atrial contractions (PACs)
64. Sinus rhythm with premature ventricular contraction (PVC)
65. Atrial flutter (AF)
66. Sinus tachycardia (ST)

CHAPTER 58: MANAGEMENT OF CLIENTS WITH MYOCARDIAL INFARCTION

1. C
2. D
3. E
4. F
5. G
6. A
7. B
8. NTG is a vasodilator that can increase circulation to the cardiac muscle
9. Light decreases the potency of the medication
10. Vasodilation causes a decrease in the blood pressure
11. Beta-blockers prevent bronchodilation
12. Calcium channel blockers slow the conduction/depolarization
13. A
14. B
15. B
16. B
17. B
18. B
19. 4
20. 1
21. 2
22. 3
23. Diagram
24. Troponin I and CK-MB
25. There is an elevation of the WBCs secondary to inflammation and tissue necrosis.
26. Decreases mortality by 23%; limits thrombus formation and progression.
27. Relieving the chest pain; medication of choice is morphine.
28. Morphine relieves pain and decreases cardiac workload.
29. Heparin limits thrombus formation and progression.
30. Nitroglycerin is a coronary and systemic vasodilator. It improves circulation to the heart muscle.
31. Oxygen is used to treat hypoxia and improve oxygenation of the heart muscle.
32. Thrombolytic therapy lyses the clot that forms part of the blockage of the coronary artery.

UNIT 13: OXYGENATION DISORDERS

1. C

2.   A

3.   B

4.   C

5.   C

6.   B

7.   B

8.   A

9.   A and B

10. B

11. A

12. B

13. B

14. B

15. B

16. C

17. C

18. A

19. B

20. B

21. C

22. B

23. B

24. B

25. G

26. E

27. D

28. B

29. C

30. A

31. H

32. F

33. B

34. A

35. C

36. B

37. C

38. A

39. B

40. A

41. Lower

42. Cilia, upper, infections

43. Rounder, air spaces

44. Emphysema, function, infection

45. Causes the two membranes to adhere, creating a pulling force

46. Diffusion is the movement from high concentration to low concentration. It moves oxygen into the capillary bed and carbon dioxide into the alveoli.

47. During inspiration intrathoracic pressure is lower than atmospheric pressure. During exhalation intrathoracic pressure is higher than atmospheric pressure.

48. The sneeze reflex is a protective mechanism of the nose to clear the upper airway. The cough reflex is a protective mechanism to clear the trachea and prevent aspiration of particles into the lower airway.

49. The sneeze and cough reflex, the mucociliary system, the inflammatory response

50. Ventilation: mucous plug atelectasis
     Perfusion: cardiac output and pulmonary embolus

51. Large bronchi: 30 minutes; bronchial tree: 2.5 hours; peripheral airway: 5.6 hours

CHAPTER 59: ASSESSMENT OF THE RESPIRATORY SYSTEM

1.   B

2.   D

3.   C

4.   E

5.   A

6.   J

7.   I

8.   H

9.   G

10. E

11. B

12. D

13. E

14. D

15. A

16. E

17. F

18. C

19. D

20. D

21. F

22. B

23. D

24. E

25. A

26. A

27. C

28. B

29. D

30. E

31. C
32. H
33. F
34. A
35. B
36. D
37. B
38. *Health perception–health management risk:* Assessment, history of respiratory problems, precipitates respiratory signs and symptoms, increases risk, slows cilia and depresses cough reflex, health promotion, prescribed and over-the-counter, identify teaching needs
39. *Nutrition–Metabolic:* Diet analysis, some respiratory diseases cause anorexia and weight loss
40. *Activity–Exercise:* Major signs and symptoms of respiratory problems
41. *Sleep–Rest:* Identify possible respiratory problems
42. *Cognitive–Perceptual:* Gas exchange
43. *Role–Relationship:* Risk for respiratory problems: working environment, type of work, living conditions, health status of household members, hazards
44. Respiratory pattern, rate and quality, ancillary muscles
45. Color changes correlate with oxygenation, especially face and lips
46. Evaluates smell
47. Chest size and contour, AP-transverse ratio 1:2
48. Color, capillary refill, clubbing indicates chronic hypoxia
49. *Sinus:* upper respiratory problems/sinus congestion; *Trachea:* chest mass, goiter, or acute injury displaces trachea; *Chest wall:* tenderness, fremitus, thoracic or chest expansion
50. Normal sounds and tone
51. Tactile fremitus, tenderness, crepitus, thoracic excursion (chest expansion)
52. Normal and adventitious sounds and voice transmission
53. *Arterial Blood Gases (ABGs):* Directly measures serum oxygen, carbon dioxide, and pH. No; circulation to hand; arterial puncture takes longer to clot.
54. *Pulmonary Function Tests (PFTs):* Measures lung volume and mechanics, and diffusion capabilities of lungs. No, but may vary with institution; accurate results depend on quality of inhalation and exhalation; interferes with test results: smoking can decrease and bronchodilators can increase.
55. *Chest X-Ray:* Illustrates anatomy and structure of chest. No; interferes with accurate x-ray

56. *Pulse Oximeter:* Noninvasive test for assessing oxygenation. No; inaccurate reading
57. *Lung Scan:* Evaluates ventilation and perfusion. Yes; test takes 30–60 minutes and is usually done in the supine position but can be done in other positions to decrease anxiety and increase compliance to test; a noniodine-based dye is used.
58. *Bronchoscopy:* Direct visualization, fluid and tissue specimens, and removal of foreign bodies or thick secretions. Yes; risk of aspiration; evaluates gag reflex, pharyngeal movement, and swallowing
59. *Sputum:* Assessment for bacteria, fungus, or cellular elements. No; decreases contamination from oral cavity; most accurate results; direct method: client coughs up sputum; indirect: sputum obtained by suctioning
60. *Thoracentesis:* Draining fluid and/or air from the pleural space and analysis for specific gravity, glucose, protein, pH, culture, sensitivity, and cytology. Yes; pleural fluid accumulates in the base of the thorax; higher concentration of peripheral nerve endings in thorax; minimizes the risk of pneumothorax, lung expansion, monitor for signs and symptoms of respiratory distress and pneumothorax, fluid is considered output.

CHAPTER 60: MANAGEMENT OF CLIENTS WITH UPPER AIRWAY DISORDERS

1. B
2. A
3. F
4. E
5. B
6. C
7. Blood is swallowed
8. Decreases the risk of aspiration; facilitates drainage
9. Hemorrhage is a complication
10. Spicy foods irritate the traumatized mucosa; soft foods easier to swallow
11. Decrease secretions from allergic response
12. Could cause rhinitis medicamentosa
13. Possibly a sinus infection
14. GERD (gastroesophageal reflux disorder) can be the cause
15. Reduce stress on inflamed larynx.
16. Voice abuse can cause laryngitis.
17. Reduce nasal edema and pressure.
18. Decreases trauma; eliminates the need for constant wiping
19. Increases pressure and traumatizes suture lines
20. Decreases pressure

21. Liquefies secretions
22. Tracheostomy, endotracheal tube insertion, cancer of the larynx, sleep apnea
23. Flange, pilot tube, open
24. Obturator
25. Tracheal necrosis, stenosis, airway obstruction
26. Tract or opening, ventilation, oxygenation
27. Deflating, plugging, breath
28. Cough, bypassed, liquefy
29. Heart rate, skin
30. Valsalva maneuver
31. Verbal communication
32. B
33. B
34. A
35. D
36. C
37. A
38. A
39. C
40. A
41. B
42. B
43. A
44. B
45. B
46. C
47. D
48. A
49. B
50. A
51. Smoking, alcohol, occupation
52. Hoarseness, difficulty swallowing, weight loss
53. Explain that the additional tests are to evaluate his health status and possible metastasis.
54. T_3 tumor: primary tumor less than 2 cm, N_2: single positive node, M_0: no metastasis present
55. Cancer has spread to lymph nodes.
56. Obstruction, hemorrhage, carotid artery rupture, fistula formation
57. *Risk for aspiration:* Semi- or high-Fowler's position, keep tracheostomy tube cuffed, suction as needed.
58. *Ineffective airway clearance:* Encourage coughing and deep breathing, respiratory assessment, vital signs
59. *Risk for impaired gas exchange:* Assess oxygenation with ABGs and pulse oximeter, maintain oxygen at prescribed rate, monitor lung sounds

60. *Altered nutrition:* Weigh daily, maintain nasogastric tube, administer feedings per orders, evaluate swallowing, teach swallowing techniques
61. *Impaired verbal communication:* Develop a temporary form of communication prior to surgery, check client often, call light within reach, refer to speech rehabilitation
62. Lost cords
63. Olfactory cranial nerve is stimulated by air passing through nose
64. The ability to close the airway and force exhalation is lost.
65. Upper airway bypassed
66. Air flows from tracheostomy opening preventing air flow through mouth.
67. Normal airway is permanently altered.

CHAPTER 61: MANAGEMENT OF CLIENTS WITH LOWER AIRWAY AND PULMONARY VESSEL DISORDERS

1. A
2. B
3. C
4. A
5. B
6. A
7. C
8. D
9. D
10. B
11. A
12. A
13. A
14. B
15. A
16. B
17. A
18. A
19. B
20. A
21. A
22. B
23. Respiratory complications and to monitor medical therapy
24. Bronchospasms cause mucus to pool
25. Liquefies and thins secretions, replaces fluid loss through rapid respirations
26. Decreases risk of infections, comfort measure
27. Beta$_2$ blockers prevent bronchodilation
28. Reduce risk

29. Increases self-care and control over disease
30. Facilitates drainage of mucus and secretions
31. Maximizes respiratory function
32. Large meal may create an excessive feeling of fullness that may make breathing uncomfortable or difficult
33. At risk for constipation
34. Leaves positive end-diastolic pressure in lungs and helps to keep airways open
35. High concentrations decrease hypoxic drive and can precipitate respiratory distress.
36. Living with a chronic progressive disease affects the client and significant others.
37. Promotes relaxation and reduces oxygen demands
38. Dyspnea and reduced energy affect sexual activity; measures to reduce physical exertion and maximize available oxygen levels improve sexual and general well-being
39. Promotes airway clearance
40. A precipitating factor
41. Common complication
42. *Keflex:* cephalosporin-type antibiotic used to treat respiratory infections or preventive treatment
43. Contraindicated for clients with penicillin allergies
44. *Gentamicin:* aminoglycoside antibiotic used to treat serious infections
45. Adverse side effect: ototoxicity damages cranial nerve VIII (acoustic)
46. *Theophylline:* bronchodilator
47. May increase blood pressure and heart rate
48. Toxicity is common
49. *Prednisone:* reduces inflammation
50. Causes GI irritation
51. Immunosuppressive effects can mask infections
52. *Benadryl:* antihistamine inhibits bronchoconstriction
53. Side effect of the medication—thickens secretions
54. Client safety
55. *Metaproterenol:* bronchodilator
56. Therapeutic effect depends on correct use of inhalers—must be taught
57. *Heparin* inhibits thrombus and clot formation
58. Monitors therapeutic range and dosage
59. B
60. C
61. A
62. D
63. A
64. C
65. C
66. C
67. C
68. B
69. C
70. D

CHAPTER 62: MANAGEMENT OF CLIENTS WITH PARENCHYMAL AND PLEURAL DISORDERS

1. A
2. C
3. D
4. B
5. D
6. D
7. A
8. A
9. B
10. C
11. D
12. D
13. B
14. A
15. Decrease pooling of secretions
16. Assessing for changes in respiratory status
17. Activity intolerance
18. Increases compliance with coughing, supports chest wall during coughing
19. Decrease spread of infection
20. Causes GI distress, taking at night increases chance of compliance
21. IV fungicidal antibiotics are irritating to vein tissue
22. High risk for lung infections
23. Sign of possible erosion of pulmonary vessels
24. Minimize the chance of infection
25. At high risk for developing pulmonary edema in the denervated transplanted lung. It is crucial that the client adheres to the immunosuppression therapy regimen to avoid rejection.
26. To monitor for signs and symptoms of rejection, compliance with immunosuppressive therapy, and progress in functional status.
27. A
28. G
29. B
30. F
31. E
32. H

33. I
34. C

CHAPTER 63: MANAGEMENT OF CLIENTS WITH ACUTE PULMONARY DISORDERS

1. B
2. B
3. B
4. B
5. B
6. A
7. A
8. A
9. A
10. A
11. A
12. *Altered respiratory function*: Fewer adventitious lung sounds, lung sounds equal, O_2 saturation greater than 92%, arterial blood gases (ABGs) and acid-base balance returning to normal levels
13. *Anxiety*: Less agitation, calm appearance, following commands, not fighting the respirator
14. *Risk for infection*: Temperature and vital signs within normal limits for client, lung sounds clear, clear sputum, WBC within normal limits
15. *Altered nutrition*: Stable weight; intake of adequate calories; no infection; and prealbumin, total protein, and transferrin laboratory values within normal limits

UNIT 14: SENSORY DISORDERS

1. See Figure U14-1C in textbook.
2. C
3. I
4. F
5. B
6. D
7. G
8. N
9. J
10. A
11. O
12. M
13. L
14. E
15. H
16. K
17. See Figure U14-4 in the textbook.

18. C
19. C
20. A
21. B
22. B
23. A
24. A
25. Eyebrows and lashes turn inward which can cause corneal abrasions and/or infections of the eyelids.
26. Decrease in tearing causes loss of the protective mechanism for the cornea. In addition the client may not be able to wear contacts.
27. Cataract formation decreases vision and perception that can be a safety hazard, especially driving.
28. Decrease in near vision is a normal part of aging, but can affect ADLs that require close vision such as reading medication labels.
29. Decreased tolerance to glare makes it difficult to see in bright sunlight and difficult to drive at night. It is often the reason that older people stop driving at night.
30. Decreased ability to adapt to light changes. It takes longer to adapt to sudden changes in light, which can be a safety hazard and may be the reason for falls among the elderly.
31. Ear hair becomes coarser which can cause a build-up of ear wax. Wax build-up can further affect hearing and balance.
32. Changes in the inner ear; loss of auditory neurons and cochlear hair cell degeneration can cause inability to hear or distinguish high-frequency sounds and diminished hearing and speech comprehension.

CHAPTER 64: ASSESSMENT OF THE EYES AND EARS

1. M
2. D
3. N
4. I
5. C
6. L
7. E
8. A
9. K
10. J
11. G
12. F
13. H
14. B
15. C

16. B

17. G

18. A

19. E

20. I

21. J

22. H

23. F

24. D

25. A device consisting of a handle, a light source, a magnifying lens, and an attachment for visualizing the ear canal and eardrum

26. A test used to assess the inner ear for balance.

27. Deposits of collagen and calcium within the middle ear that can harden around the ossicles, causing a conduction hearing loss.

28. Drugs that are toxic to the eighth cranial nerve can cause damage to the nerve and result in hearing loss.

29. The unit measure of hearing; a logarithmic function of sound.

30. A test to measure compliance (mobility) and impedance (opposition to movement) of the tympanic membrane and the ossicles of the middle ear

31. Tests to assess conductive and sensorineural hearing loss

32. The otology history is designed to obtain specific information related to the ears and hearing. See Box 64-5.

33. Being familiar with common behaviors for hearing loss alerts the nurse to identify clients with possible hearing loss. See Box 64-4.

34. Straightens out the ear canal for easier visualization of the tympanic membrane

35. Because it is semitranslucent, it can provide clues to middle ear conditions.

36. May be associated with vestibular dysfunction

37. Because the ear and the temporomandibular joint share the same sensory nerve supply

38. If pain is elicited examine the other ear first. Pain or tenderness in the tragus alerts the nurse to possible otitis externa or a furuncle. Pain or tenderness at the mastoid process may indicate a middle ear infection, mastoiditis, or lymphadenitis of the posterior auricular node.

CHAPTER 65: MANAGEMENT OF CLIENTS WITH VISUAL DISORDERS

1. Primary or secondary: a primary disease or secondary to other causes

2. *Acute* or *chronic* refers the onset and duration of clinical manifestations

3. Open (wide) and closed (narrow) describe the width of the angle between the cornea and iris.

4. A

5. C

6. A

7. B

8. C

9. A

10. A

11. B

12. B

13. C

14. Miotics constrict the pupil, which opens the Schlemm's canal to improve drainage of aqueous humor.

15. Constipation will increase the risk of straining, which would increase intraocular pressure.

16. The use of a miotic medication will cause temporary blurred vision and also decreases the eye's ability to dilate in low light.

17. Lying on the operative side will increase eye pressure.

18. Pain should be controlled by acetaminophen (Tylenol); unrelieved pain may indicate complications and the physician should be notified.

19. Both eyes

20. Right eye

21. Left eye

22. A, b

23. C, a

24. C, d

25. D, e

26. B, c

27. B   With cataracts the clouding of the lens causes blurred vision and difficulty with night driving, particularly because of the glare of headlights.

28. C   The cloudy lens blocks light from passing through, therefore, the red reflex is either absent or diminished.

29. A   To facilitate surgery, the pupil is dilated and the muscles are paralyzed.

30. A   Pain should be minimal after surgery and controlled by acetaminophen (Tylenol). Medications such as aspirin or other aspirin-containing drugs should not be taken due to their effect of increasing bleeding.

31. A   Open-angle glaucoma results from either increased production of aqueous humor or obstruc-

tion of humor outflow through the trabecular meshwork.

32. D   Pilocarpine causes the pupil to constrict and pull the muscles away from the trabecular mesh-work and Schlemm's canal for improved outflow of aqueous humor.

CHAPTER 66: MANAGEMENT OF CLIENTS WITH HEARING AND BALANCE DISORDERS

1. N
2. G
3. D
4. M
5. E
6. A
7. C
8. B
9. I
10. L
11. K
12. J
13. H
14. A
15. A
16. A
17. A
18. A
19. B
20. B
21. B
22. B
23. B
24. B
25. B
26. B
27. Straightens out the ear canal for easier visualization of the typmpanic membrane
28. Because it is semitranslucent, it can provide clues to middle ear conditions
29. May be associated with vestibular dysfunction
30. Because the ear and the temporomandibular joint share the same sensory nerve supply
31. Diuretics are used to treat the cause, which is an excess of endolymph
32. Slow movement allows the vestibular system time to regain balance and integrate messages
33. The acoustic nerve through which the electro-chemical impulse travels to the temporal cortex of the brain

34. Deposits of collagen and calcium within the middle ear that can harden around the ossicles, causing a conduction hearing loss.
35. Drugs that are toxic to the ear and can cause damage to hearing
36. The unit measure of hearing; a logarithmic function of sound
37. Benign tumor of the eighth cranial nerve
38. Prevents squealing feedback
39. The eustachian tube is connected with the middle ear; these procedures will lessen the pressure on the middle ear
40. Exposure to loud music near the speakers presents a danger to the sensorineural system; intensity drops off with distance
41.-43.   Use Box 66-2 and the Care Plan "The Client with Vertigo."
44. D   The correct technique for using the otoscope to examine the ears is to hold the otoscope in the dominant hand and rest that hand on the head so that if the client moves suddenly the otoscope will also move, lessening the danger of injury to the external canal. In the adult, the pinna is pulled up, backward, and out to help straighten the ear canal.
45. A   Running the IV antibiotic at a 60-minute rate will keep the blood level from getting too high and thus potentially damaging the eighth cranial nerve.
46. C   Presbycusis is a bilateral perceptive hearing loss, especially at high frequencies, that occurs in the elderly.
47. D   Talking directly to the client while facing him will help the client to hear, as well as provide nonverbal clues to improve understanding.
48. B   Opening the battery compartment at night will help preclude accidental drainage of the battery fluid.

UNIT 15: COGNITIVE AND PERCEPTUAL DISORDERS

1. A
2. J
3. K
4. F
5. H
6. M
7. I
8. G
9. C
10. B
11. N
12. E

13. L
14. D
15. (a) frontal, (b) temporal, (c) occipital, (d) parietal
16. C
17. A
18. A
19. D
20. A
21. A
22. A
23. B
24. (a) Receptor in skin, (b) effector in muscle fiber, (c) ventral root, (d) sensory nerve, (e) central neuron, (f) dorsal root, (g) dorsal root ganglion, (h) motor nerve
25. P
26. S
27. S
28. S
29. S
30. S
31. P
32. (a) P, (b) S, (c) P, (d) oculomotor or III, (e) facial or VII, (f) glossopharyngeal or IX, (g) vagus or X

CHAPTER 67: ASSESSMENT OF THE NEUROLOGIC SYSTEM

1. N
2. E
3. L
4. G
5. A
6. F
7. J
8. M
9. I
10. K
11. No, need cranial nerves II (optic) and III (oculomotor) to function
12. III (oculomotor), IV (trochlear), and VI (abducens) coordinate to control eye movements in all six cardinal directions of gaze; VI controls the lateral rectus muscle, IV the superior oblique, and III all other muscles
13. III (oculomotor)
14. 20%
15. Anisocoria
16. III (oculomotor)
17. V (trigeminal) and VII (facial)

18. Scratch the foot's outer aspect (outer sole) from heel toward toes
19. Forearms 40 mm and fingertips 2.8 mm (fingertips about 13 times more sensitive)
20. Parietal
21. Yes
22. No need to check temperature unless pain sensation is impaired
23. Pressure on cranial nerves III, IV, or VI, and increased intracranial pressure
24. Use the following items to determine if you have considered the major points about an MRI test and the case study in developing a thorough plan of care.
  a. Analgesia for Ms. B.'s muscle and joint pain prior to the procedure.
  b. The fact that she will have to lie absolutely still for approximately one hour for the procedure to be accurate.
  c. Assess for "claustrophobia" as she will be in a small cylindrical tube, which is only open at the ends.
  d. Inform Ms. B. about the loud rapping sounds that she will hear as part of the MRI test.
  e. Assess Ms. B. for a pacemaker or any metal implants.
  f. Remind Ms. B. to empty her bladder prior to the procedure.
  g. Assess Ms. B.'s ataxia, numbness and paresthesia, and blurred vision prior to the procedure.
  h. Inform Ms. B. about the "safeness" of the MRI procedure.
  i. Inform Ms. B. that she can maintain constant communication with the MRI technician.

CHAPTER 68: MANAGEMENT OF COMATOSE OR CONFUSED CLIENTS

1. C
2. J
3. G
4. K
5. L
6. B
7. A
8. F
9. E
10. D
11. I
12. M

13. Risk for suffocation because cannot swallow due to loss or suppression of gag and cough reflexes

14. Risk for aspiration due to ineffective airway clearance and loss of gag and cough reflexes

15. Altered oral mucous membrane related to mouth breathing and having nothing by mouth (NPO)

16. Impaired skin integrity due to immobility

17. Altered nutrition: less than body requirements because cannot eat or swallow

18. Risk for fluid volume deficit because cannot drink or respond to thirst

19. Risk for injury because cannot voice pain and may fall out of bed when regaining consciousness

20. Bowel incontinence because cannot respond to normal stimulus for evacuation of feces

21. Altered family processes related to impending death of patient

CHAPTER 69: MANAGEMENT OF CLIENTS WITH CEREBRAL DISORDERS

1. L
2. I
3. M
4. E
5. D
6. P
7. O
8. G
9. N
10. B
11. A
12. J
13. F
14. Dilantin can cause hypertrophy of the gums and good oral hygiene will help to prevent this.
15. Bradycardia and heart block could occur.
16. Dilantin should be given no faster than 50 mg/minute.
17. The drug may precipitate in other fluids.
18. Dilantin can cause agranulocytosis (lowered white blood cell count).
19. Because it initially suppresses REM sleep, phenobarbital can cause initial drowsiness. Clients will adjust to this and will no longer feel sleepy with the same dosage.
20. Sudden withdrawal of phenobarbital could cause seizures.
21. To decrease intracranial pressure when it is elevated

22. Clear fluid that dries in concentric circles (halo ring) on dressing or bed linen

23. Postoperative respiratory complications

24. 4.5; antacids and histamine-blocking agents

25. Head of bed is elevated after supratentorial surgery and head of bed is flat after infratentorial surgery. (Remember, head is up when surgery is above the tentorium.)

26. Yes, because medications could depress respirations. (The client will also need help maintaining a clear airway.)

27. Phenytoin (Dilantin) and diazepam (Valium)

28. Someone with epilepsy is viewed as being "struck down" by the gods; education of the public as well as the client with epilepsy

29. Length of seizure, where on the body it began and how it progressed, whether the client's eyes deviated, if client was incontinent or had labored respirations, type of body movements and body parts that moved

30. They are signs of meningeal irritation.

31. Headache and pain when moving the eyes, photophobia, drowsiness, weakness, painful extremities, neck and spine stiffness

32. Tumor of the vestibular nerve; prognosis is excellent with early surgical resection and preservation of the remaining cranial nerves

33. All of the tumor cannot be removed by surgery (even one cell left could grow) so other (adjuvant) therapy is needed (such as radiotherapy). The client has many needs and requires a clinical team to provide care and support from diagnosis to recovery.

34. Classic migraine headaches are preceded by an aura or prodromal phase, followed by crescendo pain with nausea and vomiting, and eyes become swollen, red, and tearing.

35. Beta-adrenergic blocker (propranolol) and tricyclic anti-depressant (amitriptyline).

CHAPTER 70: MANAGEMENT OF CLIENTS WITH STROKE

1. E
2. D
3. G
4. B
5. C
6. A
7. F
8. Clients often are emotionally labile and depressed, bursting into tears. They use profanity, regress to

childlike behavior, and exhibit inappropriate sexual behavior.

9. Respiratory infection and brain stem failure

10. Determine client's yes-no reliability; use gestures to aid communication; speak slowly and clearly; and stand within 6 feet and face client.

11. Short-term ischemia leads to temporary or transient ischemia attacks (TIAs). Long-term ischemia leads to permanent infarction (death) of cerebral cells.

12. Blood in the subarachnoid space prevents adequate cerebrospinal fluid circulation.

13. Avoid rectal temperatures. Get client a bedside commode. Give stool softeners/mild laxatives. Encourage deep breathing, but no coughing.

CHAPTER 71: MANAGEMENT OF CLIENTS WITH PERIPHERAL NERVOUS SYSTEM DISORDERS

1. D
2. C
3. L
4. B
5. F
6. G
7. E
8. I
9. A
10. J
11. H
12. K

CHAPTER 72: MANAGEMENT OF CLIENTS WITH DEGENERATIVE NEUROLOGIC DISORDERS

1. B, I, O
2. A, H, N
3. E, F, L
4. C, J, M
5. D, G, K
6. Medications result in increased muscle strength that prevents choking with meals.

7. Dosages are highly individualized based on physiologic response to the medicine.

8. Client could develop sudden worsening of condition, especially if client has infection, and may require intubation.

9. Steroids decrease mucus secretion and increase hydrochloric acid secretion in the stomach that could lead to the formation of ulcers. The antacids are given to prevent ulcers.

10. Beginning medications may temporarily worsen symptoms

11. All hormones need to be given on a strict schedule as the body is "expecting" that amount of hormone.

12. The medicine can cause orthostatic hypotension.

13. The addition of carbidopa to levodopa treatment decreases systemic side effects by preventing peripheral metabolism of levodopa, allowing levodopa to reach the brain.

14. Vitamin B_6 decreases effectiveness of levodopa.

CHAPTER 73: MANAGEMENT OF CLIENTS WITH NEUROLOGIC TRAUMA

1. D
2. B
3. C
4. A
5. Effect of nursing interventions on ICP can be monitored. The timing of procedures known to raise ICP, e.g., suctioning, can be altered to coincide with periods of "lower" pressure. The effectiveness of medical treatment can be evaluated. Delays in taking client to surgery can be avoided. Some monitoring systems allow ventricular drainage.

6. It induces hypocapnia (lowers carbon dioxide levels in the blood) that reduces cerebral blood volume and ICP (increased carbon dioxide causes dilation of cerebral blood vessels).

7. Hyperthermia increases metabolism and cerebral blood flow and thus increases ICP.

8. Seizures increase metabolic requirements, cerebral blood flow, and volume, thus increasing ICP.

9. He may be developing increased intracranial pressure. His level of consciousness is decreasing, his pulse pressure is beginning to widen, and his pupils are not equal.

10. Assess using Glasgow Coma Scale as this provides objective measurements of neuro exam. Elevate head of bed 30 degrees and avoid neck flexion as this decreases intracranial pressure.

11. Accidents, trauma (e.g., diving, motor vehicle accidents)

12. Males < 40 years of age

13. Have young people with spinal cord injuries deliver the message at school-based educational programs

14. Assessment, stabilize the neck in neutral position, use spinal board and a hard collar, tie Velcro straps around the torso and legs, assess baseline deficits

15. Greater injury and more permanent disabilities

16. Complete loss of motor, sensory, autonomic, and reflex activity below the level of injury; hypotension and bradycardia
17. Loss of sensation below the level of injury
18. Contralateral loss of pain and temperature sensation
19. Loss of motor function below the level of injury
20. The client has no phrenic nerve function and would need to be managed with a phrenic pacemaker, ventilator, and intensive respiratory therapy to prevent pneumonia.
21. Spastic
22. To immobilize the cervical spine and reduce the fracture and dislocation. The tongs are inserted through the outer layer of the skull.
23. No; logrolling to maintain stability of the spine until surgical stabilization can be done
24. To prevent urinary tract infections; the client needs between 3000 and 4000 cc of fluid each day.
25. Client with indwelling catheter
26. Pressure, which decreases blood supply to tissues
27. Active and passive range of motion exercises and positioning joints in extension
28. It varies by state. Check with your state's Spinal Cord Commission.
29. E, F
30. E, F
31. A, C, G
32. A, C, G
33. H
34. D
35. After spinal shock resolves, exaggerated sympathetic responses to noxious stimuli below level of injury produce hypertension, diaphoresis, piloerection, dilated pupils; baroreceptors stimulate parasympathetic nervous system in an effort to decrease B/P, resulting in bradycardia, flushing, and headache.
36. Kinked or clogged urinary catheter, distended bladder, or fecal impaction.
37. Elevate head of bed to sitting position; check B/P; check for possible sources of irritation and remove (if this can be done quickly); administer antihypertensive medication per physician's order or protocol; call physician if above measures do not correct problem.

UNIT 16: PROTECTIVE DISORDERS

1. Cells, plasma, heart's
2. Oxygen, nutrients, waste, lung, kidneys
3. Homeostasis

4. Bone marrow
5. Concave disc
6. Hypoxia, erythropoietin
7. Lymphoblasts, monoblasts, myeloblasts; percentage
8. C
9. A
10. A
11. B
12. E
13. C
14. D
15. D
16. D
17. A or B
18. E
19. E
20. C
21. B
22. A
23. D
24. C
25. D
26. F
27. A
28. B
29. C
30. A
31. D
32. B
33. E
34. F
35. G
36. Color: arterial bright-red, venous dark-red; viscosity: 3–4 times thicker than water; pH: 7.35–7.45; volume: 70–75 ml /kg, 4–5 L; composition: 55% plasma, 45% cells/platelets
37. *Rh positive* means the D antigen is present and *Rh negative* means the D antigen is absent.
38. B_{12}: RBC formation and maturation; normal nervous system function; folic acid: RBC formation and maturation; iron: hemoglobin formation
39. Spleen: stores RBCs for emergency use, recycles iron, removes particles from blood and removes antigens; Liver: phagocytosis by Kupffer's cells, stores iron, and breakdown of hemoglobin
40. Secretes growth factors necessary for cell replication and differentiation
41. (a) Tonsils, (b) lymph nodes, (c) spleen, (d) gut-

associated lymphoid tissue, (e) lymph nodes, (f) bone marrow, (g) thymus gland

42. Thymus gland and bone marrow

43. Thymus gland—maintenance and function of T cells; bone marrow—maintenance and function of B cells

44. Markers to recognize "self"

45. In active immunity, individuals produce antibodies following stimulation by antigens. In passive immunity, individuals receive antibodies that were not produced by themselves.

46. To rid the body of a foreign substance (antigen)

47. Monocyte

48. T helper cells, T suppressor cells, cytotoxic "killer" T cells, T memory cells

49. Antigen-activated T helper cells

50. IgG crosses the placenta and protects the newborn; IgA's mucosal immunity helps to prevent local GI and genitourinary infections; IgM reacts with blood group antigens; IgE helps initiate atopic allergy expression; and IgD's effects are unknown.

CHAPTER 74: ASSESSMENT OF THE HEMATOPOIETIC SYSTEM

1. J
2. L
3. A
4. D
5. H
6. B
7. C
8. I
9. K
10. E
11. M
12. F
13. P
14. O
15. N
16. G
17. C
18. E
19. F
20. A
21. D
22. B
23. C
24. E
25. F

26. G
27. D
28. G
29. F
30. A
31. B
32. C
33. D
34. A
35. D
36. C
37. D
38. D
39. C
40. B
41. D
42. B
43. C
44. C
45. C
46. A
47. Yes
48. Decrease risk of infection
49. Decrease hematoma/bleeding
50. Decrease pain
51. Bleeding
52. Pruritus, jaundice, pallor, flushing, petechiae, ecchymoses, delayed wound healing
53. Numbness, tingling, pain, visual disturbances
54. Fatigue, dyspnea, orthopnea
55. Tachypnea, murmurs, angina
56. Nausea, vomiting, weight loss, abdominal pain, hepatomegaly, splenomegaly
57. Timing, quality and quantity, severity and location, precipitating factors, aggravating and relieving factors, associated manifestations
58. Inguinal and popliteal nodes
59. Scratch, patch, and intradermal tests.
60. Negative results may indicate that (1) antibodies have not formed to this antigen; (2) the antigen was deposited too deeply into the skin; or (3) the client is immunosuppressed as a result of disease or therapy. Therefore, negative results may be inconclusive, indicating the need for further assessment.

CHAPTER 75: MANAGEMENT OF CLIENTS WITH HEMATOLOGIC DISORDERS

1. A
2. G

3.   H
4.   H
5.   C
6.   D
7.   I
8.   J
9.   B
10.   G
11.   B
12.   C
13.   A
14.   D
15.   A
16.   C
17.   C
18.   D
19.   B
20.   A
21.   C
22.   A
23.   D
24.   C
25.   A
26.   B
27.   E
28.   C
29.   A
30.   B
31.   D
32.   C
33.   A
34.   C
35.   Bleeding
36.   Heat causes vasodilation
37.   Increased intrathoracic pressure can cause bleeding
38.   Petechiae and ecchymoses
39.   Maintain hydration
40.   Anticalcium medication
41.   Complications
42.   A or O
43.   B or O
44.   B, O
45.   O
46.   Safety measures, "five rights" as with medication safety
47.   Prior knowledge of transfusion reactions
48.   Donor blood may be a different type
49.   Safety

50.   Decrease lysis of RBCs
51. D_5W causes lysis of RBCs
52.   Monitor for transfusion reactions
53.   Majority of reactions occur in first 10–20 minutes
54.   Blood bank policy: cannot be returned after 30 minutes
55.   Decrease contamination and temperature changes
56.   Maximum time blood can infuse
57.   Intolerance to cold temperature
58.   Ensure ample B_{12}, folic acid, iron
59.   Activity intolerance a common problem
60.   Cardiovascular system works to compensate for decreased oxygen.
61.   B   The tachycardia is an attempt by the body to supply oxygenated blood to the tissues.
62.   C   Endometriosis causes excessive blood loss during the menstrual period.
63.   D   Kidney beans, lean meat, and carrots will increase the client's iron intake.
64.   A   The iron preparation should be taken after meals since it is irritating to the gastric mucosa.

Chapter 76: Management of Clients with Immune Disorders

1.   A
2.   D
3.   B
4.   D
5.   C
6.   A
7.   B
8.   A
9.   C
10.   Penicillins
11.   Seafood
12.   Honeybees
13.   Vaccines
14.   Whole blood
15.   Skin testing agents
16.   Iodinated contrast media
17.   Take a careful nursing history.
18.   Always mark known allergies clearly on the permanent health record, front of the client's chart, nursing Kardex, and nursing care plans.
19.   Teach clients with allergies to wear special ID bracelets.
20.   If you suspect a client to be allergic to a certain medication, make sure the client has an intradermal test before giving the medication.

CHAPTER 77: MANAGEMENT OF CLIENTS WITH AUTOIMMUNE DISORDERS

1. E
2. M
3. I
4. G
5. C
6. O
7. L
8. N
9. F
10. A
11. B
12. H
13. D
14. K
15. J
16. Large doses of aspirin may enhance the actions of oral anticoagulants and heparin by competing for protein-binding sites. Even when given alone, aspirin decreases platelet aggregation and, in large doses, inhibits prothrombin formation.
17. To prevent stomach irritation and ulcers
18. Toxic levels of aspirin cause tinnitus.
19. May cause decreased creatinine clearance, nephro-toxicity, and acute renal failure
20. Since ibuprofen may prolong bleeding time in some people, the dentist or surgeon needs to know that the client is taking the medication in order to avoid potential complications of excessive bleeding with certain procedures.
21. Ibuprofen can cause GI ulceration.
22. These medications may increase risk of GI ulceration and bleeding tendencies.
23. A   The rapid onset of sharp hip pain may indicate dislocation. Notify the physician of hip pain of this type and pain that is not relieved by prescribed analgesics.
24. D   Abduction is a desirable position immediately after surgery to prevent dislocation of the prosthesis and is necessary for about 6 weeks. An abduction pillow usually is used between the legs when turning the client or getting the client in a chair.
25. C   Quadriceps-setting exercises need to be done every hour during the day, especially to prevent thromboemboli. An easy way to teach the client these exercises is to put your hand under her knee and ask her to straighten her right lower extremity while pushing your hand down "into the mattress."

She needs to do the exercises for both lower extremities.

26. B   Quadriceps and gluteal exercises will help prevent thromboemboli and pulmonary emboli. Gluteal exercises may also help prevent dislocation of the prosthesis. Teach gluteal exercises by asking her to squeeze and relax her buttocks.
27. C   Dextran is a hypertonic fluid that will draw fluid into the intravascular space thus increasing blood flow to the operative site and, therefore, increasing the drainage. Dextran is given slowly IV to prevent thromboemboli because it decreases platelet adhesiveness and aggregation (which begins the blood-clotting process).
28. B   She should also be encouraged to lie prone to prevent a hip flexion contracture. She needs to avoid sleeping on her right side for a while, usually until after her first postoperative visit.

CHAPTER 78: MANAGEMENT OF CLIENTS WITH LEUKEMIA AND LYMPHOMA

1. L
2. I
3. J
4. F
5. N
6. C
7. A
8. G
9. E
10. D
11. D
12. C
13. A
14. B
15. D
16. C
17. E
18. A
19. Decrease spread of infection
20. Neutropenic
21. Decrease membrane trauma
22. Causes bruising
23. B   Depression often causes changes in eating habits.
24. A   The physician has probably ordered the radiation therapy as a palliative measure. It will reduce the size of the liver and spleen and provide the client with an increased comfort level.

25.   A   The nurse must be careful to avoid transmitting infections to the client. Her ability to fight infections is diminished by both the disease process and the radiation therapy.

UNIT 17: MULTISYSTEM DISORDERS

CHAPTER 79: MANAGEMENT OF CLIENTS WITH ACQUIRED IMMUNODEFICIENCY SYNDROME

1.   D
2.   F
3.   G
4.   H
5.   A
6.   C
7.   E
8.   B
9.   A
10. B
11. B
12. A
13. C
14. C
15. Teach clients the basics of routine skin care and observation: daily bathing (showers are preferred if a client has fungus involving the feet or groin); the use of lotions or creams to prevent dry skin and cracking; avoidance of excessive hair washing, brushing, or dyes. Teaching proper oral, vaginal, and rectal hygiene is extremely important. Oral care needs to include brushing after meals with a soft toothbrush, daily flossing, scheduling regular dental visits, and using oral rinses, such as saline or quarter-strength hydrogen peroxide to enhance bactericidal effect. Teach clients to avoid enemas and douches or other chemicals that interrupt the normal flora, and sexual activities that may result in breaks in the mucosa. Teach clients the need for proper nutrition, adequate rest and exercise, smoking cessation, and stress reduction. In essence, you need to teach good health practices.
16. Low CD4 T-cell count (often < 200); fever; fatigue; weight loss; low oxygen content on pulse oximetry; nonproductive cough indicating *Pneumocystis carinii* pneumonia; tingling, burning and pain with lesions indicating herpes simplex; focal neurologic manifestations indicating toxoplasmic encephalitis; watery diarrhea and positive stool culture indicating infection with *Cryptosporidium*. These are examples of common opportunistic infections with AIDS.

17. Three-week course of trimethoprim–sulfamethoxazole, aerosolized pentamidine, or oral dapsone for treating *Pneumocystis carinii* pneumonia; acyclovir for herpes simplex infection; combination of pyrimethamine and sulfadiazine as treatment for toxoplasmic encephalitis; replacing fluid and electrolytes for *Cryptosporidium* infection causing diarrhea.
18. Start with a complete nutritional assessment and then educate the client on the need for routine dental care, a well-balanced diet, and multivitamin supplements containing B complex.
19. Anorexia, which leads to reduced intake, gastrointestinal diseases, etc., which decrease the amount of nutrients absorbed; infection, which increases the amount of nutrients required; excess intake of fats, which may further impair the immune system; and weight loss
20. Oral nutritional supplements
21. Assessing and assisting the client in three key areas: family support, community resources, and individual coping ability
22. Unresolved family conflicts, the client's level of functioning, and resources at home and in the community
23. Do not isolate the client; establish a therapeutic relationship. Help the client to identify support systems, including helping to arrange for those that are lacking. Instruct family, friends, and visitors about universal precautions and when they need to be used. Help the client to discuss feelings and coping skills.
24. Educating the client and his/her family; help them to maintain a realistic sense of hope
25. Functioning, current stressors and coping patterns, use of stress reduction techniques
26. Refer to counseling or support groups, appropriate nursing interventions for specific problems
27. Working with the client on discharge planning and making appropriate referrals to help prevent problems
28. Client's understanding of transmission of disease
29. More education, obtain information for follow-up of contacts

CHAPTER 80: MANAGEMENT OF CLIENTS REQUIRING TRANSPLANTATION

1.   D
2.   E
3.   G
4.   A
5.   B

6. F
7. C
8. Presence of an active systemic infection, active peptic ulcer disease, lack of sufficient financial resources to pay for surgery, hospitalization, medication, and follow-up
9. Yes, if the family gives consent.
10. No
11. Yes, if he meets the criteria for brain death and family consent. Jehovah's Witness does not encourage organ donation.
12. No, he does not meet the criteria for brain death. Consult the organ procurement organization in your state.
13. Will vary some with the type of transplant but any signs and symptoms of rejections or infections need to be communicated.
14. The goal of immunosuppression therapy is to suppress the immune response to prevent rejection without developing complications from the therapy.
15. Rejection can occur suddenly or over a period of months. Patients need to be aware of signs and symptoms and contact the primary health care provider and/or transplant coordinator immediately.
16. Infection is the leading cause of morbidity and mortality after transplant. The immunosuppression therapy and altered immune defenses can mask infections.
17. It is important to have regular mammogram and pap smears, colon screening, immunizations and regular eye and dental exams following transplant. Recipients are more at risk than the general population.
18. Recipients need both initial and ongoing education of activity—what they can and *cannot* do.
19. To alert health care personnel in the event the client is unable to give health history
20. Meticulous follow-up is required for long-term success.
21. Recognizing and preventing complications
22. Assess pancreatic function; clinical manifestations of GT are: sudden rise in serum glucose, severe graft pain, increased serum creatinine.
23. Monitor signs of heart failure/rejection, S_3 S_4, decreased ejection fraction
24. Signs and symptoms of liver failure/rejection
25. Disruption and loss of innervation results in loss of protective mechanisms: ciliary movement, cough reflex, and changes in mucus production.
26. D, T
27. NA

28. T
29. NA
30. D, T
31. D, T
32. NA
33. D, T
34. D, T
35. D, T
36. D, T
37. NE
38. D, T
39. D, T
40. D, T
41. NA

CHAPTER 81: MANAGEMENT OF CLIENTS WITH SHOCK AND MULTISYSTEM DISORDERS

1. Decreased tissue perfusion causing cell death
2. Decreased cardiac output stimulates the sympathetic nervous system. The resulting vasoconstriction and tachycardia maintain B/P for awhile. Pulse pressure tends to parallel cardiac stroke volume and provides a clue that shock is worsening, especially in young adults.
3. Respiratory failure (ARDS, aspiration, loss of neurologic control of breathing) continues to be a major cause of death in shock.
4. When bacterial endotoxins present in septic shock, or hemolysis accompanying trauma occurs, along with the stagnant, acidic blood of shock, widespread intravascular clotting occurs.
5. 1 and 3; a pulse pressure of 40 mm Hg is normal.
6. Check the airway, breathing, and circulation (ABCs).
7. To provide external pressure to the lower extremities in order to route blood flow away from the lower extremities to vital organs
8. To assist the heart by improving coronary blood flow
9. The modified Trendelenburg position is the recommended position for a person in shock. It includes elevating the lower extremities, leaving the trunk flat, and elevating the head and shoulders slightly.
10. CVP indicates the pressure in the right side of the heart and is useful as a guide in fluid administration when shock is not due to pump failure. For example, a rapidly increasing CVP may indicate that fluids are being given too rapidly. However, with cardiogenic shock, the nurse needs to know the pressure in the left side of the heart. The Swan-

Ganz catheter allows the nurse to obtain these pressure readings.

11. Size of molecules in solution: colloids have larger molecules that keep fluid in the intravascular system by increasing osmotic pressure. Colloids include plasma, albumin, dextran, and hetastarch. Crystalloid solutions include normal saline, Ringer's lactate, or half-normal saline.

12. Warm the environment, not the person in shock. Heat to the skin draws blood away from vital organs.

13. To prevent aspiration of gastric contents. During shock, there is diminished blood flow to the GI tract with resulting nausea and vomiting.

14. To detect a decrease in urinary output below 50 cc/hour so that increased fluids may be given to prevent acute renal failure.

15. To maintain adequate blood flow to vital organs

16. Cautiously, if at all. Narcotics interfere with vasoconstriction necessary to maintain B/P.

17. 0.1–0.5 mL of epinephrine 1:1000 subcutaneously every 10–15 minutes

18. (a) Bacterial toxins cause early vasodilation; (b) with increased capillary permeability, fluid shifts to the interstitial spaces; and (c) as fluid shifts to the interstitial spaces, edema results.

19. Whether a client appears to be conscious or not, always explain what is happening. Keep the atmosphere as quiet and orderly as possible.

20. Keep them informed of what is happening. Let them stay with the client as much as possible. See Client Education Guide for Shock in the text.

21. C, E, G
22. A, K, L
23. G
24. A, C, G
25. A, K, L
26. D, F, H
27. B
28. B   Ms. T. could have significant blood loss and acute hemorrhage with a fractured femur. The other signs and symptoms could result from a stimulation of her sympathetic nervous system due to the traumatic circumstances.
29. A   Bleeding resulting from her fractured femur causes hypovolemic shock.
30. C   Pulse rate will increase before B/P decreases. During the early stage of shock, Ms. T. will be anxious, but the nurse should not expect her to be confused once she has been oriented. There should be sufficient blood flow to her kidneys to produce at least 30 cc urine/hour.

31. B   IV fluid (3 mL crystalloids, such as lactated Ringer's, for every 1 mL of estimated blood loss) is given to restore blood volume. If she loses over 1250 cc of blood, she probably will need blood replacement as well.

32. C   Since shock causes inadequate tissue perfusion, the primary goal is to improve tissue perfusion to prevent death of cells that could occur as shock progresses.

CHAPTER 82: MANAGEMENT OF CLIENTS IN THE EMERGENCY DEPARTMENT

1. F
2. G
3. B
4. C
5. H
6. E
7. D
8. A
9. E
10. E
11. E
12. N
13. E
14. U
15. U
16. U
17. N
18. N
19. E
20. U

21.–30. All are examples of situations that must be reported.

31. When a client is unable to give consent or is unconscious, emergency care may be given under emergency doctrine.

32. Patent airway is the first priority in any emergency situation. The nurse must quickly assess and intervene. For airway obstruction use the Heimlich maneuver; for patent airway but no respirations begin rescue breathing and, depending on the situation, an esophageal obturator airway (EOA) or an esophageal gastric tube airway (EGTA) may be used in the field. In the emergency department an endotracheal tube is more commonly used.

33. Suspected suicides or homicides, deaths in which the deceased has not been attended by a physician within 24 hours before death, deaths caused by accidents, deaths after surgery, deaths associated

with firearms or weapons, deaths occurring as a result of a crime, stillbirths, deaths resulting from drugs, and deaths possibly associated with hazards to public safety (infectious diseases that may cause epidemics).

34. C
35. N
36. H
37. D
38. K
39. O
40. B
41. F
42. G
43. A
44. L
45. R
46. S
47. I
48. E
49. J
50. P
51. Q
52. M
53. B
54. C
55. H
56. G
57. F
58. E
59. D
60. A
61. To determine possible cause of altered level of consciousness
62. Naloxone, a narcotic antagonist, may be administered if a narcotic overdose is suspected to be the reason for altered level of consciousness
63. Given for low serum glucose
64. Prevent injury to the cervical spine until cervical injuries are ruled out
65. Decreased chance of hypoxia and increased intracranial pressure
66. Unconscious victims who recover report hearing conversations at the bedside
67. May be ordered for known diabetics to increase serum blood sugar; it has rapid onset with minimal chance of aspiration
68. Given prophylactically when history is unavailable or when alcohol abuse is suspected

69. Prevent aspiration
70. Decrease risk of injury to cornea
71. Standard protocol for trauma victims for rapid fluid administration, blood, and medications
72. To thoroughly assess the skin for injuries
73. Causes more tissue damage
74. Assume there is a spinal injury until it has been ruled out
75. High infection rate; considered a contaminated "dirty" wound
76. Clients with multiple traumas often have significant blood loss. It is better to anticipate the possible need for blood replacement and have it available than to wait until it is needed.
77. Changes in LOC could indicate a hematoma or increased intracranial pressure.
78. To discuss test results and do a follow-up pregnancy test; often the psychological impact of the trauma does not appear until weeks or months later
79. Decrease the chance of infection.
80. Glasgow Coma Scale is 12
81. Penetrating wounds are open wounds into the chest wall. Nonpenetrating wounds are blunt trauma wounds that do not pierce the skin or open into the chest wall.
82. Severe head, neck, and chest injuries; fractures
83. Lacerations and bruises of head, face, chest; abdominal injuries from lap belt; acceleration/deceleration injuries
84. Major head, chest, and abdominal injuries; fractures of upper and lower extremities; spinal injuries
85. Heel, ankle, knee fractures; compression fractures of vertebrae
86. Compression fractures of vertebrae, spine injuries, pelvic fracture, major organ injury
87. Head injuries, lacerations, bruises, major organ injury
88. Naloxone (Narcan)
89. Gastric lavage (washing) is performed to treat GI bleeding. A nasogastric tube is inserted into the stomach and cold water or saline is instilled into the stomach and evacuated. The procedure is repeated until the returning fluid is clear.
90. Initial assessment is directed toward identifying and treating immediate life-threatening conditions: ABCs (airway, breathing, and circulation); cover any sucking wounds; listen to breath sounds, quickly assess for mediastinal shift; obtain vital signs and obtain a quick history; mechanism of injury; perform a quick respiratory assessment; start two large-bore IVs; administer oxygen.

91. May cause compression of the lung in the direction of the shift and compression, traction, torsion, or kinking of the great vessels, thus, blood return to the heart is impaired. Symptoms may include marked and severe dyspnea, tachypnea, crepitus, progressive cyanosis, acute chest pain on the affected side, hyperresonance to percussion of the affected side, tachycardia, asymmetric chest wall movement, trachea shifts to unaffected side, and extreme restlessness and agitation.

92. Symptom analysis of chest pain: onset, location, duration, characteristics, aggravating factors, relieving factors, and treatment

93. Symptom analysis of acute abdominal pain: nausea and vomiting, last meal, description of last bowel movement, and menstrual history in all sexually active females of childbearing age

94. Health care providers are required to use the term "alleged sexual assault" when caring for clients who may be victims of rape. Rape is a crime that is punishable by law. Rape is considered a legal term; therefore, alleged sexual assault is used to avoid possible legal implications.

95. If it has been more than five years since the last booster, a tetanus booster is administered.

96. The usual treatment is to reduce the body's temperature rapidly (immerse or sponge with cool water, or use a hypothermia blanket); an IV line is started, cardiac monitoring, oxygen, and take frequent vital signs. Chlorpromazine or diazepam are used to reduce shivering.

97. The usual treatment is to rewarm the affected part in tepid water (about 105° F). Do not massage the affected part or debride blisters because this may result in further tissue damage.

98. A   The highest priority is to assess airway, breathing, and circulation in emergency situations.

99. C   In an auto accident without seat belts, it is likely that the person will hit the steering wheel with his/her chest resulting in bruising of the chest wall as well as other injuries to the thorax.

100. B   In an auto accident with an adult, additional injuries to consider would be cardiac contusions and facial fractures, again from impact against the steering wheel.

101. D   It is recommended to begin with a chronology of the accident rather than starting with the bad news.

102. C   Shallow, rapid breathing may be an early sign of increased intracranial pressure.

A

Classical Textbook Picture of the Medical Diagnosis

Use as a guide before clinical, listing the most pertinent information about the classical textbook description of the client's medical diagnosis. As you work with the client, use as a guide to compare and contrast the client's medical diagnosis with the classical textbook picture. You may also find this a helpful method of preparing for class as this form can be used as a note-taking outline and later as a study guide in preparing for examinations.

Name	Etiology and Risk Factors	Clinical Manifestations	Diagnostic Findings	Medical Management and Nursing Care	Surgical Management and Nursing Care

CLASSICAL TEXTBOOK PICTURE of _____

CLASSICAL TEXTBOOK PICTURE of _____

Name	Etiology and Risk Factors	Clinical Manifestations	Diagnostic Findings	Medical Management and Nursing Care	Surgical Management and Nursing Care

WORKSHEET FOR SELECTED DISORDERS OF SLEEP

Name	Etiology and Risk Factors	Clinical Manifestations	Diagnostic Findings	Medical Management and Nursing Care	Surgical Management and Nursing Care
Insomnia					
Narcolepsy					
Obstructive Sleep Apnea					

WORKSHEET FOR SELECTED DISORDERS OF SLEEP
Sleep Disorders Associated with Medical and Psychological Disorders

Disorder	Etiology	Signs and Symtpoms	Treatment
Parkinson's Disease			
Depression			
Head Injury			
Diabetes Mellitus			
COPD			
Gastroesophageal Reflux			

WORKSHEET FOR SELECTED GASTRIC DISORDERS

Name	Etiology and Risk Factors	Clinical Manifestations	Diagnostic Findings	Medical Management and Nursing Care	Surgical Management and Nursing Care

Dysrythmia Note-Taking Outline or Study Guide

Use as a note-taking outline during lecture or as a study guide to help learn specific information about each type of dysrhythmia.

DYSRHYTHMIA NOTE-TAKING OUTLINE

Type and Etiology	Rate and Rhythm	P Waves	P-R Interval	QRS Complex	Clinical Manifestations	Treatment

DYSRHYTHMIA NOTE-TAKING OUTLINE

Type and Etiology	Rate and Rhythm	P Waves	P-R Interval	QRS Complex	Clinical Manifestations	Treatment

DYSRHYTHMIA NOTE-TAKING OUTLINE

Type and Etiology	Rate and Rhythm	P Waves	P-R Interval	QRS Complex	Clinical Manifestations	Treatment